Drugs, Society and Man

A GUIDE TO ADDICTION
AND ITS TREATMENT

Drugs, Society and Man

A GUIDE
TO ADDICTION
AND ITS
TREATMENT

M. M. GLATT *M.D., M.R.C.P., F.R.C.Psych.,*
D.P.M.

MTP   Medical and Technical Publishing Co Ltd

Published by

MTP
Medical and Technical Publishing Co. Limited,
P.O. Box 55,
St. Leonard's House,
St. Leonardgate,
Lancaster, England.

ISBN-13: 978-94-011-5901-2   e-ISBN-13: 978-94-011-5899-2
DOI: 10.1007/978-94-011-5899-2

'That humanity at large will ever be able to dispense with Artificial Paradises seems very unlikely. Most men and women lead lives at the worst so painful, at the best so monotonous, poor and limited that the urge to escape, the longing to transcend themselves if only for a few moments, is and has always been one of the principal appetites of the soul. Art and religion, carnivals and saturnalia, dancing and listening to oratory – all these have served, in H. G. Wells's phrase, as "doors in the wall". And for private, everyday use, there have always been chemical intoxicants. All the vegetable sedatives and narcotics, all the euphorics that grow on trees, the hallucinogens that ripen in berries or can be squeezed from roots – all, without exception, have been known and systematically used by human beings from time immemorial. And to these natural modifiers of consciousness modern science has added its quota of synthetics – chloral, for example, and benzedrine, the bromides, and the barbiturates.

Most of these modifiers of consciousness cannot now be taken except under doctor's orders, or else illegally and at considerable risk. For unrestricted use the West has permitted only alcohol and tobacco. All the other chemical "doors in the wall" are labelled "dope", and their unauthorised takers are "fiends".'

Aldous Huxley (1959). *The Doors of Perception and Heaven and Hell*, 51/52 (London: Penguin Books).

FOREWORD

The field of Addiction Studies is often one in which highly specialized investigations in narrowly defined areas of concern, provide results which are not immediately or easily transferable to the practical problems faced in society.

The collected work of many specialists is frequently too 'specialized' for successful presentation to a wider audience.

Against such a background, Dr Max Glatt has emerged clearly as one of the better authorities on alcohol and drug problems in the world. His 'specialities' cover an extremely broad range of disciplines, approaches and interests.

When Dr Glatt writes, he does so with a brilliant command of the larger picture, the overall impact of alcohol and drug problems in society and the complexities, human and social, inherent in the development of addiction, its treatment and prevention.

'A Guide to Addiction and Its Treatment' provides further testimony on Dr Glatt's skill in weaving together the infinite number of threads on the subject area. This new volume is a most valuable resource which is sure to become required reading for all those with an interest in comprehensive approaches to this vital health and social problem.

Throughout the book, Dr Glatt strongly emphasizes the need for interdisciplinary approaches to addiction and shows clearly why such a coordinated view is necessary if societies are to respond adequately to the escalating health problems associated with the ever-increasing use and misuse of drugs.

Although traditions, values and the actual drug substances themselves may vary substantially from one country to another, the principles which Dr Glatt presents in this new volume have direct relevance and application to all societies and all situations.

I am pleased to join with Dr Glatt and invite the members of all our healing professions to learn and think more about the public health problems associated with drug use and to plan more effective health programmes.

H. David Archibald, M.S.W., D.Sc. (Hon.)
Executive Director,
Addiction Research Foundation,
Toronto, Canada.

Drugs, Society and Man

A GUIDE TO ADDICTION AND ITS TREATMENT

PREFACE

It is customary and almost obligatory to start yet another treatise on drug dependence, adding to the present epidemic of such books, by an apology and an attempt at an alibi for so doing. I have no genuine excuse except that publishers' requests to doctors to write such books, must indicate some interest by the public. Moreover, as I have been actively interested and involved in this subject for many years – as a clinician, as well as writing and talking about it – it was difficult to resist the temptation to summarize my views, when invited to do so, and given a free hand as to the contents and composition. After all, my involvement with the subject over such a long time has provided me with a greater opportunity to make mistakes than many other people – a chance of which I have undoubtedly often availed myself!

A question which gave the Publishers and me something of a headache was that of a suitable title. Since first becoming interested in the field of alcoholism and drug misuse and dependence at Warlingham Park Hospital in the early 1950's, I was struck and fascinated by the complex and multifactorial nature of the problems involved. From the beginning of the Alcoholism Unit at Warlingham Park Hospital (started in 1952), doctors, nurses, social workers, pharmacists, psychologists, hospital chaplains, patients, their families, and Alcoholics Anonymous collaborated closely in a multi- and interdisciplinary team venture and effort. Since then the necessity for a broad interdisciplinary approach has remained foremost in my mind: an approach aimed at improving or correcting any deficiencies or problems whether arising from the mental or physical make-up of the personality, from the environment, or from the pharmacological nature of the drug involved. However, as the Publishers were quick to point out, a title such as 'Drugs, Society and Man' would give little indication of the subject matter – i.e. dependence. Again, a query mark hangs over using the term 'addiction' in the title. As an old admirer of the work of the

World Health Organization, who years ago abandoned the term 'addiction', substituting the term 'dependence', I remonstrated at the term 'addiction' proposed by the Publishers. However, they pointed out that whereas everybody had heard of the term 'addiction', not everybody would know the meaning of the term 'dependence'.

Moreover, addiction or dependence is only one of the complications of excessive or faulty use of drugs, which also include, for example, overdoses, mental or physical illnesses, traffic accidents, etc. As Dr George Birdwood has rightly stressed, we ought really, therefore, to talk about drug 'abuse' rather than drug dependence alone. However, the term 'abuse' seems to imply a moral judgement (Concise Oxford Dictionary: '. . . an established unjust or corrupt practice . . .'), and therefore the term 'misuse' might be preferable, as suggested by Mark Keller. Then again, this volume deals not only with misuse of drugs but also of other substances, such as food, coffee, and tea; yet a title such as 'A Guide to Misuse of Substances' would certainly leave everyone baffled, and moreover would not include gambling. This brings us back to 'square one' – 'dependence' or 'addiction'? As discussed in the text, semantic difficulties are attached to all these definitions. For example, the infant born to a heroin-dependent mother has never had any pathological desire for heroin in the past and, as he has no 'compulsive craving' at present, surely the term 'addict' does not apply – but yet he is physically dependent, i.e. suffering from abstinence symptoms, after birth. Under the circumstances, as I could not think of any better title than the one suggested by the Publishers, I agreed somewhat reluctantly to a compromise title – namely, 'Drugs, Society and Man – A Guide to Addiction and its Treatment'.

One of the earliest lessons I learned, when dealing with alcoholics at Warlingham Park Hospital twenty years ago, was the prevalence of alcoholics' misuse of drugs other than alcohol – in particular barbiturates and, to a lesser extent, amphetamines – both drugs to become much later agents of misuse by teenagers. The great majority of the WPH alcoholics were also heavy smokers. a few were compulsive gamblers. Most of them ate little, but when recovering from their state of alcoholism the great majority regained their appetite. Exceptionally, a recovered alcoholic became a compulsive eater, but not uncommonly did recovered alcoholics develop a hankering for sweets which they had either abhorred or been indifferent to in the past. Very often, having forsworn alcohol, they also began to consume large amounts of coffee or tea. Because of these experiences, I became interested early on in the question of similarities and dissimilarities between the various substances lending themselves to misuse, and in the extent to which they could be handled administratively and therapeutically 'under one umbrella'.

Preface

The personal observations – on which this book is mainly based – were gained: at the Alcoholic Unit at WPH in the early and mid 1950's (initially a purely alcoholism unit, it also from time to time contained a number of middle-aged professional and therapeutic narcotic and 'soft drug' addicts); later on at the Alcoholism and Drug Dependence Unit at St Bernard's Hospital (and its Out-patient Clinics) started in the late 1950's (where one began to see an increasing number of young misusers of, and addicts to, 'soft' and narcotic drugs); at the Treatment Centre for drug addicts and at the Alcoholism Clinic of the University College Hospital; at the Out-patient Clinics for alcoholics and addicts at the Paddington Clinic and Day Hospital; at Hostels for alcoholics and drug addicts, respectively, working in conjunction with the St Bernard's Unit; and, throughout the 1960's from individual and group work with alcoholics, drug misusers, gamblers, etc., at Wormwood Scrubs Prison, which in 1972 led to the formation of a Unit for all these types of patients in that Prison.

However, possibly a much more important reason for discussing the old-time favourites and stand-by's of adult society in the same volume as the hashish and the heroin of the modern teenage misusers, is the need of parents and adult society in general to realise that in principle their excessive use of alcohol and nicotine is essentially not different from the youngsters' opiates and cannabis. This is notwithstanding the fact that society has accepted and legalised alcohol and nicotine but not opiates and cannabis.

As mentioned above an early lesson from the WPH Unit was the need for an integrated, multi-disciplinary team approach. For example, from the start of the Unit, nurses, social workers, psychologists, priests, probation officers, family members, Alcoholics Anonymous, etc., were involved in the work, as well as doctors. Similarly, groups were run by nurses, psychologists, priests, sociologists, as well as by doctors. Research work, too, was from the start interdisciplinary in nature, as reflected in Papers written jointly with psychologists, sociologists, pharmacists, social workers, nurses, pathologists, etc. It was clear from experiences in a therapeutic community and the success of teamwork, that the quality of caring was greatly improved by sharing the work and responsibility (though not shifting it). The vital need in this field to keep up a dialogue and communication applies, of course, not only to the relationship between staff and patients and to members of the therapeutic team, but also between research workers of various disciplines, and between workers in the different countries, in order to learn from each others' observations, experiences, and mistakes; and clearly also between adults and adolescents, and parents and children, so as to bridge the generation gap.

My thanks are due to the Editors and Publishers of books and journals for their permission to reprint extracts from my articles – in the main, the British Medical Journal, The Lancet, The British Journal of Addiction, *the* Nursing Mirror, *the* Nursing Times, The Pharmaceutical Journal, *the* World Health Organization Chronicle, *the* United Nations Narcotics Bulletin, *and the* International Journal of Addictions. *I am also grateful to the Authors and Publishers from whose works I have quoted – too numerous to enumerate here, but referred to in the text. There are a number of journals which over the years I have found very valuable and informative, as undoubtedly they will be to other readers. Among scientific journals:* The Quarterly Journal for the Study of Alcohol (*Editor, Mark Keller*), The International Journal of Addictions (*Editor, Stanley Einstein*), Alcoholism (*Editor, Vladimir Hudolin*),The British Journal of Addiction, *the organ of the Society for the Study of Addiction,*Drug Dependence, *an abstracting Journal published in the Netherlands,and the French language journal,*Toxaconamie (*published by OPTAT in Quebec*). *Among Journals written for a wider public, there are those published by the Addiction Research Foundation in Ontario* (Addictions *and* The Journal), *and the Medical Council on Alcoholism (the* Journal of Alcoholism, *Editor, H. D. Chalke). Mention must be made here of the popular journal* Drugs and Society, *which was published by the Standing Organization on Drug Abuse. Unfortunately, however, it has now ceased publication. Two other series well worth while studying are the regular publications on drug dependence (and occasionally on alcoholism) written by Expert Committees of the World Health Organization; and the Proceedings of the regular Congresses run by the International Council on Alcohol and Addictions (Executive Director, Archer Tongue).*

However, in the main, this book is based on what I have learned over a period of some 25 years from my patients in innumerable individual and group discussions – patients coming from all walks of life, and belonging to all social strata, ranging from those seen in the Drug Dependence Unit at Wormwood Scrubs Prison to those in private practice. Much of my experience also stems from talks and seminars with medical students, doctors, social workers, nurses, clergymen, probation officers, pharmacists, magistrates, police officers, etc., and the lay public. Special thanks are due to my medical, nursing, and other colleagues at Warlingham Park Hospital, St Bernard's Hospital, University College Hospital, the Paddington Clinic and Day Hospital, Spelthorne St Mary, Maidenhead Hospital, Wormwood Scrubs Prison, etc.; to Members of the National Council on Alcoholism, the Medical Council on Alcoholism, and the Society for the Study of Addiction; and to the many colleagues and friends from this country and abroad whom I have met over the years at the Conferences of the International Council on Alcohol and Addictions. I can mention here only a few individuals by name, with whom at some time or other I discussed some of the issues touched upon in the following pages: The two late Presidents of the Medical Council on Alcoholism, Professor Francis Camps and Lord Rosenheim, and its present Executive Director, Surgeon Vice-Admiral Sir Dick Caldwell; Dr T. L. Chrusciel (World Health Organization) and Professor Hans Halbach (formerly with the WHO); Archer Tongue (International Council on Alcohol and Addictions); Doctors A. D. Archibald, J. de Lint, R. D. Smart and W. S. Schmidt, all from the Ontario Research Foundation (Canada); Professor Jorge Mardones (Chile); Dr Jaroslaw Skala (Czechoslovakia); Professor Kettil Bruun (Finland); Dr Pierre Fouquet (France); Dr Lothar Schmidt and the late Professor Stefan Wieser (Germany); Dr Janos Metneki (Hungary); Professor Joshua O. Leibowitz and Dr Louis Miller (Israel); Professor W. van Dijk and Hank Krauweel (Netherlands); Sir Charles Burns (New Zealand); Dr Th. Kjolstad (Norway); Dr Leong Hon Koon (Singapore); Dr Nils Berjerok, Dr Peter Frisch and Professor Gunnar Lundquist (Sweden); Professor Raymond Battegay and Professor Hugo Solms (Switzerland); Professor Mark Keller, Professor David Pittman, Dr Stanley Einstein, Dr Donald B. Louria, and Dr Frank A. Seixas (USA); and Professor Vladimir Hudolin (Yugoslavia). I have learned and borrowed freely from all of them, but the responsibility for possibly having misinterpreted them and having come to conclusions with which some of them may possibly disagree, is completely my own.

Finally, my thanks are due to Mr David Bloomer, Managing Director of MTP, for his valuable suggestions and untiring help, in spite of his strenuous business schedule; and to my Personal Assistant, Mrs Phyllis Buffam, for her help with typing the manuscript – for some reason or other the Publishers seem to prefer her typing to my own laborious two-fingered typing efforts!

PART 1

PART 1

INTRODUCTION

'In these days of "strenuous life" with its consequent strain and worry, most of us are interested in discussions upon the moderate and immoderate use of drugs. The interest is aroused, not only on account of the many people who now treat themselves for their various aches and pains, but also because there are so many instances of the drug habit, that the baneful influence of excess is often apparent to us in a most realistic and painful manner' [1].

There is nothing very remarkable about the above statement in these days when drugs and drug 'addicts' make news and headlines, except that it was written not in the 1960s or 1970s but in a book published in London on 'Popular Drugs – their Use and Abuse' 65 years ago.

A *drug* has been defined by the psychopharmacologist C. R. B. Joyce [2] as '... any chemical which is introduced into a living organism and which leads to physiological effects ... which can be detected by objective means', whether or not such a substance is used for therapeutic reasons or not. Man has employed drugs since time immemorial in an attempt to banish pain and discomfort, to attain a state of oblivion, or alternatively, euphoria or ecstasy, or to get away from unpleasant reality into a much more agreeable state of phantasy. From time to time some drug may have been regarded as sacred by some culture, but condemned as a devil's instrument by another. Over the ages many such psychotrophic drugs (i.e. drugs that affect the mind) have gained and lost popularity. Some of the best known among them, such as alcohol, the opiates and cannabis, so popular in many parts of the world today, have been great favourites for thousands of years even though such popularity waxed and waned, and varied from culture to culture.

1

Such substances have been used and abused by millions of people the world over, although with many of them it is difficult or impossible to say where 'use' ends and 'abuse' begins.

Drug abuse

Drug abuse has been defined by a WHO Expert Committee [3] as '. . . the consumption of a drug apart from medical need or in unnecessary quantities'. Yet doctors often disagree as to what constitutes medical need, this not only at varying times in history, but also at the same age in different countries and even between doctors in the same country. (Consider, for example, present-day controversies about the advisability of or need for methadone maintenance, or the use of LSD in certain psychiatric conditions.) The nature and significance of drug abuse may be considered in terms of interaction between the drug and the individual on the one hand, and between drug and society on the other. With many drugs it may be said that moderate use may be beneficial, whereas immoderate use may be harmful. However, the effects of drugs depend not only on their pharmacological nature but also on the personality of the individual who takes them and on the environment or the total situation [2] in which the drug is taken. Again, what constitutes use and abuse, or what is defined as such, may depend not only on pharmacological factors or on the interaction between man and drug, but also on the prevalent view taken at a given time by a given society.

Besides 'The Pill', we have pills to sedate us when we are nervous, excite us when we are dull, slim us when we are fat, fatten us when we are thin, wake us when we are sleepy, put us to sleep when we are awake, cure us when we are sick, and make us sick when we are well [4]. It would seem – judging from the enormous amounts of tranquillisers and sedative-hypnotics prescribed nowadays by the medical profession and swallowed by the population – that sedation of even mild nervous states and the consumption of sleeping pills in mild states of insomnia is widely regarded as justifiable use (and certainly not as deviant behaviour) despite the risk that many people in this way may become unduly mentally and physically dependent on such drugs. In fact, taking an overdose has become so common an occurrence as to warrant its description as the modern epidemic [5] (see Section 5.2). Overdoses account for at least 10 % of acute medical admissions to hospitals in Britain. Barbiturates are the most frequently used drug for this purpose but other drugs affecting the central nervous system and commonly prescribed nowadays – such as tranquillisers, antidepressants and non-barbiturate hypnotics – contribute an ever-rising proportion [5]. In 1970 General Practitioners dispensed nearly 50 million NHS prescriptions for psychotropic drugs. The number of barbiturate prescriptions rose greatly during the 1950s and the early 1960s to over 15 million prescriptions in 1961. They reached their highest figure of over 17 million in 1965, falling gradually to 10.9 million in 1971. However the decline in barbiturate prescriptions has been paralleled by a gradual rise in prescriptions for non-barbiturate hypnotics (3.4 million in 1961, 7.1 million in 1971) and tranquillisers (6.2 million in 1961, 17.1 million in 1971) (see Section 5.2). If medical students had better training in the principles of psychological medicine and medical men more time to listen to patients (and fewer to look after), and if people were not taught by the mass-media to expect a magic pill to rapidly banish all worries and pains, then patients would not ask for so many pills and doctors would be much less forthcoming in prescribing them. In this way what is now regarded as more or less legitimate 'use', might come to be regarded as 'abuse'.

The attitude of the medical profession and society
Changes in the way doctors look at a given drug – its values and dangers – may sometimes occur fairly rapidly. Not so long ago the prescribing of amphetamines, the 'pep pills', to provide energy and euphoria, reduce obesity and keep people alert (the German term for the amphetamines is 'Weckamine' – wake-up amines) was generally accepted as good medical practice by the medical profession. Nowadays their use is frowned upon and actively discouraged, and in general, they are considered useless and often dangerous (see Section 5.1). The success of this campaign against using 'pep pills' is reflected in the gradually decreasing prescription figures of amphetamines during the past decade. Many youngsters, however, use them or rather abuse them in grossly excessive doses for stimulation, to feel 'good' and 'high' and in order to feel sufficiently energetic to roam around all night. This in the eyes of their middle-aged parents and society is obviously gross 'abuse'. However, are such youngsters completely in the wrong when they maintain that their parents' widespread use of tranquillisers and hypnotics, of alcohol and tobacco, constitutes as much drug abuse as their own indulgence in pep pills, 'sleepers', 'hash' and 'acid'.

Often fashion or the law may decide what is use and misuse. In

Western culture alcohol in moderate amounts is accepted and its use
widely encouraged, but the smoking of cannabis in the eyes of the Law
constitutes abuse – whether or not its pharmalogical properties make it
less or more harmful than alcohol. Again, some nations seem to imply
by their activities that they regard the ingestion of certain drugs by their
own citizens as harmful abuse, but as useful as far as other nations are
concerned. They therefore may ban such substances at home but continue to manufacture them for export purposes; or they allow the
manufacture of certain products and even advertisements extolling
their virtues, while at the same time issuing faint-hearted statements
warning against their abuse.

Doctors' prescribing habits regarding psychoactive drugs have been
greatly criticised (see Section 7.1) Some reasons for this state of affairs
have been referred to above, such as the lack of training in psychiatry
of the medical undergraduate and the heavy pressure on doctors' time.
Doctors themselves are also exposed to a great deal of persuasion by
the drug industry, with letters, brochures, etc. floating through the
doctor's letter box morning after morning. The doctor's lack of time
to study thoroughly the pharmacological value of the many drugs
manufactured regularly by the industry and to keep abreast of medical
and pharmacological progress, naturally contributes to his susceptibility
to the advertising campaign – the more so as there is much valuable
information included in such advertising material. Naturally the drug
industry has come in for much criticism. However, William Breckon,
a well known medical journalist, in a recently published monograph
dealing with this subject [6], concludes that the consistent attacks on the
drug industry are largely unjustified and depend on 'prejudice and
false premise'. The industry – he claims – provides a convenient scape-
goat for any deficiencies of the NHS; and '. . . politicians, overworked
doctors and the well-meaning legislators are immune from attack'.
In fact only 13 % of NHS spending relates to drugs. However, whilst
the busy G.P. certainly will obtain much valuable information from
reading the drug brochures, it seems difficult to believe that the
industry would spend so much money on this approach without
believing that the doctors' prescribing habits will be influenced in this
way. Therefore, as a safeguard against indiscriminate use of drugs
doctors are constantly encouraged to get intimately acquainted with a
limited number of preparations rather than trying out any new drug
coming on to the market.

Whatever reasons there may be for all the ambivalence towards drug abuse shown by state, society and the medical profession, etc., the questions involved are complex and do not lend themselves to simple, easy answers so often proposed by extreme partisans on one side or the other. 'Who is sick?' asks Professor Raymond Battegay, 'Is it the individual or is it the whole society?' [7]. Young drug addicts not uncommonly lay the blame for their having been 'driven to' drug abuse fairly and squarely at the doors of the non-caring materialistic society which, they claim, is concerned with technical progress only and could not care less about the value and dignity of the individual. This is clearly a gross exaggeration and oversimplification of a complex problem and obviously drug addicts cannot passively sit back and expect society to solve their personal problems for them. However, it behoves society to attempt to discover what factors and defects there are in modern society that may contribute to so many of its younger members looking for relief in deviant forms of behaviour, such as delinquency and drug abuse. Some sociologists question whether the interest taken by the community today in the drug abuse of youngsters may not have its origin in the guilt feelings of society which has found a convenient scape-goat in youngsters' drug abuse [8]. Yet doctors coming across numerous cases of youngsters who have gone to pieces physically and mentally as a consequence of such behaviour, may be forgiven for feeling that there are other, more obvious reasons why society must take an interest in, and care about, drug abusers.

There is a vital need for objective, fact-finding research in all aspects of the problems of alcohol and drug abuse, research that must be multi- and interdisciplinary in nature and scope. Doctors are clearly important members of such a multidisciplinary research team. Yet at the same time, doctors – and other professional workers – cannot be content with just observing and researching; they must also actively render help, they must care and become involved. Moreover, often action cannot always be postponed until research has settled and answered all or most of the outstanding questions; casualties may require help urgently. As far as possible, facilities for planned research should form part and parcel of all new therapeutic facilities for addicts and alcoholics, but where treatment facilities are urgently needed they should be started, even if the possibilities for research are meagre for the time being. At a time when, for example, it is unknown whether it might be a help or a hindrance to mix alcoholics and addicts to other drugs in the same treatment facility, it would seem wise to start a number of facilities with different programmes. It would then be possible to learn from a comparison of the findings and observations obtained under such varying conditions. This is surely preferable to waiting until a definite answer (if there is a definite answer to such a question) is forthcoming.

Abuse of 'other drugs'
The vastly increased interest shown by the British public in the last decade in the problem of 'other drugs' (i.e. drugs other than alcohol) has probably been triggered off by a number of factors, such as:

(a) The increase of abuse of narcotics (a problem of many years standing in the USA), and the epidemics of soft drugs abuse not only in the UK but also in Sweden, Holland, the Netherlands etc.

(b) The fact that drug abuse and addiction are occurring in younger and younger individuals. Cases of drug dependence in the late teens are common nowadays, and of those in the early teens are no longer exceptional.

(c) The earlier more familiar types of middle-aged therapeutic and professional addicts have been replaced by the non-therapeutic and non-professional addicts [4] who started drug misuse for reasons such as pursuit of kicks, and among whom drug abuse spread has sometimes been likened to the contagiousness of infectious diseases [9], and

(d) The widespread rise in the use of the various types of cannabis all over the world, hailed by its users and protagonists as a drug much less dangerous than alcohol. It has been estimated that 24 000 000 Americans have now smoked marijuana [10].

In view of such developments, it is little wonder that governments have been forced to take more and more notice of the increasing drug menace. For example in the UK, whereas the first Interdepartmental Drug Addiction Committee in 1961 issued a report indicating that the drug situation was more or less under control, its Second Report only four years later had to admit that the situation had worsened rapidly and seriously, necessitating far-reaching new recommendations [4]. In the USA, in March 1972, President Nixon signed the Drug Abuse Office and Treatment Act which appropriates $1.1 billion over a period of three years providing the means to attack the nation's drug abuse problem through the White House Special Action Office for Drug Abuse Prevention [10].

Likewise, the increasing number of International Conferences reflects the concern over the widespread rise of drug abuse in many countries. To give only a few examples: in Basel, Switzerland, of pupils aged 13–16 years, attending intermediate schools without school-leaving examination, 8·3 % had had experience with drugs; of pupils attending schools with school-leaving examinations, 13·5 % had had experience with drugs and in a training school for clerks with pupils between 15 and 19 years the figure was 27·3 % [11]. In Italy, a country little heard about in connection with drug abuse, the percentage of students using drugs has been estimated to be up to 2 % of the student population [12]. As regards CNS stimulants, Japan had an epidemic of amphetamine abuse in the 1940s affecting 6 000 000 persons which was brought to a halt following energetic intervention by the Japanese authorities. However another intravenous amphetamine epidemic has more recently affected Sweden, the number of such addicts estimated at 10 000 [13]. In Denmark, up to 25·3 % of the student population has been reported to experiment with hashish [14].

The approach to alcoholism and drug dependence
In view of the great interest in recent years shown by the mass-media in the problem of abuse of drugs it is important to stress that in all Western countries the greatest drug menace – the one still creating the greatest and most widespread harm – is alcoholism. In the UK, for example, the number of narcotic addicts may perhaps be in the region of 3–4000 (if one were to include the black market users). The numbers of those dependent on amphetamines and barbiturates – although of course even approximate estimates are impossible – were thought a few years ago to be in the region of 80 000 and 100 000 respectively [15]. In comparison the most widely accepted estimate of alcoholics in the UK is approximately 350 000 [16]. This is one reason why in this volume a chapter on alcoholism precedes the chapters dealing with the other drugs (see Part 3). Another reason for this arrangement is that a few years ago an Expert Committee of the World Health Organisation (1967) [17] recommended a *combined approach* to alcoholism and dependence on other drugs in view of so many factors similar to both these problems. (The author feels that 'coordinated' is perhaps a better term than 'combined'.) Therefore, in spite of certain dissimilarities, it was recommended that national public health authorities should, in principle, approach these conditions 'under one umbrella', i.e. under the same organisational structure [18] (see Section 3.1).

An earlier WHO Expert Committee (1957) had named four features as characteristics of, and as distinguishing features between, what was

then called *habituation* and *addiction* respectively (terms later replaced by
the more embracing term *dependence*). Features of addiction were:
  (a) A desire or compulsive need to continue taking the drug and to
      obtain it by any means.
  (b) A tendency to increase the dose.
  (c) A psychic (psychological) and a physical dependence on the
      effects of the drug.
  (d) A detrimental effect on the individual and society [19].

Drug habituation was said to be characterised by a desire but not a
compulsion to continue taking the drug, little or no tendency to
increase the dose and some degree of psychic dependence but absence
of a physical dependence and hence of an abstinence syndrome.
Detrimental effects, if any, were primarily on the individual. *Drug
addiction* was said to be characterised by 'craving', tolerance and psychic
and physical dependence – as shown by the development of psychological and physical abstinence symptoms respectively. These old
definitions often gave rise to difficulties but in the following chapters
these terms will still have to be referred to repeatedly. Alcoholism for
example, seems to fall midway between these definitions of habituation
and addiction. Sometimes one comes across the term *pharmacological
dependence*, occasionally employed as synonymous with *physical
dependence*. However, as O. J. Kalant [20] rightly points out, 'There
can be psychological dependence on the pure pharmacological effects
of the drug, even in the absence of physical dependence as shown by
the lack of withdrawal reaction'.

Drugs affecting the central nervous system have been classified in
various ways; for example as those producing psychic dependence
only, as those producing physical as well as psychic dependence, or as
CNS-stimulating and CNS-depressing drugs, as soft and hard drugs
etc. All these terms – some of which have been strongly criticised – will
be discussed later. It has often been pointed out, and rightly so, that the
term soft drugs – applied for example to amphetamines, barbiturates,
cannabis, and LSD – might wrongly give the idea that such drugs may
be more or less harmless. The history of alcohol and drug abuse has
been beset with many highly emotionally-charged controversies and
arguments, which left the contestants hot and bothered, but which were
often highly irrational and strongly biased. For example, thousands of
articles were written prior to the emergence of the modern, 'scientific'
approach to alcoholism in the early 1940s; but research by Jellinek
and Keller in 1939 [21] revealed that of the voluminous literature only a

relatively small proportion was really founded on an objective, rational basis and that the great majority could not be relied on as the subject was approached in a preconceived emotionally biased way. Over the centuries and up to the present time battles have been fought between the 'wet' and the 'dry', and even among the 'dry' themselves; between the prohibitionists, who wanted to eliminate the liquor industry and the moral persuasionists, who wanted to educate the people to renounce the use of alcohol on the basis of moral arguments; between those who see the answer to drug problems in relying on a strong law (aiming at prohibition or restriction) and those who would prefer to rely mainly on education (see Section 7.2); between those who want resources mainly used to finance research in order to prevent abuse and dependence, and those clamouring for the establishment of better therapeutic facilities to treat today's addicts; between those in favour of the British system of drug approach (i.e. allowing certain doctors to prescribe narcotic drugs to addicts) and the punitive American approach (under which doctors do not prescribe heroin to addicts) (see Section 6.2); between the protagonists of the chemical treatments (e.g. methadone maintenance and antagonists) and those in favour of self-help organisations; between the 'legalise pot' lobby and their opponents etc. Such controversies are often very bitter and acrimonious and lead to passionate counter arguments [22].

Two further examples can be quoted. The first refers to the famous 'Battle of the Barbiturates' [22] which was fought out in the twenties and thirties in the conference halls of British medical societies and in the correspondence columns of the 'Lancet'. The Home Office pathologist, Dr William Willcox, possibly the first to recognise the addictive nature of barbiturates but bitterly attacked by other doctors who described them as ' . . . one of the great gifts . . . offered to suffering humanity', felt it necessary to defend his views about the barbiturates when opening a discussion in a scientific debate:

'What I shall tell you is very controversial, but I stand by my statements. I know what I am telling you is true and is not the result of reading, but of tragedies which have come to my notice from the many cases I have seen and treated personally. There can be no doubt that the very large group of barbituric acid derivatives occupies the foremost place amongst the drugs of addiction. The need for care in their use cannot be too strongly emphasised . . . The members of the medical profession should exercise care in the prescription of these drugs . . .'

Many doctors at the time rebelled against what they called 'the absurdities of Willcox' teaching' on the barbiturates. Clearly later developments fully bore out Willcox' warnings.

The second more recent example refers to the current debate as to whether alcoholics may occasionally learn to drink in moderation, a controversy that evoked the comment from two American research workers [23], 'It might be proper logically and clinically to question or challenge the permanence or stability of this benaviour, but to deny its existence for a stated period of time is merely prejudice, not science'.

Emotional prejudice and bias rather than objective findings and scientific research have all too often dominated (and bedevilled) the approach to problems on drug dependence. The 14th WHO Expert Committee [17] dealing with alcoholism as well as dependence on other drugs expressed the hope that the *combined* approach might also assist the *scientific* approach to questions of dependence on other drugs, just as 30 years ago the scientific approach to alcoholism began to supersede the former more prevalent emotional approach. Until fact-finding research provides some of the answers, one has to admit openly that frequently definite answers can not be given today. One should not confuse hypotheses so often based on prejudice – even if put forward with great confidence and vigour – with objective facts.

Types of dependence-producing drugs

With the approval of the WHO Expert Committees, Eddy *et al.* [24] have listed the following main types of dependence-producing drugs according to the agent or class of agents involved:

Alcoholic type (which because of many close similarities, and of marked cross-tolerance, is often coupled with the barbiturates into a barbiturate –alcohol type)

Barbiturate type

Morphine type

Amphetamine type

Khat type

Cocaine type

Cannabis type

Hallucinogen type

It must be constantly kept in mind, however, that in contrast to former years, drug addicts nowadays, particularly those in the younger age group, commonly misuse several types of drugs at the same time. It is not unusual to meet young drug abusers who take any drug they can get hold of, often without bothering to ask what type of drug it is, whether it has sedative or stimulating effects, or even of what strength are the tablets they buy on the illicit market. In England, at the present time, youngsters attending the Treatment Centres where they receive heroin and/or methadone, may also at the same time be buying on the illicit market the so-called Chinese heroin (containing, apart from heroin, caffeine and sometimes also quinine or barbiturates), amphetamines, the non-barbiturates (e.g. mandrax), cannabis (usually in the form of the resin hashish) and LSD. In addition some drink heavily or they may also obtain some proprietary cough mixture preparations. Often they manage, by attending various doctors as temporary patients, to obtain barbiturate tablets which they dissolve and inject intravenously, often together with heroin or methadone. The result therefore is a mixed type of dependence. The doctor who is called upon to treat a young drug addict must therefore take great care to elicit by careful history taking, not only from the patient but also, if possible, from family and friends, which combination of drugs have been involved, for how long and in what amounts. This should be followed by physical examination and laboratory tests (chemical analyses of blood or urine), and by close observation after the treatment has started.

In the chapters that follow the individual groups of dependence-producing drugs will be discussed but this modern pattern of multi-drug involvement must not be underemphasised. To comprehend one of today's most disturbing problems it is not the single drug, not the individual patient and not the isolated community's subculture pattern that must be appreciated alone, but the whole spectrum of drug abuse in modern society – a spectrum that emerges from the following chapters. As will be seen, in considering the complex area of modern drug use, the interacting triad of man, society and drugs must be considered together and the effects of drugs perceived and approached in appropriate perspective [25].

REFERENCES

1. Hiller, S. (1909). *Popular Drugs – their Use and Abuse*, 9 (London: T. Werner Laurie).
2. Joyce, C. R. B. (1966). *New Horizons in Psychology*, 271 (B. M. Foss, editor) (London: Penguin Books).
3. WHO Expert Committee (1965). *Tech. Rep. Ser.*, **312,** 7, 8.

4. Glatt, M. M., Pittman, D. J., Gillespie, D. G. and Hills, D. R. (1969). *The Drug Scene in Great Britain*, Revised 1st ed., 1 (London: Edward Arnold (Publ.) Ltd.).
5. Matthew, H. (1972–1973). *Medicine*, **4**, 273.
6. Breckon, W. (1972). *The Drug Makers*, 211–212 (London: Eyre Methuen)
7. Battegay, R. (1972). *Vom Hintergrund der Süchte*, 2nd ed., 7 (Blaukreuz Verlag, Bern; Blaukreuz Verlag, Wuppertal-Barmen).
8. Wiener, R. S. P. (1970). *Drugs and Schoolchildren*, 165 (London: Longman).
9. Bejerot, N. *Addiction and Society*, 91 (Springfield, Illin.: Charles C. Thomas).
10. National Co-ordinating Council on Drug Education (1972). *Drug Education Report*, **II**, No. 4. Washington D.C.
11. Battegay, R. and Ladewig, D. (1972). *Int. Symp. Drug Abuse, Jerusalem* (Abstracts), 4.
12. Frighi, L. *ibid.*, 16
13. Bejerot, N. *ibid.*, 66.
14. Manniche, E. *ibid.*, 72.
15. Bewley, T. H. (1966). *Bull. Narcot.* (*U.N.*), **18**, 1, (4).
16. Glatt, M. M. (1970). *The Alcoholic and the Help He Needs* (London: Priory Press).
17. WHO Expert Committee (1966). *Tech. Rep. Ser.*, 363.
18. Glatt, M. M. (1970). *A World Dialogue on Alcohol and Drug Dependence*, 311 (E. D. Whitney, editor) (Boston: Beacon Press).
19. WHO Expert Committee (1957). *Tech. Rep. Ser.*, **116**, 9.
20. Kalant, O. J. (1966). *The Amphetamines*, 98 (Toronto: Univ. Toronto Press).
21. Keller, M. (1972). *Brit. J. Addict.*, **67**, 153.
22. Glatt, M. M. (1962). *Bull. Narcot.* (U.N.), **14**, 20, (2).
23. Gerard, D. L. and Saenger, G. (1966). *Out-Patient Treatment of Alcoholism*, 110 (Toronto: Univ. Toronto Press).
24. Eddy, N. B., Halbach, H., Isbell, H. and Seevers, M. H. (1965). *Bull. WHO.*, **32**, 721.
25. Chrusciel, T. L. (1973). Personal communication.

PART 2

WHAT MAKES AN ADDICT?*

2.1 DRUG DEPENDENCE

The problems of drug addiction or dependence – complex in themselves – are subject to added confusion because of the often quite different meanings attached to them by different observers. The following discussion refers to the question of aetiology of dependence and not merely of physical addiction. Some drugs produce psychological dependence only, others produce physical as well as psychological dependence. Contrary to widespread popular misconception, it is psychological rather than physical dependence which in the long run may be much more difficult to overcome. At any rate because of continual confusion in using the terms addiction (physical plus psychological dependence) and habituation (psychological dependence), the World Health Organisation in 1964 [1] suggested dropping these terms in favour of the more embracing term dependence.

Drug dependence was defined by the 1964 WHO Expert Committee [1] as, '. . . a state arising from repeated administration of a drug on a periodic or continuous basis'. All dependence-producing drugs are capable of creating a state of mind in certain individuals which is termed psychic dependence . . . a psychic drive which requires periodic or chronic administration of the drug for pleasure or discomfort. Drugs producing psychological dependence only include cannabis, the hallucinogens and the CNS-stimulating drugs, such as cocaine and the amphetamines. (There seems to be no evidence that a physical abstinence syndrome has ever been observed in clinical practice

* This chapter is based in part on an article published in the *Nursing Times*, 4th November 1971

3

following amphetamine withdrawal, though research workers in Scotland have described certain physical withdrawal symptoms [2]. Other drugs can induce physical and psychological dependence. Physical dependence is an adaptive state or physiological change in the body which manifests itself by the development of frequently very severe physical disturbances if the drug is suddenly withdrawn. Such drugs include alcohol and those drugs which depress the CNS – the hypnotic sedatives (e.g. the barbiturates), certain tranquillisers and the narcotics (such as the opiates).

Whilst the new terminology regarding drug dependence is, in many ways, clearly superior to the old one, unfortunately semantic problems still remain and will probably always be with us. For example, fenfluramine, one of the modern appetite-reducing drugs, and imipramine, a popular antidepressant, are generally regarded, in the light of present-day knowledge, as being non-dependence-producing drugs, but scottish research workers (Oswald *et al.* [3]) described them recently as '. . . drugs of dependence though not of abuse'. However, the Scottish observers' terminology was later criticised by H. A. Wendel [4], because their patients had no compulsion (an irresistible drive to commit irrational acts) to take the two drugs and drug dependence had been defined by a WHO Expert Committee in 1969 [5] defined drug dependence as '. . . a state, psychic and sometimes also physical . . . characterised by behaviour and other responses that always include a compulsion to take the drug . . .'. Lack of compulsion thus meant also absence of dependence, and Oswald *et al.* were not justified in equating the presence of withdrawal symptoms with physical dependence.

Wendel claims that physical dependence is no more than an accidental feature of drug dependence, so that withdrawal symptoms or physical dependence may, or may not, indicate drug dependence. As we will see shortly, Canadian observers have recently described the presence of physical abstinence symptoms after severe drinking bouts in individuals who are not drinkers of long-standing [6].* Similarly, in our experience, publicans are often heavy drinkers who may show physical abstinence symptoms, such as DT, without necessarily having ever exhibited the phenomenon of compulsion; yet, physical abstinence symptoms denote

* On the other hand, Schuster and Balster [8] define physical dependence as, '. . a state which is produced by chronic drug administration and is revealed by the occurrence of signs of physiological dysfunction when the drug administration is abruptly discontinued. In other words, after prolonged exposure to the drug an organism's physiological functioning is dependent on the presence of the drug at certain receptor sites in the body . . . these withdrawal symptoms are readily reversible by the administration of the drug'

a bodily need for the presence of the drug, and are therefore described by Jellinek as evidence of the presence of physical addiction or of disease in strictly pharmacological terms [7]. Wendel refers to the finding that the narcotic antagonists nalorphine and cyclazocine, produce marked withdrawal symptoms after prolonged administration but no desire or compulsion to continue with them. And he finally points to the pathetic cases of babies born by heroin-addicted mothers. Such an infant may show obvious narcotic withdrawal symptoms (e.g. constant tremblings and convulsions), but he could hardly be called a heroin addict or a heroin-dependent individual. Similar to the drinker in DTs, where alcohol in Jellinek's view has become a temporarily required metabolic constituent, the infant's body temporarily needs the drug apparently in the absence of psychological desire or compulsion. Possibly the term physical dependence may not be the most fitting description for states such as the abstinence symptoms following the withdrawal of fenfluramine and imipramine, or those seen after withdrawal of alcohol after a severe bout in occasional drinkers or heavily drinking publicans, or those observed in infants born to heroin-addicted mothers. None of these individuals exhibiting physical abstinence symptoms seem to be psychologically dependent on the drug, although their body seems temporarily to require it for adequate physiological functioning, somewhat similar to, for example, the more prolonged need of the diabetic's body for insulin.

On the other hand, the pharmacologist H. O. J. Collier [9] comes to the conclusion that, 'Psychic and physical dependence can conveniently be regarded as subjective and objective manifestations of the same state, with the neural mechanisms involved in these two aspects of dependence not very different,' Physical dependence, in Collier's view, is most satisfactorily explained on the basis of a hypothesis of 'autonomic hyperreactivity' put forward by Himmelsbach 30 years ago. According to this theory, which defined physical dependence as '. . . a condition of autonomic hyperreactivity induced by opiates' (nowadays of course it is well-known that other drugs too, can produce physical dependence), the predominantly depressant effect of morphine leads to a greater excitability or reactivity, by inducing a compensating homeostatic mechanism in the autonomic nervous system. As long as morphine is present, this compensating mechanism is kept in check; once morphine is withdrawn, the way has been cleared for the excitability to manifest itself in the form of the abstinence syndrome. Nowadays autonomic hyperreactivity is ascribed to an interaction between the drug and endogenous neurohumoral factor(s). A number of hypothetical mechanisms have been proposed, most of which regard tolerance as a necessary precondition for physical dependence to develop.* As regards psychic dependence, in Collier's view, the danger of abuse is determined more by a drug's liability to induce psychic dependence than a tendency to induce physical dependence (a view, with which probably most clinicians would concur). He states that, 'The essential psychopharmacological action of a drug that leads to its abuse is that of enhancing pleasurable excitement, escape or relaxation – in a word, "reward" – and of lessening painful boredom, anxiety or defensiveness – in a word, "punishment".'†

The relationship between psychological and physical dependence
The relationship between psychological and physical dependence remains unclear. The characteristics of any state of dependence (see Part 1, page 8) include:
(a) Craving or pathological desire for the effects of the drug.
(b) A state of tolerance. (This necessitates increasing the dosage to obtain the same effect.)
(c) The supervening of psychological and/or physical abstinence symptoms on sudden cessation (or even too rapid reduction of the dosage) of the drug.

The length of time that has to elapse between onset of drug taking and the development of psychological and/or physical dependence may vary and may be related to any one of a number of factors, e.g. to the pharmacological nature of the drug concerned. Dependence in general arises more rapidly with the opiates than with the barbiturates, and with the latter more rapidly than with alcohol. This time interval also depends on the dosage employed and the speed and route of getting the drug into the system, the predisposition or emotional vulnerability of the drug taker's personality, and the interaction of psychological and environmental factors (e.g. ready availability and such socio-cultural

---

* However, according to J. E. Villarreal [10], 'The fact that severe abstinence syndromes cannot be produced with strong central depressant drugs to which tolerance of a high order is developed (i.e. cyclazocine-like drugs) shows again that tolerance and physical dependence are not necessarily associated'
†Many alcohol and other drug abusers are intolerant of frustration so that drugs bringing about relief or gratification rapidly carry a probably much greater risk of abuse than long acting drugs. As A. W. Peck put it, 'The abuse liability of a compound. . . is likely to be related, at least to some extent, to the immediate reward of a desired subjective effect' [42].

factors as social attitudes, and fashionability of the drug in a given locality).

Psychological dependence can certainly occur without physical dependence but can physical dependence occur without psychological dependence? Recent work carried out at the Addiction Research Foundation in Ontario [6] suggests that it can, and that, 'The physical dependence aspect of alcoholism is not, as previously thought, the cumulative result of years of abuse; instead it can be brought on by repetitive drinking over a few weeks and can be reversed when drinking stops'. Thus, as Archibald [6] remarks in his paper describing these findings, 'One does not have to become a socially or psychologically deteriorated alcoholic in order to experience physical dependence; one simply has to drink large enough quantities during a short period of time'. This conclusion fits in well with the present author's experience of very heavy drinkers who sometimes exhibit physical withdrawal symptoms at the sudden end of a severe bout, even without their having been long-standing alcoholics. Similarly one may mention in this connection the well-known finding that drinkers may develop definite physical and mental complications (chronic alcoholism) without necessarily having been psychologically dependent on alcohol, but just as a consequence of habitual heavy drinking (e.g. 9 ounces of whisky or 21 ounces of wine or $5\frac{1}{2}$ bottles of beer per day, every day in the year [6]). Naturally other factors, such as nutritional status, inadequate food intake, etc. may also be closely involved. To what extent such findings are also relevant to drugs other than alcohol, is not yet clear. In view of many other similarities between alcoholism and other types of drug dependence, there is at least the possibility that similar factors may also be at work in the case of some other drugs. This is yet another example showing the need for much further research in the field of dependence on alcohol and other drugs.

The aetiology of drug dependence

Regarding the importance or otherwise of physical dependence or abstinence symptoms in the aetiology of drug dependence, it should not be overlooked that there may be a difference between those aetiological factors that initially put the drug user on the road to drug abuse, e.g. psychological and social factors, and those that tend to maintain the state of dependence once it has been established. Clearly the fear of, and the distress caused by, physical abstinence symptoms can be important factors in maintaining a state of dependence. For example, many addicts give the fear of the 'cold turkey' as a reason for their not entering hospital for withdrawal treatment (although this may often be no more than a rationalisation). Other addicts trying to get off drugs give up in despair after a day or two of physical suffering. As regards alcohol, in Jellinek's view [7], the withdrawal symptoms following abrupt withdrawal or very rapid decrease of consumption indicate a true physical demand for alcohol (i.e. an adaptation of cell metabolism to that substance) and the demand for alcohol gives rise to the idea of 'craving'. This demand seems to be two-fold. First, the necessity to allay the distressing withdrawal symptoms, i.e. a physical demand, and second, the obsessive belief that sufficient alcohol ingestion will ultimately bring about the desired tension reduction. In a working hypothesis Jellinek suggests that, '. . . enzyme and vitamin anomalies, liver injuries, adrenal factors, and many biochemical lesions . . . may . . . weaken the resistance of nervous tissue to the integration of a noxious substance into its metabolism and to becoming dependent upon it. . . . Such anomalies and injuries could be products of heredity or of the stresses which prolonged heavy alcohol intake exerts'.

In a recent review, Van Dyjk [11] stresses that dependence is not a separate entity, but the final stage of a process, the earlier stages of which consist of contact, experimentation and excessive use. As regards the aetiology of dependence, Van Dyjk distinguishes between generating factors and factors maintaining the process after contact with the drug. His generating factors include the pharmacological effects of the drug, the personal factors of the user, the social meaning and value of a drug and of drug taking, and the environmental influences on the user. Among the factors that maintain dependence he discusses a number of relevant vicious circles: the pharmacological, the cerebro-ego weakening, the psychic and the social vicious circle. One additional reason given not infrequently by the modern type of young mainlining drug addict is the dependence on the 'needle' and on the act of 'fixing', described by some such addicts as a kind of orgiastic experience.

'I was mentally more dependent on the needle than on the drug', said an intelligent 23 year old methadone addict who had been 'fixing' 30–35 ampoules per day, injecting six ampoules with a 5 ml syringe several times a day. 'The needle fulfilled a sado-masochistic complex in me: hunting to find the elusive vein was a terrible hang-up. I searched masochistically for the vein for half an hour, and when I eventually hit the vein and pushed the stuff in, the relief when I saw the blood coming into the syringe was fantastic. By then, getting the drug into my body had become a secondary consideration. Shooting the stuff in was just an obvious conclusion after hitting the vein. The relief came when I hit it'.

There is no such person as 'the' addict. Different types of personalities use drugs of greatly varying chemical composition for different reasons under different conditions and in different situations. Among drug abusers one finds all kinds of personalities, and it would seem highly unlikely that there is any such thing as 'the' cause of drug dependence. Two aetiological factors were described by a WHO Expert Committee in 1952 [12] which divided drugs into three classes, on the basis of the user's psychological make-up, on the one hand, and the pharmacological property of the drug, on the other. In the first group of drugs, it is the pharmacological nature of the drug that is paramount whereas the user's individual reactions are no more than an adjunct. Sooner or later addiction (i.e. physical dependence) will develop in practically every user of this group of drugs. In the second category of drugs, their pharmacological nature plays no more than a subsidiary role whereas the user's individual reactions are decisive. Such drugs never produce addiction or an irresistible need for the drug, but lead to habituation (psychological or emotional dependence) in vulnerable personalities. Finally, with the third group of drugs, their pharmacological action is intermediate in kind and degree between the addiction-producing and the habit-forming drugs. Their pharmacological role is significant but the predominant factor is the mental make-up, so that addiction may develop in psychologically vulnerable personalities. The 1952 WHO Committee thus drew attention to two important aetiological factors, but failed to point to the significance of a third namely the social factor.

While the exact causation of drug dependence is still not clear, at the present state of knowledge it would seem that in a given individual at least three sets of factors are involved to bring about, in dynamic interaction with each other, a state of drug dependence. Drawing a rough analogy with the infectious diseases the person-to-person spread of the drug abuse habit among the young has often been likened to the contagiousness of infectious diseases. It is possible to discuss the causation of drug dependence under three headings: The 'host', i.e. the mental or physical personality make-up; the environment; and the 'agent', i.e. the pharmacological nature of the drug concerned [13].

2.2 PERSONALITY: THE ROLE OF THE 'HOST'

The importance of the role of an individual's psychological make-up in the causation of alcoholism and drug dependence, at least in initiating the abuse, is widely accepted. The role of a predisposing physical make-up though often postulated, and rightly the subject of much research, seems as yet unproven. It is of course very difficult, or even impossible, to draw conclusions from the condition of the long-established and advanced chronic alcoholic or drug addict as to his pre-addictive personality. If, for example, one finds certain physical abnormalities in a long-standing alcoholic, these could be just as likely (or in fact more likely) to be the consequence of his drinking behaviour, rather than their cause.

Pre-addictive personalities

A great many investigations have indicated fairly conclusively that there is no uniform pre-addictive or pre-alcoholic personality make-up which predisposes inevitably to the development of dependence. The picture of a fairly similar personality shown by advanced alcoholics on the one hand, and drug addicts on the other, seems due to the influence of secondary features which appear during the lengthy course of the developmental process of dependence. Yet if one compares the personality features shown by a great many alcoholics and drug-dependent individuals as described in the literature, or seen in one's own practice, one is often struck by their resemblance. Thus, emotional immaturity, a strong wish to turn one's back on reality, a low frustration tolerance, an unwillingness or inability to endure and to cope with tension, or to stick for long to a given course of activity (low staying power), etc. are features which occur frequently in many alcoholics and addicts.

It would seem that the choice of symptom in the individual with low frustration tolerance is largely accidental, and determined not so much by qualities inherent in the host, but in the environment (see Section 2.3), such as the availability of a suitable escape route at the time when the individual feels in need of one. The route, however, must be acceptable to his personality, and not incompatible with his outlook, attitudes, and values. Many alcoholics also tend to misuse other drugs which have an effect on their central nervous system. These are the predominantly *psychogenic* patients (whose alcoholism is due to under-lying personality factors) rather than the predominantly *sociogenic* ones (whose alcoholism is due to socio-cultural factors). This seems to refute the hypothesis of a specific predisposition to alcoholism (at least in most types of alcoholism). It possibly points to an unspecific tendency on the part of certain emotionally vulnerable individuals to look for ways and means of obtaining relief from discomfort and pain or, alternatively, for a higher degree of satisfaction than they have hitherto experienced. The degree of emotional and physical discomfort, the individual's ability to enjoy it, and the strength, character, and direction of internal controls of behaviour (consequence and ego control) are all important factors in the personality of the potential addict, and in the development of drug dependence [14] as well as of alcoholism.

In psycho-analytic literature, drug dependence, alcoholism, and habitual smoking, are frequently seen as phenomena resulting from 'oral fixation'. Another suggestion, put forward by Wikler [15] is the existence of certain differences between individuals and societies that prefer alcohol to opiates and *vice versa*. Alcohol releases the aggressive drive, opium weakens it. Alcohol, therefore, may be more likely to be popular with, and opium likely to be condemned by, individuals and such (for example, Western) society that value manliness and competitiveness – whereas opium would be preferred by more placid individuals and societies. It may not be irrelevant to note that this hypothesis was put forward more than twenty years ago and one might perhaps query whether these types of drugs were not taken by such societies long before they became either passive and placid, or competitive and aggressive respectively.

Genetic influences
Does inheritance play a role in causing alcoholism and drug dependence? Some drinkers claim that they are born alcoholics because they found it difficult to stop drinking practically from the time they took their first drinks. Again, the finding that so often there are several other problem drinkers in an alcoholic's family, is often quoted as an argument favouring an inheritance theory. However, most observers would tend to ascribe such occurrences to early environmental influences. For example, the disturbed and unstable home atmosphere created by an alcoholic's unpredictable behaviour is not the best breeding ground for a growing child's emotional security. Later on in life psychoneurotic or psychopathic tendencies arising on a foundation of emotional insecurity, may predispose to excessive drinking, drug taking etc. Conscious or, perhaps more often, unconscious identifica-

tion with a drinking father may then, in such cases, determine drinking as the choice of symptom, and it is interesting in this connection to note the not infrequent finding that a young drug taker's parent was in fact an alcoholic. This might be an example of rebellion on the youngster's part against his parent's behaviour. Similarly, not infrequently one comes across examples of fanatic teetotallers amongst children of alcoholics, and occasionally these teetotallers' sons may again turn out to be alcoholics.

However, the possible role of genetic factors, in particular as regards alcohol dependence, is being actively investigated in a number of countries. For example, Professor Jorge Mardones, in Chile [16] a pioneer in this type of research, points to the wide individual fluctuations not only in normal 'physiological appetency' but also in pharmacological appetency (i.e. drinking for the effect of alcohol), pathological appetency (characteristic of the loss-of-control and inability-to-abstain drinker), and in susceptibility to medical complications. In theory, such fluctuations may originate from genetic or from environmental influences. The environmental factors such as accessibility of the drug, and cultural rules concerning its use, act on everybody, and yet there are important individual fluctuations. These must be the result of genetic factors which would influence the progress of dependence from one step of its evolution to the next. Mardones quotes three examples where, in his view, genetic influences have been demonstrated:

(a) The genetic origin of individual fluctuations in alcohol preference of rats preferring alcohol solutions to water. Such fluctuations are probably related to the physiological appetency for alcohol.

(b) The existence of a typical alcohol dehydrogenase of an activity six times higher than the typical one [17].

(c) The discovery of a significant correlation between colour blindness, liver cirrhosis, and alcoholism. This correlation has not been confirmed by observers in other countries.

Such findings, Mardones believes, encourage further studies in order to establish whether genetic factors are involved in the step-by-step development of alcohol dependence. As regards other forms of drug dependence, such as dependence of the morphine or barbiturate type dependence, the transition between drug use and physical dependence is less influenced by individual fluctuations than in alcoholism. Nevertheless, in his view, the influence of genetic factors here, too, cannot be excluded definitely. This could possibly be shown by studies in populations where the abuse of the drug concerned is widespread.

At present the majority verdict as to whether there exists a genetically-determined predisposition to alcohol and other-drug dependence is probably one of 'Not Proven' – which does not exclude the possibility that it might yet be shown to be important in at least certain types of dependence.

Inherited factors may obviously play a role in those relatively infrequent examples of symptomatic (alpha) alcoholism or drug abuse which occur in individuals suffering from schizophrenia, manic or depressive episodes of manic-depressive psychosis, mental subnormality and possibly also in some psychopaths.

Relief drinking and drug taking

Individuals with marked personality problems are more likely than other more stable persons to look for emotional relief and to try to find it in relief drinking or drug taking. It is therefore also likely that among alcoholics and even more so among other drug abusers one may find a higher proportion of inadequate, immature and insecure personalities than among the general population [13]. However, even relatively 'normal' or average personalities can in time develop alcoholism or drug dependence, either when having to face conditions of prolonged special strain and stress or after continual occupational exposure and temptation, e.g. alcoholism among publicans and drug dependence among members of the helping professions – the 'professional addicts'. Similarly, in a society, where the habit of smoking is accepted more or less by a majority of the population, quite 'normal' or average personalities can become dependent smokers. Other smokers may have developed the habit mainly because of inner needs [18], having discovered early in their smoking career that relief smoking helped to mitigate their anxiety, tension or irritability [19].

In Western culture, alcohol, in contrast to other drugs, is widely accepted socially. It is therefore likely that the proportion of immature and insecure personalities is much higher among abusers of other drugs than among alcoholics (see below). On the other hand, the reasons often given by young takers for having been initially attracted to drug taking [20] do not generally apply, to the same extent at least, to drinkers. Thus many youngsters claim that curiosity was behind their first experiments of taking drugs – such curiosity whetted either by what they had been told by friends, or by glamorising and sensational stories they read or heard in the mass-media, leading to the feeling, 'I would like to find out what it is in drugs that makes so many other youngsters take them'. Some youngsters indeed may be more attracted to drug taking initially not so much because of ignorance but rather because of a feeling of bravado, or because of the lure of the unknown and of the excitement of taking a certain risk, the gravity of which they usually underestimate. The search for stimulation and excitement ('buzz', 'high', 'kicks') for relief from feelings of hopelessness, frustration and monotony, for consciousness expansion, for a conscious or unconscious spirit of rebellion or for a desire to adopt the values held by the adolescent's peer groups, may all be factors which influence drug taking. It has been said that youngsters may start to take drugs in order to express their revolt against parents, whereas they may begin to drink (and perhaps also to smoke tobacco) to emulate their parents' habits [21], but often such situations must be very complex. It would seem that the reasons why young addicts have started on their drug-taking career are often quite different from the frequently quasi-therapeutic ones which made adults first go to drugs. Middle-aged female barbiturate addicts, for example, often begin to take drugs for relief of tension, depression etc., or amphetamine-dependent women may have originally taken these pills as a slimming aid. Thus drug-taking by adults often starts for similar reasons to those which first launch many alcoholics on their excessive drinking career (relief drinking, see Part 3, Figure 1), i.e. some kind of self-medication. These are reasons quite different from those given by young drug takers.

2.3 THE ROLE OF THE 'ENVIRONMENT'

Social dependence
Reference was made above to the fact that the 1952 WHO Committee had drawn attention to only two of the main aetiological sets of factors – the psychological and the pharmacological ones – but had failed to refer to a third, i.e. the importance of environmental and social factors.

Not infrequently one comes across drug-dependent individuals who revert to drug taking long after their physical dependence has disappeared. These individuals show no obvious evidence of a psychological dependence (i.e. a desire to resume the drug in order to gain pleasure or avoid discomfort), but apparently relapse mainly because they maintain contact with their former friends, their old subculture, one of whose features was the abuse of drugs. In such examples it might be reliance on, or an attraction to, such a subculture, a form of social dependence which perhaps was the main reason for the relapse into drug taking. At times such resumption of contact with former friends may have been accidental or unavoidable, e.g. when there was no other place for such an individual to go to after leaving hospital. On other occasions, the individual returns to his old subculture despite other available accommodation and non-drug taking friends. This return is caused by a feeling of belonging to this subculture. The individual shares their values and ideals, which may not necessarily be directly connected with drug taking.

The failure of the WHO Expert Committee to refer to social factors when replacing the terms addiction and habituation by dependence, has been criticised on the basis that its definition ('drug dependence is a state, psychic and sometimes also physical, resulting from the interaction between a living organism and a drug . . .') overlooks the social context of drug use. In the view of the sociologist, Jock Young (1971), the social context of drug use necessitates a 'socio-pharmacological' classification of drug use and dependency [22]. He argues that one cannot generalise about drug use without consideration of the specific cultural context. Drug users will have to be divided into categories describing patterns of drug use involving similar social beliefs as well as of drugs with closely related pharmacological effects. Young's examples include cases of dependence on opiates in doctors and members of allied professions which occur in most advanced industrial countries, and cases of marihuana dependency in bohemians which occur chiefly in Britain, North America, France and Holland. In Young's view the social person's dependence on a drug is related to the degree to which his self-conception involves viewing himself as a drug taker. The role of the bohemian for example, involves smoking marihuana, just as the role of the merchant seaman involves heavy drinking. Whereas the absolutists, who see society as an organic entity, regard legal drug taking (alcohol, nicotine, caffeine, as well as amphetamines and barbiturates prescribed by the doctor) as behaviour in line with society's values, they see illegal drug taking as inimical to these values. Young as a relativist (seeing society as a multitude of sometimes agreeing, sometimes disagreeing groups) regards drug-induced behaviour as '. . . interaction between the physiological effects of the drug and the norms of the group of which the drug taker is a member. . . . Drugs are vehicles, in which, in the majority of cases, alternative values are realised in the form of behaviour rationally comprehensible in terms of these norms'. One should try to explain '. . . the origins and content of the culture the drug taker belongs to and then, and only then, the role drugs play in it'. The drug taker is not usually 'seduced' into drug taking by corruptors (e.g. pushers), but he voluntarily and willingly joins certain cultures which seem meaningful to him. For example, Young explains – 'The drug taker often embraces cultures which contain notions of hedonism or of transcendental experience . . .'.

In spite of Young's many strictures on the views of psychiatrists and drug experts, who allegedly completely fail to acknowledge the contribution of social factors to and the responsibility of society for the problem of drug abuse, the importance of such factors has been widely recognised for many years. For example, Young himself quotes the widely accepted division, proposed by Jellinek [7] in 1960, of alcohol addicts into gamma and delta alcoholics (see Section 3.2) with widely differing life styles and symptomatology. This partly originates from the fact that the French delta alcoholic, unlike the Anglo-Saxon alcoholic, is not exposed to rejection and ostracism – a difference which has been often referred to by the present writer (as by many others) in a number of publications [13, 23, 24]. (The following exposition, dealing with the environmental and social causes of drug dependence, was very largely written long before the present writer read Young's book criticising the alleged neglect of such social causes by psychiatrists and drug experts.)

The influence of socio-cultural factors
The role of environmental factors (such as ready availability of supplies, social, cultural, religious factors, etc.) in the aetiology of the dependence on alcohol and other drugs can be illustrated [13]. For example, the proportionately much lower incidence of female as compared to male alcoholics is probably largely a reflection of the social taboo on heavy drinking among women. Connected with this may be the relatively higher incidence of barbiturate abuse among women, who may prefer getting their emotional relief from these (socially acceptable) pills rather than from heavy drinking (which may be all too obvious to the outsider). Not unlikely, socio-cultural reasons may also be responsible for the finding that the ratio of female to male alcoholics seems to be higher in the UK than anywhere else, and for the gradual rise in the proportions of numbers of female alcoholics in many parts of the world (female emancipation, women taking over roles, occupations and

responsibilities previously held by men only, etc.). Socio-cultural as well as religious factors probably also help to explain the relative infrequency of alcoholism among Jews, in particular orthodox Jews [25]. That alcoholism should be relatively rare among this group, may seem initially the more surprising as one finds hardly any teetotallers among them. But drunkenness is rejected and the ability to hold drink does not carry a status symbol. Moreover the imbibing of alcoholic drinks may from childhood onwards become, among Jews, associated with the notion of a ritual. Jewish ritual drinking has been contrasted with the secular or hedonistic drinking of the Irish, who lack clear-cut, consistent attitudes towards drinking and among whom alcoholic rates are high. On the other hand, there are no clear-cut restraining attitudes and value system amongst Jews against drug taking (or for that matter gambling, or overeating). Abuse of other drugs and gambling seems relatively much more common amongst Jews than is abuse of alcohol again probably largely for socio-cultural reasons [26]. Studies of the relative infrequency of Jewish alcoholism, especially if compared with the more common abuse of other drugs, may tell one a great deal about the causation of such problems in general. They certainly seem to point clearly to the importance of socio-cultural factors in connection with alcoholism and, as very recently stressed by James Willis [27] may have a 'bearing on efforts to prevent alcoholism'.

The influence of economic factors
The role of economic factors is reflected in the very high incidence of alcoholism in France with its high wine production, strong vested interests and the popular belief that wine drinking is necessary for good health. Economic influences are also at work in today's 'affluence alcoholism', as they were in the 'misery' or 'poverty alcoholism' of the 18th and 19th centuries, and are reflected in the predominance of drug dependence among America's underprivileged and slum dwellers (a picture that has now begun to change). They were also reflected in the emergence of the heroin/cocaine epidemic in Britain in the early 1960s, when youngsters who left school early and obtained a job with high wages that made them independent of home, who had money in their pockets, time on their hands, and no inner resources for spending their leisure time constructively, readily drifted into London's glittering West End. Here they were tempted into buying drugs from the so called registered addicts [28].

The relatively high incidence of alcoholism among people having easy access to alcohol is well known, e.g. among publicans and their wives – and likewise among occupational groups where drinking is widely accepted and expected such as merchant seamen, journalists, certain sections of industry, and retired army and naval officers.

Similarly, the high proportion of professional addicts (doctors, pharmacists and nurses) to other drugs is readily explained on the basis of easy access and availability, rather than on the (unlikely) hypothesis of an abnormally high percentage of emotionally vulnerable personalities among such professional groups.

Subcultural influences

Social factors also play an important role in explaining the influence of the young addicts' subculture on the spread of drug abuse. What matters to such youngsters often much more than the attitudes and beliefs of their elders and society at large, are the ideas and ideals of their drug-taking peers and their subculture with its own moral standards. The participation by youngsters in activities not approved of by their parents and condemned by society, such as the smoking of cannabis, mainlining heroin, or buying and pushing drugs, alienates them even further from general society and socially approved (largely middle-class) values, such as steady work, maintenance of family ties, and the acquisition of further education and vocational skills. Similarly, subcultural influences are also at work in the life of Skid Row drinkers in American cities and the much less common surgical spirit drinkers in large British cities. Here the homeless and inadequate drifting drinkers congregate, establishing a way of life for themselves that is utterly at variance with the standards set by society at large, but in which the habitual down-and-out drinker may feel accepted and to a certain extent at home.

The widespread drug misuse among today's youngsters causes increasing worry and anxiety among parents, teachers, the general public and governments. Rather than putting the blame on the weak personalities of the young drug abusers or on the strongly addictive pharmacological properties of the drugs, many sociologists and the affected youngsters themselves often put the blame chiefly at the door of today's 'sick society'. Old family and religious ties have either been greatly weakened or have vanished; old standards have largely disappeared, without the modern, permissive society erecting any clearly discernible new ones in their place. Adolescents are thus left floundering, insecure, bewildered and perplexed, without clear yardsticks.

Adolescent drug taking may often be no more than one aspect of the difficulties in adjustment at that period in life. The vicious cycle of insecurity leading to anxiety may further produce aggressive feelings (towards oneself as well as against others) and actions, resulting in delinquency, 'dropping out' and a search for security by affiliation to subcultures and drug taking etc. The real cause, says the American psychiatrist Joel Fort [29], '. . . is the alienating character of our society itself. Repressive family life, meaningless schools, pointless jobs, bigotry, wars, and intolerance everywhere'. These are the reasons often given by drug-taking youngsters for their dropping out from a society and culture that fails to give them hope, comfort, satisfaction and spiritual sustenance [30].

Young drug abusers often claim that society is too much preoccupied with materialistic aims and technological progress to take sufficient notion of the value of the individual. In despair over the chaotic state of the world, frustrated and disillusioned with what they regard as the false and hypocritical values of their elders and with the communication problems arising out of the generation gap, they turn their back on society. Thus happenings such as 'students' revolt' are symbolic of the questioning by the young of long cherished, familiar, old values. Not finding satisfying solutions in the ways accepted by society, such youngsters look for new ways to gain satisfaction. As Young [22] puts it, 'When there is a disparity between people's aspirations and their means of achieving them a situation occurs which sociologists term anomie. People may then create new means of achieving their aspirations. . . . For example a group of boys may crave a measure of excitement and fun in their lives but find their work repetitious and boring, and the leisure activities available in their area staid and uninteresting. As a result, in certain circumstances, they may develop a subculture which involves delinquency and vandalism. That is, they create their excitement in illicit ways'. Or, a youngster unable to resolve his problems in ways approved by society, may '. . . adopt illicit drug taking as a solution'. Again the interplay between social, psychological and pharmacological factors should be stressed. For example, students may signal their disapproval of society by smoking cannabis – a readily available drug which is within easy reach even of the average student who is not moving in social circles, and which moreover he regards as much less dangerous than other illicit drugs. Psychologically more disturbed personalities may go out of their way to obtain Chinese heroin on the black market, thus running the risk of becoming

4

rapidly dependent psychologically and physically.

Thus the abuse of drugs other than those approved of by society (such as alcohol, coffee, tea, and those prescribed by the doctor) has become a symbol of turning away from society: 'Drugs such as LSD and marihuana are, rightly or wrongly, in the forefront of the war between freedom and repression, youth and age, powerless and power...' [31].

The interaction between psychological and social factors
The close interaction between psychological and social factors in the aetiology of dependence forms the background to Jellinek's hypothesis, referred to above [7], that in countries (or socio-occupational groups [23]) where heavy drinking is not only tolerated but widely accepted, even psychologically 'normal' individuals may acquire the habit and thus run the risk of progressing in time towards alcoholism. Such largely sociogenic alcoholics are common in countries like France. But in countries or social groups where heavy drinking is taboo, it will be in the main people with more than their fair share of personality difficulties who may defy the social taboo directed at heavy drinking, and in such countries and groups the mainly psychogenic type of alcoholic is likely to predominate. Similarly, in the case of drugs, even the average young college or art student may be strongly tempted to start smoking cannabis if he happens to find himself among a group of students whose subculture includes the custom of smoking hashish. In general, it would therefore seem that the more widely accepted a certain drug is in a given society, the greater the proportion of relatively 'normal' personalities who may in time start to use this drug regularly.

It thus makes sense that social factors rather than inner needs are often given as an explanation of the development of the tobacco habit by many smokers. The so-called *consonant smokers* who may be quite happy about their smoking often mention social circumstances as reasons for their habit, in contrast to the *dissonant smokers* who may have developed their habit mainly for psychogenic reasons and are worried about it [18].

For such reasons it would therefore seem more likely that the proportion of 'normal' personalities is highest among tobacco smokers and relatively small among abusers of drugs (other than cannabis which must have many 'normal' adherents). The proportion of 'normal' personalities among alcoholics probably comes midway between tobacco smokers and drug addicts. As the hypothetically average pre-addictive personality is thus likely to be a more stable one among alcoholics than among drug addicts, the outlook for the average alcoholic can be expected to be better than for the average drug addict (given other factors being equal). Prognosis (see Section 6.3) for similar reasons, would seem better for the professional addict than for the non-professional addict, for the therapeutic than for the non-therapeutic addict (who had to gain access to the drug in spite of many social and legal obstacles) and for the consonant, sociogenic smoker than for the dissonant mainly psychogenic smoker. All this applies of course, only if such people can be motivated to face up to the problem, and it is made much easier when some change in the harmful social environment is feasible. This in the case of professional addicts may often not be possible. However, it would seem that a basically more stable personality would still have better chances of recovery despite having to continue working in hazardous surroundings, than unstable individuals moving into a safer environment.

Again, whilst in general the mainly sociogenic smokers, alcoholics and drug addicts can be expected to have a better prognosis than their mainly psychogenic counterparts, the strength of the stranglehold kept by a given drug (with the pharmacological nature and potency varying from agent to agent – see Section 3.3) must obviously also play an important part in this connection. Moreover, wide availability and widespread social acceptance of a drug, encourage not only its abuse by the relatively 'normal' but even more so by the emotionally vulnerable and insecure. Because of easier access and constant temptation, these individuals may be more inclined to use such a drug more regularly and in larger doses, and thus come to grief. This consideration should perhaps not be overlooked in the current cannabis controversy. O. J. Kalant has pointed out, that whilst the use of the stimulant khat (an amphetamine-like drug) is a normal ingredient of Middle Eastern culture, it nevertheless causes widespread harm to the whole society. This illustrates the principle that, 'While a society may incorporate the widespread use of naturally occurring stimulants into its culture, it may none-the-less suffer serious consequences' [32].

The possible or probable influence of widespread use of alcohol and other drugs in a given population on the development of heavy use (with resulting complications) among a minority has in recent years been studied by workers at the Ontario Research Foundation. J. de Lint and W. Schmidt quoting S. Lederman's earlier findings of a '. . . quasi-mathematical connection between reasonable consumption and unreasonable consumption' (of alcohol), have shown that rates of alcoholism tend to rise and fall with the overall level of alcohol use in a population and that there is '. . . an apparently fixed relationship between consumption averages and alcoholism prevalence' in a given population [33]. Similarly, large scale surveys of drug use carried out in Canada by Smart *et al.* indicated a log normal distribution, i.e. a smooth distribution with no discontinuities, so that most numerous in such a distribution were the infrequent users, with the moderate drug users being less numerous, and the heavy users the least numerous [34]. These findings of a relationship between *per capita* use of alcohol and other drugs and the frequency of alcohol and drug problems would obviously have an important bearing on prophylaxis and the type of preventive programmes (see Section 7.3).

2.4 THE ROLE OF THE 'AGENT'

Pharmacological influences in the development of drug dependence

Some years ago, a WHO Addiction Subcommittee [12] divided drugs affecting the CNS into three classes, on the basis of the interaction between the individual personality make-up and the pharmacological nature of the drug (see Section 2.1). Often the pharmacological properties of a given drug play a decisive role. For example, the great majority of individuls introduced to the opiates for even a relatively brief period, however stable their underlying personality, will become psychologically and physically dependent, and this even with the (initial) use of small, therapeutic doses. Most users of even small amounts of opiates may become dependent in a matter of weeks. Among those who misuse barbiturates a relatively much smaller proportion may become dependent after taking them for, roughly, a period of a few months in slightly above therapeutic dosage. In the case of alcohol, an even smaller proportion of drinkers (perhaps up to 5–6 %) may develop dependence after imbibing grossly excessive amounts for several years. From the aspect of dosage, length of administration, and proportion of users developing dependence, as referred to above, the opiates would thus be more serious dependence-producing agents than the barbiturates, and these in turn more serious than alcohol.

Other factors naturally enter into the picture, such as the method of administration. Drugs that can be injected (in particular, intravenously) produce dependence more readily than those which can only be taken by mouth. However, certain predisposed people can become dependent on orally taken drugs which are consumed with impunity by the great majority of the population; for example, certain cough syrups (see Section 5.4) – Dr Colles-Brown's Chlorodyne (containing chloroform and morphine), chlordiazepoxide and diazepam etc. All these with prolonged administration and in high dosage, have led to dependence. This dependence is not uncommon in the case of Chlorodyne [35], but is rare in the case of the benzodiazapines. There are however certain drugs which, apparently have not (as yet) been reported to have caused dependence, such as the phenothiazine class of tranquillisers and the hypnotic nitrazepam. These seem to have proved exceptions to the rule that sooner or later all CNS-affecting sedative or stimulating drugs will be found to be dependence-producing agents, at least in certain emotionally vulnerable personalities, such as inadequate and immature individuals, certain types of alcoholics or individuals who formerly had abused other drugs, etc.

At any rate, the role of the agent itself in producing drug dependence must not be overlooked. Take, for example, the popular and superficial attractive slogan: 'Alcoholism does not come in bottles, it comes in persons.' This is by no means an adequate description of the process. The pharmacological nature of the agent – alcohol – in interaction with the host may produce not only psychological but also physical dependence, and may thus play an important role in the developmental process of alcohol addiction [7] (see Section 3.3). Cannabis, despite its reputation of being a relatively weak drug, has been known to induce a strong degree of psychological (though not physical) dependence even in emotionally fairly stable individuals when smoked habitually and heavily at times of stress [28]. The dependence of the ordinary tobacco smoker is attributed to the pharmacological action of the agent nicotine. Many smokers are said to crave tobacco for the sake of the nicotine content present, and the craving is regarded as probably having a pharmacological basis [18].

Probably in all cases of dependence a number of factors are at work, acting in dynamic interaction with each other though their relative importance may vary from individual to individual. Factors responsible for initiating the abuse or the onset of dependence are not necessarily the same as those involved in maintaining the state of dependence, and different factors may be responsible for inducing psychological and physical dependence. Psychological and social factors, for example, may initiate the habit of alcohol and drug abuse, and may be mainly responsible for inducing psychological dependence and for triggering off a relapse after the habit had been discontinued for a period, but by themselves they can hardly explain physical dependence. As regards ordinary smoking, social factors are described as the dominant influence in starting the activity, but as taking the second place to pharmacological factors in its maintenance.

Interaction between personality make-up and social environment seems mainly responsible for social dependence. This alongside psychological dependence may be mainly responsible for resumption of drug taking or drinking after a drug- or alcohol-free interval. Interaction between personality and the pharmacological nature of the drug seems mainly responsible for psychological and physical dependence. One example is the opiates. There are, of course, various reasons for starting their use. A persistent hunger or craving for narcotics has been suggested as constituting a major factor in perpetuating their use, and in producing relapses. Two kinds of hunger for drugs have been described. Firstly, the drug user's desire to re-experience the initial effects which he had obtained in the past from the use of the drug – such as a feeling of euphoria or a relief from discomfort or pain. Secondly, the desire of a user who has been physically dependent because of a persistent feeling of emptiness and of 'not being physically normal' after withdrawal, to re-establish his feeling of 'normality' by resumption of narcotic use [36]. The hunger for narcotics has been attributed by Dole and Nyswander [37] to drug-induced metabolic change that could persist long after withdrawal.

Social and pharmacological reinforcement

Some hypotheses attribute the perpetuation of opiate use and the relapse into drug use to a set of conditioned responses. Drug-seeking behaviour is here explained by conditioning; drug taking rewards the user by reducing his tension, or by producing a more positive feeling of euphoria (e.g. in the case of the stimulating amphetamines or cocaine), or perhaps by improved perception or pleasant illusions (in the case of cannabis or LSD). With each subsequent success or reward following the use of the drug, the drug-seeking habit is *reinforced*. In the case of those drugs which produce physical dependence, alleviation of the distress of the abstinence syndrome may be yet another reinforcing fact or.

Reinforcement can be social and pharmacological in nature. According to a recent exposition by Professor A. Wikler [38], the leading research worker in the application of conditioning theory to the field of drug dependence, the pattern of using psychoactive drugs is started by means of social reinforcement. This occurs under the influence of factors such as peer groups, prevailing drug-cults, and mystiques about the effects of such drugs propagated by folklore and literature. Once such drug use has been initiated, there arises, in the case of certain drugs, the responsibility and the danger that drug-using behaviour will be strengthened by pharmacological reinforcement. For example, the effects of the drug may interact with primary pre-existing 'organismic variables' (psychic dependence) which had not been induced by the drug (*direct pharmacological reinforcement*). In the case of certain drugs, after tolerance has developed to such direct reinforcement, it may be replaced by *indirect pharmacological reinforcement*, i.e. interactions between the effects of the drug and drug-induced organismic variables (physical dependence). Relief of abstinence symptoms as a consequence of taking the next dose, now augments operant conditioning of such drug taking behaviour. Concomitant classical and operant conditioning* can produce secondary pharmacological reinforcement when there happens to be contiguity in time between certain stimuli and the direct and indirect (primary) pharmacological reinforcement described above. Clearly, such hypotheses put forward in the case of narcotics can also be more or less readily applied to the tobacco habit, alcoholism, or other drug abuse, and to a certain extent, to compulsive gambling. The fact that in gambling (unlike in the case of alcohol and other CNS depressing drugs) there is only psychological and no physical dependence should prove important and very illuminating for the purposes of research into the whole subject of 'addiction'.

* Reflexes can be conditioned (*a*) by the Pavlovian or classical type of conditioning, or (*b*) by making use of Skinner's technique of operant conditioning. In Pavlovian conditioning, simultaneous presentation of a second stimulus (e.g. ringing of bell) with an unconditioned stimulus (placing meat in the mouth of the dog) in time leads to the response of salivation. Originally this response could only be elicited by the unconditioned stimulus of placing meat in the mouth of the dog. Eventually the salivation response could be elicited on presentation of the condition stimulus (bell) alone. Skinner's operant technique brings about conditioning through *positive reinforcement* (rewarding a response) or through *negative reinforcement* (e.g. punishment by electric shock when no appropriate response is made). The term operant is applied because the animal has to operate upon its environment in order to be reinforced, having to give specific responses in order to produce the reinforcement. Therefore, in Pavlov's experiments, given time, a previously neutral stimulus (bell ringing) could eventually lead to anticipatory food-taking reactions (i.e. salivating). Skinner, on the other hand, waited for an animal to make a specific response spontaneously and then stepped in with a reinforcing agent such as food [39]

What causes abuse and dependence?

In concluding Part 2, an attempt will be made to describe briefly current knowledge and certain hypotheses in the field of causation of abuse of drink, drugs and tobacco. As outlined, there are certain differences between them but also quite a few similarities – so much so that the author in the past few years has found it possible to attempt group sessions and, more recently, the establishment of a therapeutic community (in a London prison) composed of addicts to various drugs, i.e. compulsive drinkers, drug abusers, compulsive smokers, and even gamblers and an occasional excessive eater. To a certain extent these individuals though dependent on the different agents were able to identify with each other and to form a common therapeutic community.

The question, 'What causes abuse and dependence?' is of much more than academic interest. A rational, comprehensive and preventive therapeutic and rehabilitation programme will only be possible after it has become known what produces misuse of and dependence on certain potentially noxious agents. This demands an understanding and knowledge of the socio-cultural circumstances and personality types involved. The answers to these questions – if they can ever be fully given – will require a great deal of integrated multi- and interdisciplinary research. What can be said today is that it is highly unlikely that there is anything such as 'the' cause but rather a multiplicity of factors, pertaining to host, environment and agent and acting in dynamic interplay with each other.

Why does society accept some drugs and reject others?

To a certain extent related to the question, 'What makes an addict?' is one as to why society says 'yes' to certain drugs and offers a more or less firm 'no' to others. This, as we have seen, has indirect consequences on the individual's chances or risk of becoming dependent on one drug or another. In groups or countries where certain drugs are widely accepted even the average, 'normal' individual could more readily become dependent. With drugs rejected by a certain culture only the more vulnerable run such a risk.

Clearly there is no simple answer to this question. Sydney Cohen [40] names three factors that might be involved: seniority, delayed morbidity, and economics. As regards seniority, he feels that substances with which society is on a familiar footing tend to retain their place, whereas strange substances are distrusted. Delayed morbidity and mortality, affecting a minority of users only, are not a bar against acceptance. Finally, drug customs are often initiated and perpetuated by economic factors (e.g. ready regional availability at relatively little expense) and possibly also by socio-cultural aspects if the pharmacological effects of a given available drug reinforce the basic values or at least do not interfere with the aims and goals of such cultures (e.g. with their work ethic as against the hedonistic aims of certain subcultures). Although drugs that become accepted by society were naturally at first considered beneficial or at least harmless, Cohen feels, surprisingly enough, that potability or safety frequently do not play a decisive role.

However, not infrequently it may take a very long time before all the possible risks attached to a given substance come to be fully appreciated. Tobacco for example, regarded for so long as a relatively harmless habit, has only in our times been found to be definitely harmful. By now however, the habit has become so widely ingrained and accepted, that it may require much more than the hesitant official steps, taken at the present time, to make inroads into the wide acceptability of the habit. Moreover, revenue from tobacco, as from alcohol, has long become one of the sheet anchors of the country's economy. For many years now, drinkers and smokers between them have financed the National Health Service [41]. In 1963, revenue from taxation of alcoholic liquors amounted to £481 million and from tobacco to approximately £900 million; the NHS at the time cost the state about £1000 million per annum. In 1964, Britain's consumer expenditure on alcoholic drink amounted to over £1300 million and expenditure on tobacco to just under £1350 million. In 1970, expenditure on drink had almost doubled, nearly £2500 million, and expenditure on tobacco had risen to nearly £1700 million. Duty on alcohol in 1969/1970 amounted to £863 million. In 1970 duty on tobacco amounted to £1141 million (i.e. nearly 70% of the consumer expenditure). Together duties for alcohol and tobacco – £2000 million – almost paid for the NHS bill, which by now had risen to about £2500 million per year.

One could argue that had the risks of tobacco and alcohol been known before these drugs had gained a firm foothold it might be doubtful that society would in fact have adopted them as part of the acceptable, daily 'fare'. With the more powerful new chemical agents, whose dangers become known more rapidly, society is now much quicker in imposing regulations. Initially hailed as harmless, barbiturates, amphetamines and synthetic opium-like products, such as pethidine etc., were soon put under more or less strict restrictions. Thus safety after all, does play a role in determining whether a given substance stands a good chance of becoming accepted. On the other hand it may be the excitement of the 'walking a tightrope' feeling that often makes the more dangerous (e.g. mind-bending) drugs attractive to rebellious, adolescent subcultures. Once a drug has become accepted, safety naturally only plays a subordinate role – just as it is in general of little help to attempt to persuade an addict to abstain from his drug merely by telling him about the risks he runs. As the history of attempts at prohibition of alcohol have shown, once a drug has been definitely accepted by a culture (and this may happen before there has been sufficient time to fully assess its possible danger), attempts to dislodge it from its pedestal are often doomed to failure. However, matters could possibly be different if such attempts were made when only a minority had become attracted to a new drug. Moreover, although alcohol is undoubtedly a dangerous drug, over the centuries mankind has learned to live with it. This may be because only a minority of drinkers come to grief and then – as in the case of tobacco – usually only after a more or less lengthy period of misuse.

As regards safety as a factor in determining the acceptability or otherwise of a drug, it is only fair to point out that of the widely accepted drugs in Western culture – alcohol, tobacco, coffee and tea – the latter two are in fact comparatively harmless (see Section 5.1). Cohen makes the interesting point that in time society has often progressed from less harmful to more harmful forms of a drug, e.g. from beer to wine and spirits, or from opium smoking to intravenous heroin injection. Possibly after large segments of a population have developed a certain tolerance for, and perhaps have become somewhat bored with a given drug, there may be a certain temptation to search for and enjoy somewhat stronger forms of the same drug – once these had become available. At this stage the factor of safety may indeed have taken a back seat. This would be similar to the progress in individual drug abusers from milder to stronger drugs, and from sniffing to intramuscular and later to intravenous injection, or from beer to spirits. Initially, for example, the young drug abuser may have started to sniff cocaine or heroin and may have been afraid to start taking the drug intravenously; but once the abuser becomes familiar with such drugs, the temptation of greater thrills often leads him to intravenous injections, despite the greater risk to body and mind.

With respect to the point of accepting the familiar and excluding the exotic substances, it is interesting to recall that originally – about half a century ago – it was in fact countries familiar with the effects of cannabis (i.e. Turkey and Egypt) that pressed for putting the drug onto the category of dangerous narcotic substances. Countries such as the UK and France – where cannabis was at that time a largely unknown quantity – were not particularly interested in forbidding it. However, nowadays it may be true that a society in which a large segment of the population has 'sold its soul to the devil', and has, despite certain drawbacks and dangers, learned to live with this situation, may prefer the devil it has come to know to a new one it knows less well. On the other hand, rebellious adolescents, rebelling against the customs of their elders, may prefer those drugs which are newcomers – unfamiliar, unexplored, uncharted and untried, surrounded by an aura of mystery, their use carrying the excitement of immediate danger – to those drugs which are familiar to their parents.

But, as we shall see in a later chapter, despite important differences between the drug abuse fashions of the young and their elders, and in spite of the 'generation gap', the drug habits of the middle-aged may nevertheless have an important bearing on the drug abuse patterns of their children (see Section 7.3).

REFERENCES

1. WHO Expert Committee (1964). *Tech. Rep. Ser.*, **273**, 9.
2. Oswald, I. and Thacore, V. R. (1963). *Brit. Med. J.*, **2**, 427.
3. Oswald, I. *et al.* (1971). *Brit. Med. J.*, **2**, 70.
4. Wendel, H. A. (1971). *Brit. Med. J.*, **2**, 766.
5. WHO Expert Committee (1969). *Tech. Rep. Ser.*, **407**, 6.
6. Archibald, D. (1970). 3rd Leonard Ball Oration, Melbourne. Reprinted in 29th *Int. Congr. Alcoholism and Drug Dependence* (L. G. Kiloh, editor) (Australia: Butterworths, 1971).
7. Jellinek, E. M. (1960). *The Disease Concept of Alcoholism*, 146, 154 (New Haven, Conn: Hillhouse Press).
8. Schuster, C. R. and Balster, R. L. (1972). *Agonist and Antagonist Actions of Narcotic Analgesic Drugs*, 243 (H. W. Kosterlitz, H. O. J. Collier and J. E. Villarreal, editors) (London: Macmillan).
9. Collier, H. O. J. (1971). *Biochemical and Pharmacological Aspects of Dependence and Reports on Marihuana Research*, 45 (H. M. Van Praag, R. De Erven and R. Bohn, editors) (Holland: Haarlem).

10. Villarreal, J. E.: *ibid.*, 73.
11. Van Dyk, W. K. *ibid.* (Ref. 9), 6–17.
12. WHO Expert Committee (1952). *WHO Tech. Rep. Ser.*, **57,** 9.
13. Glatt, M. M. (1972). *The Alcoholic and the Help He Needs,* 2nd ed., 47 (London: Priory Press).
14. Reichard, J. D. (1947). *Amer. J. Psychiat.*, **103,** 721.
15. Wikler, A. (1952) *Psychiat. Quart.*, **26,** 70.
16. Mardones, J. (1970). *A World Dialogue on Alcohol and Drug Dependence,* 367–383 (E. D. Whitney, editor) (Beacon Press).
17. Von Wartburg, J. P. *et al.* (1965). *Can. J. Biochem.*, **43,** 889.
18. Report of the Royal College of Physicians (1971). *Smoking and Health Now* (London: Pitman Med. and Scientific Publ. Co. Ltd.).
19. Glatt, M. M. (1971). *Nursing Times,* 4th Nov.
20. Glatt, M. M. (1966). *Adolescent Drug Dependence,* 167–176 (C. W. M. Wilson, editor) (Oxford, London: Pergamon Press).
21. Maddox, C. L. and McCall, B. C. (1964). *Drinking among Teenagers* (New Jersey: Rutgers Center of Alcoholic Studies).
22. Young, J. (1971). *The Drugtakers,* 95 (London: MacGibbon and Kee).
23. Rose, H. K. and Glatt, M. M. (1961). *J. Ment. Sci.*, **107,** 18.
24. Glatt, M. M. (1967). *WHO Chronicle,* **21,** 293.
25. Snyder, C. R. (1958). *Alcohol and the Jews* (New Jersey: Rutgers Center of Alcoholic Studies).
26. Glatt, M. M. (1970). *Brit. J. Addict.*, **64,** 297.
27. Willis, J. (1973). *Addicts, Drugs and Alcohol Re-examined* (London: Pitman Publ.).
28. Glatt, M. M., Pittman, D. J., Gillespie, D. G. and Hills, D. R. (1968) *The Drug Scene in Great Britain* (Revised Reprint) (London: Edward Arnold).
29. Fort, J. (1970). *Playboy,* **17,** 53.
30. Burroughs, W. S. (1970). *ibid.*, **17, 53.**
31. *Playboy* (1970). **17, 53.**
32. Kalant, O. J. (1966). *The Amphetamines,* 98, 136 (Univ. Toronto Press).
33. de Lint, J. and Schmidt, W. (1971). *Brit. J. Addict.*, **66,** 97.
34. Smart, R. G. and Whitehead, C. (1972). *Bull. Narcot. U.N.*, **24,** 39 (1).
35. Glatt, M. M. (1964). *Addiction to Chlorodyne. Brit. Med. J.*, **2,** 308.
36. Jaffe, J. H. (1969). *Drugs and the Brain,* 351 (P. Black, editor) (Baltimore: John Hopkins Press).

37. Dole, V. P. and Nyswander, M. E. (1968). *Res. Publ. Assoc. Nerv. Ment. Dis.*, **46,** 359.
38. Wikler, A. (1972). *2nd Int. Symp. Drug Abuse, Jerusalem* (Abstracts), 27.
39. Thomson, R. (1968). *The Pelican History of Psychology*, 230 (London: Penguin Books).
40. Cohen, S. (1971). *Docum. Geigy* ('*Acceptable Addictions*') (Basle).
41. Glatt, M. M. (1967). *New Aspects of the Mental Health Services*, 115 (H. Freeman and J. Farndale, editors) (Oxford, London: Pergamon Press).
42. Peck, A. W. (1973). *Lancet*, **ii,** 1209.

PART 3

ALCOHOLISM AND ITS RELATIONSHIP TO OTHER TYPES OF DEPENDENCE

3.1 THE COMBINED APPROACH

There are several reasons why this book, which deals with dependence on psychotropic drugs, includes a brief (but by no means comprehensive) chapter on alcoholism. Many books on drug dependence say very little about alcoholism. This possibly helps to strengthen the relatively widespread erroneous idea that alcohol is quite a different substance from those other drugs which can lead to addiction. Thus, not infrequently, one encounters alcoholics of many years standing who proudly proclaim that they have hardly ever in their life taken a drug. There can of course be no doubt that alcohol is a drug even if it has become traditionally and culturally widely accepted and domesticated [1], and that although it can be freely bought over the counter without requiring a doctor's prescription, it is a potentially very dangerous drug that can produce physical as well as psychological dependence. Moreover, although the mass-media nowadays pay much less attention to alcoholism than to other forms of drug dependence, it is only fair to point out that, second to the other freely available dangerous dependence-producing drug, nicotine, alcohol is responsible for a much larger number of individual cases of dependence than any other dependence-producing drug (see Table 1 in Appendix). Today there may be a few thousand heroin and methadone addicts in this country and possibly up to 100 000 or so individuals dependent on barbiturates and amphetamines, whereas the number of alcoholics in the UK may be in the region of 300 000–400 000 and it is probable that this figure is rising steadily. Why relatively little interest has been shown in the problem of alcoholism is not quite clear. Some claim that drug addicts have been pushed into the limelight by the mass-media as a kind of scapegoat because society feels guilty about so many of its own shortcomings; others claim that society wants to keep attention off the widespread abuse of the legal drugs, alcohol and tobacco, indulged in by so many 'respectable' members of the community. However, in the interest of prophylaxis of a dangerous and widespread affliction, and in order to improve the lot of so many victims of the condition, it is necessary to reduce the stigma associated with alcoholism. This can only be done by making the facts about the condition, e.g. the illness concept and the possibility of bringing help to the great majority of the sufferers, as widely known as possible. This will end the conspiracy of silence. This silence has certainly contributed to the stigma and misconceptions associated with alcoholism despite the progress made over the past ten years or so, but recently there has been increasing recognition of alcoholism as an important national and international health problem.

There is at least one other important reason why alcohol dependence should be included in a book dealing primarily with drug dependence. Certainly there are a number of dissimilarities between alcoholism and dependence on other drugs – quite apart from the fundamental difference that as a rule dangerous drugs are available on prescription only whereas alcohol is available legally to anybody (over a certain age). On the other hand, there are many similarities between alcoholism and other forms of drug dependence, for example, as regards aetiology and developmental progress [2]. The existence of many similarities was surprisingly but very clearly brought home to the author nearly fifteen years ago. Findings and impressions gained after treating middle-class English alcoholics who had voluntarily entered a psychiatric hospital were compared with the findings of Dr Leong Hon Koon in treated Chinese opium addicts, who after arrest had been compulsorily sent to and treated in a Singapore prison addiction unit. It was concluded at the time [3] that, 'In spite of the differences arising from the nature of the different drugs and the differences in personality and in socio-cultural backgrounds, in a large number of points, the findings resembled each other'.

Although, as stressed above, there is still a long way to go, there has been in recent years a welcome change in professional, lay and governmental attitudes towards alcoholism, and gradually the concept of the alcoholic as a sick man in need of understanding and assistance is gaining acceptance. Such a development in the case of dependence on other drugs is in many countries still in its infancy.

Many of the methods under investigation and those methods already used in the prevention, treatment and rehabilitation of alcoholism, might also be valuable for use (with certain modifications) in cases of dependence on other drugs [2]. Approaching alcoholism and other forms of drug dependence basically as problems belonging under one umbrella [4], might therefore in time contribute towards improving the public image of the drug addict. Because of considerations such as these, a WHO Expert Committee on Mental Health that met in 1966 recommended that, 'Problems of dependence on alcohol and dependence on other drugs should be considered together, because of similarities of causation, interchangeability of agent in respect of maintenance of dependence and hence similarities in measures required for prevention and treatment' [5]. The extent to which approaches to different types of dependence should be combined (a better term might perhaps be 'coordinated') would vary with local factors and was to be left to national and local authorities. Although the question, 'To combine or not to combine' [6] alcoholism and other forms of drug dependence was initially hotly debated both at the WHO meeting and elsewhere, in practice many leading organisations in the field soon opted for combining them; and the leading international organisation in the field of alcoholism, the International Council on Alcohol and Alcoholism, decided in 1968 to change its name to International Council on Alcohol and Addictions. In Great Britain many years earlier, in 1946, the Society for the Study of Inebriety – founded in 1884 – had changed its name to The Society for the Study of Addiction to Alcohol and other Drugs, and its journal, the *British Journal of Inebriety* became *The British Journal of Addiction* (to alcohol and other drugs). Similarly in Canada the Alcoholism Research Foundation in Ontario established in 1949, and developing rapidly into one of the world's leading establishments in this field, altered its name in 1961 to The Alcoholism and Drug Addiction Research Foundation, and that of its journal from *Alcoholism* to *Addictions*.

As indicated above, the following discussion will touch only on certain aspects of the problem of alcoholism, mainly those that are often not given sufficient attention (e.g. its social complications), and those that are of interest in their comparison with conditions present in other types of drug dependence.

What is alcoholism?

The number of proposed definitions indicates that none of them is quite satisfactory. The most widely quoted definition is the one given by a WHO Expert Committee in 1952; 'Alcoholics are those excessive drinkers whose dependence on alcohol has attained such a degree that it shows a noticeable mental disturbance or an interference with their bodily and mental health, their interpersonal relations, and their smooth social and economic functioning; or who show the prodromal signs of such developments. They therefore require treatment' [7].

The pharmacological nature of the drug alcohol
In the view of WHO Expert Committees in 1954 [8] and 1955 [9], alcohol is a drug with '. . . a pharmacological action intermediate in kind and degree between addiction-producing and habit-forming drugs, so that compulsive craving and dependence can develop in those individuals whose make-up leads them to seek and find an escape in alcohol'. Here, the individual's personal make-up is the determining factor, but the pharmacological factor is also significant The Committees did not put alcohol into the same group as the opiates for a number of reasons:

(a) tolerance increase in the case of alcohol amounted to only 3–4 times the original inherent tolerance, compared to a 25–100-fold rise in the case of opiates;

(b) addiction to alcohol occurred only in a small fraction of drinkers, compared to a nearly 100% occurrence in heroin users (nowadays the proportion would be estimated to be somewhat lower than this) and 70% of morphine users, and

(c) addiction developed in excessive drinkers after about 3–20 years, whereas in morphine users it developed after an interval of only 3–4 weeks when ordinary therapeutic doses were taken.

Unlike the CNS stimulants and the hallucinogens, the CNS depressant, alcohol, like the opiates and other CNS-depressant drugs, can produce physical dependence (see Table 1 in Appendix). There exists a close functional relationship between alcohol and the barbiturates (see below). Whether alcohol and the barbiturates taken together are merely additive or potentiating, is as yet undecided. According to the pharmacologist R. D. Laurence, 'All cerebral depressant (hypnotics, tranquillisers, anti-epileptic drugs, antihistamines) can either potentiate or at least synergise with alcohol' [10], a risk which may be of importance not only with heavy drinkers but also in the case of car drivers after a moderate alcohol intake.

As regards the intensity of psychological dependence in alcoholics, it may occasionally be as severe as in the case of barbiturates although less strong than with the opiates, cocaine and amphetamine-barbiturate mixtures. The psychological dependence in the case of users of tobacco (nicotine) apparently occurs in a much higher proportion of smokers, and sets in much more rapidly, than is the case with drinkers.

The *aetiology* of alcoholism has been discussed in Part 2.

3.2 TYPES OF ALCOHOLISM
(AND OF DEPENDENCE ON 'OTHER DRUGS³)

The most widely accepted classification is the one suggested by Jellinek [1] who prefers talking of the 'alcoholisms' rather than of 'alcoholism'. There may be more than the five types described by Jellinek in detail. To a certain extent Jellinek's classification might also apply to other forms of dependence.

(1) Alpha alcoholism
This is a purely psychological continual dependence or reliance upon the effect of alcohol to relieve bodily or emotional pain. Such undisciplined drinking is symptomatic of the '. . . pathological conditions which it relieves'.

Clearly many other forms of drug abuse and drug dependence may start as symptoms of underlying bodily or emotional (or social) disturbance. For example, barbiturates are often initially taken to relieve insomnia or anxiety, amphetamines in order to slim or to overcome depression, opiates to alleviate pain and varying drugs are taken by youngsters to relieve boredom or frustration. In compulsive smokers, gamblers or eaters, the dependence may often originally have started with the search for relief from tension, anxiety etc. (symptomatic gambling, relaxation smoking, etc.). The progress from relief drinking or drug taking to psychological dependence is gradual, and in practice it is often difficult to decide whether such relief use has already progressed to alpha alcoholism [11].

(2) Beta alcoholism
Here '. . . such alcoholic complications as polyneuropathy, gastritis and cirrhosis of the liver may occur, without either physical or psychological dependence upon alcohol'. Heavy drinking in such individuals may have been due to '. . . customs of a certain social group in con-

junction with poor nutritional habits . . .', and may in turn lead to
further impairment of the nutritional state and of the family budget,
lowering of productivity, earlier death etc. [1].

Clearly, many similar examples can be quoted of definite organic
complications following abuse of other drugs in spite of the absence
(at least initially) of dependence. For example, an individual's habitual
sociogenic drug abuse may arise on the basis of his belonging to a
certain subculture, or of prevalent regional or national drug-taking
patterns. This may lead to septic complications and serum jaundice in
the case of youngsters who 'mainline' heroin, methylamphetamine
or barbiturates (even before they may have become dependent) and
insomnia and loss in weight in the case of regular amphetamine
abusers. Similarly, in certain regions of South America, Africa and the
Middle East, the widespread customary use of cocaine and khat among
the poor, may impair the family budget and be responsible for under-
nutrition. Again, purely social, habitual overeating may lead to obesity
with its dangers for health and habitual excessive smoking, even in the
absence of dependence and which may have initially arisen out of the
social climate that favours smoking, may ultimately be responsible for
the well-known complications, such as lung cancer, chronic bronchitis,
emphysema and ischaemic heart disease. Even self-indulgent or
socially-induced heavy gambling may, by draining the family budget,
indirectly lead to neglect of nutrition.

(3) **Gamma alcoholism** (loss of control) ⎫ the addictive types of
(4) **Delta alcoholism** (inability to abstain) ⎭ alcoholism.
Apart, possibly, from epsilon alcoholism, gamma and delta alcoholism
are in Jellinek's view, the only types which constitute addictions or
diseases in the strict pharmacological sense, since it is the adaptation of
cell metabolism, acquired tissue tolerance and the (physical) withdrawal
symptoms which bring about craving and loss of control or inability
to abstain [1]. Jellinek assumed that,'Anomalous forms of the ingestion
of narcotics and alcohol, such as drinking with loss of control and
physical dependence, are caused by physiopathological processes and
constitute diseases'. Whether there is in fact a biochemical factor
responsible (at least partially) for the alcoholic's loss of control, has
not yet been proven. In the case of addicts to drugs other than alcohol
it sometimes seems that they cannot always be certain of being able to
discontinue the drug on a given occasion once they have started to
take it. Yet much more often the drug-taking behaviour of many

addicts seems to resemble that of the delta (inability to abstain) alcoholic. They often cannot or will not start the day without taking their drug and they then keep 'topping up' intermittently throughout the day. Also, many narcotic addicts live 'from one fix to the next'. This continual repetition of drug taking throughout the day, may be due to minor physical abstinence symptoms, such as those experienced by delta alcoholics.

(5) Epsilon alcoholism
The nature of this (periodic) type of alcoholism is often obscure. In some drug-dependent people, drug abuse may occur only from time to time. This may be associated not only with the individual's state of mind or emotional and physical health, but also with environmental and social factors; e.g. drug availability. It may also be due to the conflicting influences and pressures exercised on the young drug abuser by his peers on the one hand, and by his parents on the other. Recurrent depression or mania can be a (probably not very common) cause of periodic alcoholism. Depression, as well as states of tension and anxiety, can easily cause recurrent drug abuse, for example the use of amphetamines or barbiturates by middle-aged women (not only at the time of the menopause) or by younger women in the premenstrual phase. Episodes of gambling, overeating or heavy drinking, could easily arise from periods of abnormal emotional stress, depression etc. The occasional or regular 'binges' of gulping down large amounts of food (followed by induced attempts to vomit it all back immediately afterwards) sometimes occurring in compulsive eaters, usually were – in the few cases known to the present author – of relatively short duration only, though sometimes occurred day after day. Such occasional addictive eating binges are described as being invariably involved with anxiety, whether manifest or not, and are frequently initiated by hurt pride, humiliation and feelings of rejection or isolation [12].

3.3 THE DEVELOPMENT AND PROGRESS OF ALCOHOLISM (AND OF DEPENDENCE ON 'OTHER DRUGS')

The development of alcohol addiction was well described by Jellinek 20 years ago [13], and although the sample on which he based his description may have been rather unrepresentative (2000 recovered alcoholic members of AA in the USA), later studies elsewhere tended to bear out his findings [14]. The left side of the chart of 'Alcohol Dependence and Recovery' (see Figure 1 in Appendix) is based largely on Jellinek's findings; the right side – referring to 'the way back' – arose out of regular group discussions with male and female members of the alcoholic unit at Warlingham Park Hospital from 1952 to 1954. Originally the chart was prepared for 'home consumption' by War- lingham Park patients only, but it continually aroused the interest of outside visitors who kept on asking for copies, and it is now in use in many parts of the world. Its main value has been found in the fact that the alcoholic (and his family and friends) can determine very rapidly which 'phase' he has reached. Moreover, looking at the chart, a heavy drinker, hitherto clinging to the rationalisation that he was not an alcoholic, would find it very difficult to maintain this attitude when confronted with so many reflections of his own experiences and activities. The right side of the chart indicates clearly that alcoholics (or their relatives) cannot hope for a miracle cure, but that 'the way back' requires a persistent effort over a long period of time, and that although progress is gradual there is every hope for ultimate success. Finally, former notions that alcoholics have no chance of giving up drinking successfully, until they have reached 'rock bottom' in every aspect of their adjustment, have fortunately been proved wrong. As the (revised) chart indicates, the alcoholic can take 'short cuts' leading directly from any point on the 'way down' across to 'the way back', provided he realises that a continuation of his drinking is likely to lead to a further slipping down towards 'rock bottom'.

The chart requires little further explanation. Jellinek divided the development of alcohol addiction into four phases (which of course are not sharply demarcated from each other).

(a) Pre-alcoholic phase
(b) Prodromal phase, starting with alcoholic memory gaps
(c) Crucial phase, beginning in predominantly spirit drinking (e.g. Anglo-Saxon) countries with the loss of control
(d) Chronic phase, characterised by the occurrence of prolonged drinking bouts, the 'benders'.

The average duration of the whole process in men was formerly found to last from a few to as many as twenty years, although women and younger people 'travelled' the whole distance, once they had start- ed to drink heavily, in a much shorter period [14]. In recent years the average age at which people start to drink socially, has been dropping steadily and so has the hypothetical average age of male and female alcoholics. One now comes across a much higher proportion than before of young alcoholics in their early twenties, and even occasionally in their late teens. The hope that the rise of drug abuse in the young would be accompanied by a drop of heavy drinking and alcoholism has therefore not materialised.

As regards the developmental progress of dependence, there are many similarities between alcoholism and other types of dependence, although in some of the latter, as already discussed the pace is much more rapid, e.g. in dependence on opiates and barbiturates. The potential alcoholic usually starts with social drinking from which he gradually proceeds to relief drinking – at first only occasionally; but when his drinking activity rewards him with relief, the activity is thereby reinforced and he learns to drink regularly whenever confronted with any subjective stressful situation (see Part 4). Cannabis, too, is usually taken in the company of others, but, as already mentioned, the aim of the majority of cannabis smokers is probably from the beginning to obtain a definite change of feelings or a mild intoxication (high); this may also be the unconscious goal of some social drinker.

Somewhat similar to the progress from social to relief drinking, is the way in which individuals to whom a doctor originally prescribed barbiturates for insomnia or amphetamines for slimming purposes gradually begin to take these drugs to rid themselves from anxiety and tension or alternatively, to achieve a supernormal euphoric state of feeling. In other cases, excessive drinking or drug abuse may have originated not in the search for emotional satisfaction or relief, but in continual occupational temptation such as experienced by publicans, waiters, journalists etc. in the case of drinking, and by doctors, nurses, pharmacists etc., in the case of other drugs. The greater the degree of emotional pain or distress and the more often and effectively the drinker's or drug user's search for relief or for enhancement of pleasure is rewarded by obtaining the desired result, then the greater becomes the hold of the drug on the individual and his tendency to repeat the successful activity (pharmacological reinforcement) (see Section 2.4) With alcohol as with other CNS-depressing and some stimulating drugs, increasing tolerance necessitates the intake of increasingly higher amounts.

Tolerance
Tolerance has been defined by Eddy *et al.* as an '. . . adaptive state characterised by diminished response to the same quantity of a drug' [61].The irregular, incomplete tolerance increase in the cases of alcohol and the barbiturates is much less marked than with the opiates. Tolerance increases slowly and markedly with the amphetamines but not with cocaine. With LSD, tolerance may develop and disappear rapidly. In the case of cannabis the question of tolerance is as yet not clear. Tolerance has been said not to occur with cannabis and it is often pointed out that many cannabis users after some time are satisfied with a smaller number of joints than when they started to smoke the drug. However, over the years, the present author has also come across cannabis users who stated that after smoking reefers for a certain length of time, they subsequently failed to obtain the former 'high' or satisfaction from it, and because of this they occasionally began to search for more potent drugs, such as LSD. Recent animal experiments [15] have shown (in some animals) a rapid development of tolerance to Δ9 THC, the cannaboid probably largely responsible for the pharmacological activity of cannabis and cannabis extracts (see Section 5.3). A WHO Scientific Group in 1970 concluded that further investigation was required to answer the question of tolerance to cannabis [16].

Progressive psychological dependence
Gradually a state of emotional dependence develops in which the alcohol- or drug-dependent individual continually or periodically yearns and searches for satisfaction and gratification by means of alcohol or drug consumption. Progressive psychological dependence leads to increasing preoccupation with alcohol or the drug concerned (e.g. the heroin addict who cannot rely on a regular legitimate supply may spend all his day hustling for the drug). It also leads to neglect of obligations toward family, employer, and society, even though the addict may often feel very guilty and remorseful about it all and make well-meant promises to himself and others that he will mend his ways. There is increasing alienation from family and society and possible involvement in antisocial activities. Neglect of personal care, hygiene and nutrition, and lack of resistance to intercurrent infections or to the effects of the drug itself may lead to mental or physical complications. Self-respect dwindles away and there may be serious behavioural changes in the direction of irresponsibility, so that even erstwhile respectable and ordinary people with a high moral and ethical code of

behaviour come to behave as if they were irresponsible psychopaths. One has, however, to be careful not to confuse the apparently fairly uniform personalities of many long established alcoholics and drug addicts, with their often strikingly different pre-addictive personalities. Factors such as intellectual, emotional and ethical deterioration which are to a large extent the consequences of the pharmacological action of the drugs taken, of the user's need to get 'his' drug at any price and of his defensive reaction to the increasing hostility and ostracism by society etc., may all have been responsible for bringing about a marked, though often reversible, personality change. This can lead to the misconception that there is a uniform pre-drug use personality.

To a certain extent, just as after some time, beer drinkers may no longer feel satisfied with this drink and may turn to the more potent spirits, so a minority of amphetamine takers may be tempted, especially when moving in a subculture using hard drugs, to try opiates and cocaine or the hashish smoker searching for greater awareness or even more heightened perceptions may move on from cannabis to LSD. One essential difference between alcohol and certain other drugs is in the possible progress of the drug abuser from initial oral use (or 'sniffing') to hypodermic and later intravenous injection providing him with a more rapid and more intense result – although the drinker, too, may achieve a more rapid and stronger effect by gulping his drink. On the other hand, with progressive impoverishment, just as there is a gradual decline in the quality of the alcoholic's beverage (in men the decline is seen from whisky to cider and surgical spirits, and in women from gin to cheap wine), so the poor Chinese opium addict in Singapore may have to make-do with dross, the residue obtained after the first smoking of opium [3].

Progressive physical dependence

Alcohol and other CNS depressants may also induce a state of physical dependence. Psychological and physical withdrawal symptoms may in time become important reasons for continuing or resuming the consumption of alcohol or other drugs respectively. In the case of alcoholics and barbiturate and narcotic addicts, physical dependence may become an important factor inducing the individual to continue his alcohol and drug abuse (see Part 2). For example, a conditioning process (unpleasant withdrawal symptoms in the past having been relieved by further drug consumption) may contribute to a dependent individual continuing with his drinking or drug taking during a 'bout' when he experiences the first inklings of minor withdrawal symptoms. This conditioning process may also contribute to a relapse [17], although it is psychological and social dependence rather than physical dependence which seem to be the most important reasons in inducing relapse after alcohol or drugs have been withdrawn completely. At any rate, with progressive dependence, the drinker and drug taker become increasingly preoccupied with the drug (or drugs) concerned, to the exclusion of other activities, with progressive lowering of ethical, moral, occupational and social standards, and with harm ensuing both for the individual and for society.

Factors influencing regression

The extent of an individual's regression will depend on factors resting with the host, his socio-economic environment and the pharmacological nature of the given drug. Thus the more integrated and stable the drinker's or drug taker's original personality make-up, the greater the resistance which he may be able to muster in stemming the tide of the downward progress. This will be made easier for him when he is still anchored in a helpful, understanding family or has the stabilising influence of an interesting, meaningful job and helpful employers. The pace of the downward process will also be affected by the pharmacological nature of the drug involved and the extent to which it can erode the individual's psychological and physical functioning. For example, many alcoholics fortunately never slip down to the final or chronic phase of the alcoholic addiction process, with its prolonged periods of intoxication and its irreversible mental and physical complications, such as dementia or liver cirrhosis. The reason may be, at least to some extent, that the psycho- and physiopathological destructive process has not been strong enough to destroy all the original resistance of the personality, in particular when this individual still has the benefit of good communications with his family and employer. On the other hand, predominantly psychopathic or very immature personalities may reach the chronic phase relatively quickly, as illustrated for example, by the rapidity of the downward progress in many drinkers who became alcoholics at a very youthful age [14]. Similarly the downward progress of the young, unstable drug abuser (and for that matter even an initially, relatively stable youngster) will probably develop more rapidly, the more he loses all communication with his family and the more alienated he becomes from school or work. His downward progress will continue when, perhaps partly because of this alienation and lack of communication, he takes to mainlining pharmacologicically stronger agents, such as barbiturates or methylamphetamine. These in turn by undermining the user's mental and physical health will accelerate his downward path.

Likewise, in the case of the alcoholic, other factors being equal, spirits will lead to a more rapid downward path than wines and beer. However, the commonly heard remark that a drinker is safe as long as he sticks to beer is obviously no more than a wishful dream–similar perhaps in some aspects to the notion that keeping to soft drugs and avoiding hard drugs will keep a drug abuser out of trouble. Neither sticking to beer or wine nor sticking to soft drugs is a passport to avoidance of dependence and other complications. The excessive beer or wine drinker can become dependent in the same way as the heavy user of cannabis, LSD, amphetamines and hypnotics (i.e. the soft drugs). In general, however, dependence may develop more slowly with the less concentrated alcoholic beverages than with spirits, and more slowly with the soft drugs than with the opiates.

In order to prove to themselves that they can get on top of their drinking problem and that they have not lost their willpower (which many alcoholics regard as the main reason for their inability to control their drinking), alcoholics often go 'on the waggon' – i.e. abstain from alcohol altogether for a certain period. Alternatively they change their pattern of drinking, e.g. by switching from spirits to beer or wine (see below). Both these devices usually fail to stem the downward process for long and the drinker usually resumes his previous pattern of alcohol consumption with even greater intensity and destructiveness.

Alcoholism in different countries

There is, however, the interesting point that Jellinek [1] and the WHO Expert Committees (1954 [8], 1955 [9]) have linked the relative predominance of different types of alcoholism in various countries with the relative prevalence of drinking different types of alcoholic beverages, i.e. spirits or wine. In (e.g. Anglo-Saxon) countries where spirits predominate, the gamma type of alcoholism is said to be more prevalent, characterised by the loss of control (LoC). In predominantly wine-drinking countries (such as France), the delta type of alcoholism is said to be more common, characterised by the inability to abstain from drinking. Unlike the LoC alcoholic, a delta drinker does not necessarily or commonly end up drunk after starting to drink. Whereas the gamma drinker can abstain from alcohol altogether for varying periods (i.e. 'go on the waggon') the delta alcoholic is unable to do so; he has to 'top up' intermittently every hour or so throughout the day (so as to keep up a certain blood alcohol level) and day by day. As discussed later (see page 66), in Jellinek's view, these differences between gamma and delta drinkers may be connected with the (quantitatively) different pharmacological effects of spirits and wine.

However, they could also be associated with the different social attitudes to habitual heavy alcohol consumption in Anglo-Saxon countries and France [1,18]. In Anglo-Saxon countries heavy drinking is generally frowned upon. In France, for various (partly economic) reasons (including vested interests, a large proportion of the French population deriving their livelihood from the production of wine), it is widely accepted. These different social attitudes have, moreover, important repercussions on the symptomatology which in various aspects differs in the gamma and delta types.

As indicated in Figure 1 (in Appendix) – which refers in the main to the gamma (LoC) variety – the alcoholic begins to feel guilty about his drinking behaviour fairly early in his drinking career; he realises that it is different from the way in which the majority of his friends and neighbours take their drinks. Because of these vague guilt feelings he has to bolster up his drinking with feeble excuses and alibis (rationalisations), or he overcompensates for his growing failure to control his drinking by grandiose, or unreasonably resentful and aggressive behaviour. He may often be full of remorse, especially in the hangover condition the morning after a drinking spree, and may make no end of well meant resolutions and promises to himself and others to leave drink alone or to drink in moderation only. Usually these resolutions fail abysmally sooner or later; the drinker feels more and more guilty and begins to avoid contact with friends and even with members of his family, who in turn – unable to understand his strange and unpredictable behaviour – may exclude him more and more from their circle. Ultimately he may separate from his family or more often his wife in desperation may walk out on him, as may his friends, and he will find himself in utter isolation. Depressed, devoid of family, friends, job and hope, usually his only remaining ally is the bottle. Indirectly therefore the attitude of family and friends – well meant as it usually is – and the mutual misunderstanding between the alcoholic and his family and friends, may contribute to his social decline and to his retreating more and more to the bottle. Such hostile family attitudes lead to a process of 'deviance amplification' [19]. In fact, because the general social attitude in such countries is one of rejection of habitual heavy drinking, it is more often (but by no means exclusively so) people with more than their fair share of personality problems who expose themselves to the risk of social ostracism arising out of a habit of excessive drinking. A relatively high proportion of alcoholics in such countries may therefore be predominantly psychogenic alcoholics, i.e. have originally started to drink heavily for relief from personal problems (see Figure 1, top left, in Appendix). Moreover, as often noted in international conferences, representatives of such countries regard alcoholism mainly as a problem arising on the basis of psychological problems.

Thus the alcoholic in such countries, feeling that family and friends reject his drinking behaviour, will tend to drink secretly, and, as he does not want to be caught drinking, may tend to gulp his drinks. Once having started he then tends to go on drinking as much and as quickly as he can. There may also be a social aspect of LoC. The drinker may after all never be sure that there will be another opportunity for him to drink in one or two hours time without strong objections from his family, business associates or friends. In the case of the average French alcoholic the matter could be quite different. Here a high proportion of the population drink heavily (France leads the table listing countries according to the proportion of alcoholics) and there is a great deal of tolerance and acceptance of heavy drinking. Under such circumstances the alcoholic may not need to drink as much as he can in a LoC bout, as he knows he will be able to drink again in one or two hours. Thus, he probably will not have the same tendency and need to feel guilty, to rationalise his drinking behaviour to himself or to others, to feel remorseful or depressed, to make resolutions which he knows he will be unable to keep, to overcompensate by grandiose or aggressive behaviour or to avoid friends and end up in an isolated position which would then become a motivation for further drinking, as happens regularly in his counterpart, the Anglo-Saxon LoC alcoholic. In fact, whereas in the Anglo-Saxon countries social ostracism of the alcoholic is common and until very recently practically the rule, the French delta alcoholic is less exposed to social complications but may be much more prone to such physical complications as liver cirrhosis. Alcoholic cirrhosis is extremely common in France whereas it is seen much less frequently in England. Cirrhosis in England, in fact, is much more often caused by conditions other than alcoholism, in particular by virus hepatitis.

As already discussed in the previous chapter (see Section 2) in a country (and also in social subcultures or occupations) where heavy drinking is widely accepted, even the average type of individual by becoming a heavy drinker may thereby run a risk of becoming an alcoholic. In countries such as France, for example, there may be a much higher proportion of alcoholics who originally started their drinking career by falling in with their friends and national habits and customs of habitual heavy social drinking (see Figure 1, top left, in Appendix) and not by relief drinking. Because of the high number of sociogenic alcoholics in such countries, the main causation of alcoholism may be ascribed to socio-cultural and not to psychological conditions.

The effect of society's attitude
How far does this discussion also apply to other drugs? Middle-aged professional or therapeutic addicts, who basically accept the norms of society, often feel ashamed and guilty about their drug-taking be-haviour: e.g. about the need to take drugs to which they have pro-fessional access but which they of course realise is against their pro-fessional code of ethics; or about obtaining extra supplies by telling lies to their own GP or by running to a number of practitioners at the same time. Their behaviour and attitudes may therefore resemble in many aspects those of the Anglo-Saxon LoC addict, and, as discussed later on, such patients may fit in well with therapeutic groups consisting mainly of alcoholics. Young drug addicts moving in their own sub-cultures, on the other hand, may not feel guilty at all about their drug taking which, they may maintain, is their private affair. The middle-aged drug addict in principle may accept society's evaluation of him as a deviant and feel ashamed of it, although often he, or she (e.g. in the case of barbiturates) takes drugs to excess in order to keep up with the demands of society, e.g. to enable him to go to work. The young drug addict, on the other hand, does not necessarily regard his drug use as abnormal – after all, he sees his parents drink, smoke cigarettes and frequently take tranquillisers or sleeping pills. Moreover, his drug taking may be the thing to do in his subculture. He does not accept that the fault is with him (unlike the middle-aged addict) but blames the 'sick' and unfair society. However, as his drug taking is illegal, he too will have to take care to keep his secret but without feeling guilty about it. In time he may, however, accept society's valuation of himself as a deviant. It is argued by some sociologists that society's attitude to the young drug abuser may lead to an amplification of deviance [20]. Often indeed seeing himself labelled as a deviant and regarded as

antisocial by society he may live up to this label by behaving accordingly, thereby justifying and confirming such a label (self-fulfilling prophecy).

Much (but by no means all) of the young drug abuser's behaviour nowadays may be a reaction against society's attitude (or what he perceives it to be). This attitude is often one of hostility to the drug abuser – as it is to the LoC alcoholic and it may be further aggravated by their behaviour. Such attitudes of society tend to become reflected in the symptomatology of alcoholism and drug dependence. The rejected LoC alcoholic feeling more and more isolated retreats wholly to the bottle, possibly ending up in the chronic phase in a state of more or less continual drunken 'benders'. The young drug abuser, feeling alienated from home, school, work and the community, may seek solace in joining up with a social subculture. This may reinforce his feeling of being rejected by adult society and of his attempts to find an answer in drug taking. Thus taking society's labels of deviancy as a yardstick, both the middle-aged drug addict and the gamma alcoholic as well as the young drug abusers may show symptoms arising from their reactions to such labelling. The French delta alcoholic, however, would not be regarded by his community as a deviant nor would he look at himself as a deviant, and therefore will not develop additional symptoms.

The foregoing describes only a few of the many possible permutations and models of such behaviours and reactions from the vast number of permutations that may occur when different types of personalities living in different societies take drugs with varying pharmacological properties for different reasons. The examples chosen indicate however once more that the behaviour (and the symptomatology) of alcoholics and drug abusers depends on socio-cultural as well as on psychological and pharmacological factors.

The loss-of-control phenomenon
The loss of control with further alcohol intake is as we have seen one of Jellinek's cornerstones in his description of the developmental progress of gamma alcoholism, heralding the crucial phase. Loss of control has commonly been misunderstood in the past to mean that such an alcohol 'addict' has invariably to continue drinking once he has started to consume alcohol – a view also reflected in AA's famous slogan: 'The first drink is fatal.' Mark Keller – editor of the *Quarterly Journal on the Study of Alcohol*, the leading journal in the world in the field of

alcohol problems – recently pointed out [21] that this use of the term 'loss of control' had never been Jellinek's intention. The observation – by no means infrequent in our clinical investigation of the LoC phenomenon over the past ten years – that a high proportion of LoC alcoholics do not necessarily get drunk on the first occasion of drinking, but are often able to postpone drunkenness for a few days, weeks or even months [11, 18] – does not necessarily prove that the loss-of-control phenomenon is a myth [22]. Nor is this necessarily indicated by the occasional reports of a few LoC alcoholics who have managed to revert to moderate or normal drinking.

In our own investigations a proportion of more than 30 % of alcoholics managed to avoid getting drunk on the first occasion – as a rule only to end up drunk a few days or weeks later when the effort of trying moderate drinking had proved too much [18]. They managed to stick to moderate drinking for a period by being careful about such items as the type of drink (e.g. beer or wine rather than spirits), the venue of drinking (e.g. not drinking at home by oneself), considering their mood (drinking when in a cheerful but not when in a depressed state) and where possible, radical changes in their domestic or occupational set-up [11].

On reflection, it would seem that the LoC phenomenon may be influenced not only by the activity of the agent alcohol (e.g. concentration of the beverage, the speed with which it is gulped down etc.) but also by the underlying personality (host) and socio-environmental factors, working in close interaction with each other. Personality and environmental conditions as well as the pharmacological action of alcohol itself and possibly biochemical changes arising from the interaction between host and agent may affect the LoC phenomenon. Therefore a physiopathological process – as hypothesised by Jellinek (see above) – might be at work but it is not necessarily in full charge. An emotionally stable personality, supported by favourable domestic and occupational conditions might withstand the psychological or biochemically induced urge to continue drinking at least for a certain period. However should the LoC alcoholic in an undisciplined way set off by gulping several concentrated drinks on the first occasion, the resultant high blood alcohol level will probably compel him to continue immediately. In our experience the rule seems to be that, '. . . the first drink may be fatal on the first occasion, but anyhow will usually prove fatal sooner or later'.

Stabilised addicts

The question arises whether any similar processes can be observed in the case of drugs other than alcohol. There may be some similarities between such LoC alcoholics who are temporarily able to drink in moderation, and the relatively rare examples of stabilised addicts. Occasionally one encounters a previously uncontrolled heroin addict who achieves at least temporary, though rather insecure stabilisation on a given dose of heroin. This may happen e.g. (a) as a result of a greatly changed outlook and attitude or of finding a different, meaningful purpose in life (i.e. an alteration of the host factor), or (b) after finding happiness in marriage or landing a congenial job (i.e. a change of environment), and perhaps also after gaining self-confidence and obtaining helpful psychological and social support from regular attendance at a Treatment Centre, in this case, change of host and environment, perhaps coupled with (c) a marked lowering of the addicts regular dosage or a switch to a pharmacologically perhaps slightly less potent agent (e.g. from heroin to methadone). Stabilised addicts seem to be as a rule middle-aged, more mature, professional or therapeutic addicts, often supported by their family circle and the interest in their job (e.g. jazz musicians) [18]. Examples given by the Interdepartmental Committee in their (first) Report on Drug Addiction (1961) [23] in support of their belief that stabilisation on a given drug dosage was a feasible proposition, were all middle-aged drug takers. On the other hand young, inadequate, immature, possibly psychopathic non-therapeutic drug users may find such stabilisation difficult or impossible to achieve. However, in the last few years there have been cases of drug addicts in their mid-twenties who with support from the Treatment Centre staff, are able, with certain ups-and-downs to stick to a relatively stable, fairly low dosage of approximately 20–30 mg of heroin or 30–60 mg of methadone. Again these are mainly individuals who seem to have matured in their attitude a great deal since one first met them 5–7 years ago; they keep on working and may have fairly stable homes. Stabilisation is probably also easier to achieve in addicts sniffing heroin or cocaine – formerly one saw quite a few sniffers of cocaine among jazz musicians who claimed they had been doing it for years – or in those taking methadone by mouth (as in the American Maintenance Programmes) rather than in those injecting these drugs i.v. There might be a certain parallel here to the difference between the slowly drinking alcoholics and those gulping their drinks. Those of our alcoholic patients who achieve temporary success in drinking moderately usually do so by 'nibbling' at their drinks. Once they resume their former gulping pattern they usually soon revert to uncontrolled drinking.

This discussion may also be of some relevance as regards the alleged success of the old British System of narcotics control prior to the 1960s and its subsequent decline. The old system seemed to work well with the type of relatively stable and mature, often therapeutic and professional, middle-aged addict prevalent at the time [24]. Here a constellation of relatively favourable host and environmental factors may have successfully outbalanced those effects of the pharmacological agent which in interaction with other factors might tend to push the dosage up (e.g. increasing tolerance) [18]. However with the emergence in the early 1960s of the modern, young and immature, non-therapeutic hedonistic type of addict no such counteracting motivations were at work. They just desired the pharmacological effect of the agent, whilst lacking the stabilising factors in their personalities and often in their homes and jobs, which were either no longer existent or lacked cohesion, meaning and interest [18].

Diagnosis of types of alcoholism and addiction

Reverting once more to the alcoholic LoC phenomenon the question is further complicated by the difficulty in many cases of being sure about the diagnosis of gamma (i.e. LoC) alcoholism. Often one cannot be certain whether on a given occasion the drinker, as he usually claims, never wanted to stop, whether he continued drinking on a given occasion because of underlying psychological and social factors, i.e. alpha alcoholism, or whether in fact he could no longer stop, i.e. he had reached the LoC stage. Often it seems impossible to decide whether in an individual drinker, alpha (symptomatic) alcoholism has already progressed to gamma alcoholism or not – particularly since such a development is often insidious and gradual. The question as to whether the individual excessive drinker may present as the gamma or the delta type (inability to abstain) of alcoholism, may likewise be related to environmental (see page 59) and social, as well as to pharmacological factors. Delta alcoholism is more common in countries which favour drinking wine, a less potent beverage than spirits which are prevalent in countries where the gamma type predominates. Spirits as described by Jellinek [1] produce possibly a more shock-like effect, unlike the more severe abstinence symptoms following spirit drinking which may demand immediate relief by further drinking (loss of control), whereas the much less severe abstinence symptoms of the delta type may require relief only intermittently every hour or so. However, there may be another explanation: the LoC drinker living in Anglo-Saxon countries where social tolerance of excessive drinking is low, is thereby forced to drink in a hurry unlike the French delta drinker; the wide acceptance of heavy drinking in France allows him to proceed at leisure and intermittently throughout the day, and there is no need for him to gulp his drink down rapidly. Thus it may depend on environmental factors too whether a man exhibits the gamma or delta variety. Among our own patients there were quite a few who sometimes drank in a gamma fashion and at other times in a delta fashion. This depended on such circumstances as whether they had pressing business engagements ahead (preventing further drinking), or whether their wives were away from home. These men were able to store supplies safely in the knowledge that they could top up unhindered all day long. Finally it has been suggested that there are also certain differences between personalities of gamma and delta alcoholics [25]. Anyhow some types of personality may find it more difficult to tolerate psychological withdrawal symptoms (whilst drink is available) and would thus tend to drink in a LoC fashion. Others might be better able to delay their desire for further drinking for an hour or more. It thus seems possible that the triad of personality, environment and 'bottle' in interaction with each other, may greatly influence the form in which an individual's alcoholism presents itself.

Again there may be similarities here to the drug-taking behaviour of addicts. For example, some narcotic addicts, are apparently unable to refrain from finishing practically all the supplies in their possession in one go. Others are able to space their drug taking more evenly throughout the 24 hours. Thus some addicts could be trusted with a prescription enabling them to pick up three days' supply, whereas others given such a prescription would invariably turn up at the Treatment Centre the next day with stories of having lost, or having been robbed of their supplies. Personality attributes, e.g. the ability to tolerate minor withdrawal symptoms for a few hours rather than immediately having to satisfy the pharmacological demand (the strength of such withdrawal symptoms partly depending on the pharmacological nature of the drug), the social setting, etc., may all be of importance. Likewise it may often be difficult or impossible to determine in the earlier phases of an individual's drug abuse whether he takes the drugs mainly because of psychic dependence (alpha type) or whether meanwhile there has also been added a physical dependence with physical abstinence symptoms demanding relief (gamma or delta types).

Just as there are often difficulties in deciding whether the symptomatic varieties (alpha) have already progressed to the gamma or delta types, and just as the progress from alpha to the gamma and delta types is gradual, so also is the development of psychic dependence an insidious process. Sometimes it may be impossible to say whether a person has already become psychologically dependent or not. Where individuals use alcohol or other drugs for social, recreational or ritual purposes only, they are clearly not dependent. Neither are those drug takers who merely 'play around' and experiment with them. Psychic dependence probably sets in where occasional relief drinking and drug taking are gradually replaced by continual relief alcohol and drug abuse, with increasing tolerance necessitating gradually increasing amounts of the drug (see Figure 1 in Appendix). Whether or not in a given individual psychic dependence has already set in, can, in the view of Dr Dale Cameron [26], be ascertained by looking into the question, 'To what extent does the use of the drug appear to be a life-organising factor, or take precedence over the use of other coping mechanisms?'

Quite clearly our knowledge of the problems of psychic and physical dependence leaves many unanswered questions, and is a field wide open for multi- and interdisciplinary research.

3.4 SOCIAL COMPLICATIONS

Apart from the often disastrous effects of alcohol and drug abuse on the health and life of the individual, the harm to society may often be considerable.

Complications of alcoholism in the social sphere [11, 27] – which usually precede medical conditions such as cirrhosis of the liver, peripheral neuropathy and KorsaKoff's syndrome, often by a great many years – are regular features of the disorder. They are therefore worthy of the closest consideration.

Alcoholism and the family unit

The disastrous effect which alcoholism often exercises at home is well known. Very early in his drinking career the alcoholic comes to rely more and more on his favourite defence mechanisms, including, apart from outright denial and rationalisations, the mechanism of projection, namely the ascribing of his own defects to others. Thus everything and everybody is wrong – especially the members of his family circle who may already suffer at the alcoholic's hands at a time when his friends still think of him as quite a decent and reasonable person. For some time the family members will have tried to reason with and to work with the alcoholic, and to keep the 'skeleton in the cupboard', hidden from the outside world, whilst they themselves may feel very ashamed or guilty. Later however, they detach themselves from the alcoholic and begin to build up a life as if he were not there, and gradually the wife assumes the duties, responsibilities and the rights of the house-holder. This, incidentally, is one of the difficulties when the alcoholic, having decided to give up drinking, and having had treatment, returns home and assumes that he will immediately be back in charge. His family, on the other hand, will remain wary and cautious for a long time. Both family and the alcoholic will require a lot of patience and understanding of each other's difficulties during this phase. Often the alcoholic may be treated by his family as if he no longer belongs to the circle, and finally there may be separation and divorce.

It is often amazing, on the other hand, how much an alcoholic's wife can stand. Sometimes she seems to be a veritable glutton for punishment. Her pathetic attempts to help her husband usually only lead to further quarrels and sometimes to blows. For example, she may try to deal with the problem of hidden bottles which she finds in some ingenious hideout, by pouring the contents down the sink. This will probably aggravate the situation, and it is also usually completely ineffective. Naturally enough the alcoholic in turn very often puts the blame for some of his symptoms on the attitude of his wife. For instance, he may claim that her allegedly fanatical teetotal attitude forces him, in self-defence, to such measures as hiding bottles and drinking secretly before parties. The masochistic behaviour of some wives seems to indicate that not infrequently they may have married the alcoholic for the sake of satisfying unconscious personality needs of their own. At any rate, in our experience, although separation and divorce is frequent both in male and female alcoholics, it is more common among women alcoholics.

The higher divorce rate of alcoholic women then probably stems both from the wife's higher tolerance of her alcoholic husband's behaviour than *vice versa*, and from the greater destructiveness of a woman drunkard's conduct. In favour of the latter hypothesis is the finding that the average woman alcoholic – once she has embarked upon her alcoholic career (usually many years later than the average male alcoholic) – develops more serious symptoms and may have to be admitted to a hospital relatively more rapidly than the man [14].

In a survey carried out by the present author in the 1950s at Warlingham Park Hospital, the average male alcoholic had first shown suspicion and jealousy of his wife's behaviour (possibly as a projection and as a consequence of his own drinking behaviour with diminution of his sexual potency, his extramarital adventures, etc.) at the age of 33. He had first been reproached for his drinking behaviour by his wife at the age of 34. He had shown unreasonable resentment chiefly at home, between the ages of 35 and 36, and a little later, at the age of 37, he felt guilty about his behaviour at home. However, at this stage he managed to rationalise his guilt feelings about neglecting his family, as he had already felt for several years that his relatives lacked consideration for him. His family began to change their habits (e.g. giving up inviting friends to the home, etc.) when the alcoholic was aged 36. All this happened at least 5 years before at an (average) age of 40, he was first admitted to hospital for some physical complication of his drinking [14].

By the time the alcoholic finally comes for treatment, his wife, too, is also in such a nervous state that she requires treatment herself. Statements such as, 'I cannot stand it any longer' are almost the rule, and on quite a few occasions we came across cases where in utter desperation the wife of the alcoholic attempted suicide. The manner of some of these attempts indicated that they were far more than just a cry for help.

With all these statistics relating to the effects of alcoholism in causing marital disharmony, one has of course, to keep in mind that to some extent this disharmony may be partly due to the underlying personality instability of the alcoholic, and not wholly to the superimposed alcoholism. But on the other hand, the great majority of the alcoholics studied in the survey were basically not psychopathic personalities. In fact, no more than one-third were classified as psychopaths.

Children of alcoholics

A parent's alcoholism must often have far-reaching effects on the personality development of his children. The alcoholic's unpredictable attitude and behaviour necessitates a continual readjustment by all those living close to him. The child of an alcoholic will often experience disturbed emotional relations with both his parents as he is so often torn in loyalties between the parents when the mother takes over control of the household in place of the drinking father. The risks threatening the emotional development of the growing child stem not only from the drinking parent, but also from the reaction of the alcoholic's spouse to the drinker. Feeling, for example, embittered, frustrated, or angry, the alcoholic's wife may attempt to satisfy her own unfulfilled emotional needs by overattaching herself to the child, or alternatively may reject him. Therefore, the fundamental disturbance of marital and parent-child relationships, with associated maternal and/or paternal rejection, deprivation, inadequacy and broken homes, makes it very difficult for the child to undergo normal emotional and social development and to acquire the capacity of experiencing satisfactory emotional relationships. Among children of alcoholics one might, therefore, not infrequently expect evidence of emotional insecurity. This may manifest itself, for example, in the shape of neurotic symptoms, behaviour disorders, delinquency, and also alcoholism in later life. The fact that not uncommonly the son or daughter of an alcoholic father may themselves become alcoholics, despite all their bad childhood experiences and memories arising from the father's drinking behaviour, is of some interest. It may denote that such a child still identifies with the drinking father rather than with the mother who may have been driven to nagging and similar undesirable behaviour as a reaction to her husband's activities. On the other hand, the author over the past 10 years has come across many young abusers of other drugs where a parent – usually the father – has been an alcoholic. Apart from the frequently present alienation from the family, the choice of other drugs in place of alcohol – which such youngsters often blame on their father's aggressive and violent behaviour – may reflect their protest against the father's behaviour.

In the case of young, as a rule, single, drug abusers and addicts, it is most frequently their parents who will suffer emotionally, and only relatively rarely their wives and children. This is different from the case of the older alcoholics (unless of course one deals with middle-aged barbiturate or professional or therapeutic drug addicts). A young drug abuser's parents are often very shocked and surprised that this could have possibly have happened to their child. In retrospect they often admit that there had been an insidious behaviour change noticeable for some months or even years. Possibly the event of drug abuse did not occur to the parents because they may have thought that this could occur only in very underprivileged, disrupted homes to emotionally very disturbed children, and not in a respectable home with respectable children. They forgot or never knew, that in particular in the UK such drug abuse among the youngsters, since its emergence in the 1960s, has never respected social class, and often emotionally relatively stable children, even from good homes, have taken to drug abuse. Frequently however, unsatisfactory home circumstances – disharmony and unhappiness in the parental home, or what the adolescent may have perceived as a repressive home atmosphere – may have contributed to the development of his drug abuse. At any rate, both alcohol and drug dependence are often either symptomatic of, and/or lead to, family disruption. They both constitute family illnesses, and their management is not complete without including other family members in the treatment situation.

The importance of family relationships and of *family therapy* was recently well illustrated in a description of a 17 year old female drug abuser by Dr J. Gomersall [28]. In his view the basic aspects of most family problems in such situations are that someone or everyone in the family becomes concerned, worried and frightened about the problem, which leads to tension when an attempt is made to discuss it. Thus, the family may enter a non-communicating danger zone. The original issue may then fade into the background, family cooperation in general may suffer and other problems may distort the picture. There is increasing polarisation, bitterness and hostility between the two sides. In the case described, the youngster in an attempt to escape from the tense family situation sought friends outside, achieving acceptance from them by sharing their drug taking. The rest of the family too sought friends and allies by turning to other relatives, the family doctor, the minister of religion and local policemen. In this way the gulf between parents and daughter became even wider. Management in such cases aims at ending the underlying family discord by trying to restore the communication between the members of the family. This leads to a state of cooperation – although Gomersall stresses that the aim of family therapy lies in prevention and full rehabilitation other than in mere withdrawal of drugs from an established addict.

Alcohol, drugs and sex

By removing inhibitions and dissolving the superego, alcohol may contribute to sexual acting out, with its implication of illegitimate pregnancies, spread of VD etc. One occasionally comes across alcoholics suffering from sexual deviations who state that they had only been able to muster up sufficient courage to go to a prostitute for the purpose of indulging in sadistic–masochistic activities etc, when they were to some extent under the influence of alcohol. An occasional alcoholic, possibly of an obsessional personality type, may admit that he drinks to excess in order to obtain an alibi appeasing his own conscience when indulging in his deviant sexual activities. One in five of a sample of male sex offenders, investigated in 1957, had been drinking at the time of the offence [29]. Among our own patients, such acts include exhibitionism and sexual offences committed on children. This is more in line with the usual finding, known already in Shakespeare's time, that alcohol may increase the desire but impair the performance. As already mentioned, the decreased potency of the male alcoholic may be one of the reasons for the often paranoid jealousy shown by alcoholics who, by a mechanism of projection, become convinced of their wives' infidelity. This feeling may be further enhanced by the refusal of the alcoholic's wife to go to bed with him when he staggers home in the early morning hours strongly reeking of alcohol.

Regarding the relationship between other drugs and sex, as in other aspects, there are important differences between the various drugs. Contrary to the common misconception that the narcotic user is a person prone to violent and aggressive sexual behaviour, the average opiate addict is more likely to be passive, quiet and often sexually impotent and disinterested. It has even been suggested that some such individuals initially started on heroin as an alibi excusing them from having to try sexual intercourse. Again a lot will depend on psychological factors and the social setting. We found among addicts seen at St Bernard's Hospital that in general the psychological and physiological effects of narcotics make a normal sex life impossible for most addicts. Both male and female addicts report loss of sexual desire, and in males impotence is commonly found [24]. Samples of heroin addicts seen at St Bernard's Hospital, and by other observers in General Practice [30] showed the great majority to be single (obviously the young age of many such addicts must be taken into account). Nevertheless problems can arise from the finding that infants born to a narcotic addicted mother may exhibit severe physical abstinence symptoms (usually starting within 72 hours of birth); and recently there have been reports of deaths of babies born to mothers whilst on a methadone maintenance programme [31]. This of course necessitates much further research.

The question is often raised as to the relationship between drugs of the cannabis and LSD type and sex. Drug users with whom the present author discussed this question usually stated that such drugs reinforced their mood – 'If I was in the mood for sex it strengthened it; if not I remained disinterested'. Such replies seem to be in accord with many other reports on the subject. 'If one is sexually bent (writes A. Trocchi [32]), and it occurs to one that it would be pleasant to make love, the judicious use of the drug marihuana will stimulate the desire and heighten the pleasure immeasurably; for it is perhaps the principal effect of marihuana to take one more intensely into whatever experience . . .'

Writing in more sober terms but nevertheless expressing a somewhat similar viewpoint, a WHO Scientific Group, discussing the relationship between cannabis and sexual gratification, notes that at the subjective level, cannabis (a) often enhances touch and other senses (b) generally prolongs the perception of time, and (c) sometimes imparts novelty to familiar objects and activities. All these may enhance the sense of gratification experienced by some people during the sexual act, although this enhancement of sensations or of performance is difficult to verify by objective measurement [16]. The report makes these points in order to illustrate that, 'Objective measurements of performance are not necessarily relevant to the existence of reported subjective experiences', or the apparent reality for the person experiencing the sensation.

Alcoholism and drug abuse in industry [11]

In England, the contribution of alcoholism to impaired factory output, absenteeism, industrial accidents, etc. has attracted little attention. This lack of interest is partly due to the fact that the alcoholic problem in industry is probably mainly presented by the alcoholic who is still in the relatively early phases of his drinking career. Such a man may still be able to carry out his functions, although often as a 'half man' only, for many years before finally coming to the attention of the management. Problem drinking affects all levels – the shop floor workers through all grades of the management to the top.

It is not really surprising that alcoholism should be found to strike so much at top executives. Two main sets of factors responsible for alcoholism are the individual's psychological make-up and environmental conditions (see Sections 2.2 and 2.3). The ambitious, driving, worrying individual may often feel the need for a relaxant during his drive to the top, and later on, whilst trying to stay there. Moreover, he moves in circles where drinking is a widespread pastime and drink is a generally accepted social and business lubricant. In such a group, where heavy drinking is an acknowledged and accepted custom, even the psychologically less vulnerable personality may readily drift into excessive alcohol consumption with its accompanying risk of alcoholism (see Section 2.3). Thus personality make-up, environmental strain and stress, in combination with accepted customs among this group may all tend to make alcoholism something of an occupational hazard among top executives. Moreover, it stands to reason that a high executive's bad temper, irritability and frayed nerves – engendered by his alcoholism – do not make for a healthy atmosphere and good relationships at work. This further impairs efficiency among those working with and under him. If relatively little attention has so far been directed at the problem of alcoholism in industry, even less attention has been paid to the problem of misuse of other drugs.*

Clearly, as drug abuse has so often started whilst the adolescent is still at school there must be many drug abusers in industry. Because of their young age they are likely to be found on the shop floor rather than among the executives.

The middle-aged barbiturate addict may present similar problems in industry to the alcoholic. Among young drug abusers the cocaine takers usually stated that once you are hooked on the drug, work was virtually out. Apart from a minority of relatively stabilised heroin addicts, most 'H' abusers will probably be unable to work. Hashish taken in moderation (and even less so the weaker marihuana) will often present no problem, but when taken in larger amounts and more regularly, states of relaxation and lethargy often remove any interest in one's occupation. In the case of amphetamines, deterioration of school and work record and lack of interest in school or work may be early features. Moreover, insomnia and a dopy feeling in the morning often make it impossible for the amphetamine user to get up in the morning and turn up at work. In all such cases the type of underlying personality, the reasons why the individual started to take drugs in the first place, the social setting, his involvement with the subcultures, his preoccupation with drug-oriented activities etc. may often be more important factors than the pharmacological actions of the drug concerned. For example, the youthful drug user may express his belief in a hedonistic philosophy of life, and that he is not interested in work but keen on

---

* However, some aspects in relation to drugs, youth and the work world have been discussed in a recent book by M. Trico and P. M. Roman [33]

enjoying himself. Society has no right to force him to work and he would gladly leave this activity to those people who like work.

Where alcohol and drug abusers are still employed, this would in theory offer industry a chance at a preventive approach, by constructive programmes starting with early identification of such individuals and encouragement to seek treatment, whilst their jobs are kept open for them. Where people are not employed, the chances of early identification are naturally much smaller. However, in this country the problems of alcohol and drug dependency in industry have so far attracted little attention – a situation that one hopes may soon be changed.

Crime [11]

Alcoholism releases aggression which may be directed against oneself as well as against others. Nearly half the male alcoholic patients seen in the Warlingham Park Hospital in the 1950s and more than one-third of the women, admitted that whilst drinking they had behaved aggressively or had endangered others or themselves. This had happened at average ages of 33 and 40 years in men and women respectively, i.e. quite a few years before they finally sought help for their alcoholism [14].

In the history of alcoholics (of any type), appearances in court or prison sentences are not uncommon. Thus, of these patients (mainly middle class) 20% had been in prison, chiefly for minor offences, and one-third had been before the court. Of a sample of 40 homeless alcoholics and excess drinkers, who had been admitted to a London Observation Ward in the 1950s, 40% had been in court or prison. Of a group of 27 homeless alcoholics and excess drinkers living in a London Reception Centre for the poor (and chiefly belonging to the lower Occupational Classes IV and V), approximately 45% had been in prison [34]. Finally, of a number of male alcoholics admitted to a London Observation Ward – with a home of their own, and mainly coming from Class III (skilled workers, etc.) – one-third had been before the courts. In a more recent investigation, Dr Griffith Edwards and his co-workers at the Addiction Research Unit, found among a sample of approximately 500 prisoners that alcoholism was present in approximately one third. The long-term prisoners had the lowest rate of alcohol problems, the short-term prisoners convicted for drunkenness offences had the highest rates [35].

It is interesting that among the male alcoholics investigated by us [14], the great majority of those who had shown social or antisocial conduct had not done so until after a decade of excessive drinking. Frequently drunkenness had started at an average age of 25 years and social and antisocial conduct not until 34 years. Such social tendencies in the majority of these drinkers were thus clearly a consequence of heavy drinking and not its cause. The majority of alcoholics probably never get into trouble with the law, and the contribution of alcoholism to serious crime has in the past probably been greatly exaggerated. However, there can be no doubt that alcoholism in itself is in a certain proportion of cases, responsible for antisocial conduct. Again, this often occurs years before the diagnosis is made and treatment instituted. The very important, possible connection between the parent's alcoholism and the juvenile delinquency of his offspring has already been mentioned.

Aggression directed against oneself, in the form of *attempted suicide* is quite common amongst alcoholics. Thus, of our male alcoholic patients at Warlingham Park Hospital over 40% (at an average age of 36 years) had seriously contemplated suicide. One-third of the women (average age, 39 years) had considered it. 24% of the men and 26.5% of the women had in fact attempted it. Of homeless alcoholics admitted to a London Observation Ward, 20% had attempted suicide. Many of the suicidal attempts of the alcoholics are exhibitionistic, or in the nature of a cry for help. Nevertheless suicide is a very real risk in alcoholics as is accidental fatal overdosage of drugs, chiefly barbiturates (often in a state of automatism), in drug addicts.

An important difference as regards involvement with the law between problem drinkers and drug abusers arises because alcohol consumption is legal, other drugs – unless prescribed by a doctor – are illegal. One of the most common social consequences of drug use is possible trouble with the Law for being found in possession of drugs. Cannabis smokers never fail to point out how unfair it is that to be found in possession of such a 'harmless' substance could land one in serious difficulties, whereas possession of such dangerous drugs as heroin and cocaine did not – provided one had in the past received them on prescription from one of the few prescribing doctors, or since 1968 from the Treatment Centres. A feeling of hope, justified or not, that the Police might deal with one more leniently if one is registered with a Treatment Centre – even if one is found to be in possession of drugs not prescribed by the Centre or having more than the Centre had prescribed – is sometimes one of the reasons why young drug abusers originally register with such a Centre.

Antisocial activities may arise directly or indirectly from the pre-occupation of the drug user with drugs and out of his need to obtain them at any price. This may lead to disturbed relationships with others and increasing isolation, economic loss and the inability to obtain his drugs legitimately. Thus he takes to selling 'stuff' on the black market. This may be in the form of *dealing*, which is regarded by many drug consumers as acceptable, or in the form of *pushing*, a more professional business, frowned upon by many drug takers. He may also take to crime. This occurs most commonly in the United States and mainly involves crimes against property. The young amphetamine abuser may be inclined to give up work and to peddle drugs, and through his psycho-motor impairment, coupled with his reckless attitude, he may be involved in accidents. Problems may also arise from his paranoid and sometimes overtly psychotic state – a not uncommon complication – and out of his aggressive behaviour. The LSD user may also sometimes feel persecuted, for example, whilst on a 'bad trip' or in an acute psychotic condition, which may be responsible for dangerous be-haviour, such as attacking people in self defence. A well known case of this sort occurred a few years ago when a man, returning during an LSD 'trip' from orbit to earth, felt attacked by snakes. He defended himself against them and during this fight, killed his girl companion who had also taken LSD. The danger of accidents arising out of the occasional omnipotence feeling of the LSD user, such as flying out of a window, or stopping a moving car by stepping in front of it, is well known, as are the panics and the risk of suicide.

Suicide and accidental death

Suicide and accidental overdosage are important dangers in narcotic [24] and barbiturate addicts [36]. From a study of Home Office records referring to the decade 1955–1965, Dr P. James [37] calculated the mortality rate of male non-therapeutic narcotic addicts over a mean period of risk of four years, as 27 (deaths)/1000/year. This is 20 times as high as the total mortality rate which could be expected for an ordinary male population of similar age composition. An analysis of 31 deaths, showed that 5 had certainly committed suicide and 4 were suspected suicide cases all having taken a large overdose of a drug to which they were not actively addicted. Compared to a normal popula-tion corrected for age, the suicide rates among these male addicts were over 50 times as high. Twelve individuals died from an apparently unintentional overdose of the drug to which they were addicted, i.e.

usually heroin, alone or in combination with cocaine. In 4 cases, death was a consequence of septic conditions arising out of the neglect of the most elementary precautions regarding sterile needles, cleaning up the injection areas, etc. Not one died as a consequence of hepatitis during the period in question, though hepatitis follows an infection transmitted through the use of non-sterilised syringes, and jaundice from this cause is not uncommon in addicts who are in the habit of sharing syringes and needles. Three addicts died a violent death, two through falling from heights, one in a motor accident. A similar proportion of causes of death among London addicts was reported by Professor F. E. Camps in 1968 who found 54 % of such deaths to be caused by drug poisoning or overdose [38]. The mean age of death of these addicts was 31·5 years – a shortening of life span of perhaps 30 to 40 years. Our own calculations [24] showed that in the three years (1965–1967) which followed those covered by Dr James' study, the mean age of death of male narcotic addicts had dropped by another two years to 29·4 years. In the case of British-born addicts it had dropped to 27·3 years. This was in the time before the advent of the Treatment Centres in 1968. Since 1968, risks of accidental overdosage whilst in a state of chronic or acute barbiturate intoxication may have increased due to the newer custom of narcotic and other addicts of mainlining barbiturates (see Section 5.2). There has also been a gradual rise in the number of deaths involving methadone, following its increased use and popularity (see Section 5.4). rise in the number of deaths involving methadone, following its increased use and popularity (see Section 5.4).

Elsewhere more will be said about the great danger of self-poisoning – accidental and intentional – in the case of barbiturates [36]. In 1967 the number of barbiturate deaths in England and Wales exceeded 2000, a figure twice as high as the figure for 1960, five times as high as the figure for 1950. The 1967 figure means that each week nearly 40 people killed themselves with barbiturates either accidentally or intentionally [29]. In 1970, the number of deaths by poisoning with barbiturates had fallen to 1895. However, barbiturates are still the main cause of suicidal and accidental deaths from drug poisoning, followed by methaqualone and aspirin. Among non-barbiturate hypnotics, a proprietary drug containing methaqualone and the antihistamine diphenhydramine (mandrax) is most frequently responsible for self-poisoning. The benzodiazepines – commonly used as minor tranquillisers – are in spite of frequent occurrence of overdosage, much safer than the barbiturates.

7

Alcoholic and drug-dependent criminals
How much the pharmacological effect of the drug itself is responsible
for criminal behaviour, how much is due to the user's underlying
personality, and how much of a drug user's life style is associated with
drug taking etc., is difficult to say. However, two types of alcoholic
or drug-dependent criminal can be recognised [39]. The first is basically
antisocial and often drinks a lot and misuses drugs. The second is
driven to breaking the law as a consequence of his drinking or drug
abuse; e.g. because of the pharmacological effects of the drugs, or
because of strong psychic or physical dependence. Naturally, there is
no sharp dividing line between these two types—the alcoholic or
drug-dependent criminal on the one hand, and criminal alcoholics on
the other. A certain proportion of excessive drinkers or drug-dependent
individuals commit anti-social actions before becoming involved with
alcohol or drugs. Hawks (1970), for example, showed that half the
known addicts in Great Britain committed criminal offences before
receiving opiates on prescription [40]. Among male young addicts,
seen by the author in prison over the past 10 years, a very high proportion started their delinquent behaviour before beginning to use drugs,
and James (1969) found that of 50 addicts in prison almost half (44 %)
had appeared before a juvenile court, and threequarters had been
convicted in court before becoming addicted [41]. It is only fair to add
that among the addicts seen by us in prison often such offences had
first occurred at a very young age. However, in many offenders there
were often quite a number of juvenile and other court appearances
before drug abuse started.

Similarly, one finds that many of one's patients seen at a Treatment
Centre continue to commit relatively minor offences. Also one comes
across a high proportion of notified drug addicts among drug abusers
referred to one from a remand home or court, for some occasionally
relatively trivial offence. In this country, at least, the offences committed
by opiate (heroin or methadone) addicts are often petty ones, and such
drugs seem to make largely for passivity and not for aggressive behaviour. For example, a 26 year old male narcotic addict seen by us in
the mid-sixties, had been convicted and sent to prison five times. His
convictions were for altering dates on prescriptions, forging prescriptions and for breaking and entering chemists shops. Another addict of
that period, as quoted in 'The Drug Scene in Great Britain' said,
'Invariably the addict doesn't have enough "bread" to make the scene.
I mean he's always hustling for money, begging and stealing. I always

stole little stuff like art books, car radios, you know, man, all junkies do this. You gotta live, man' [24].

Cannabis and crime

Finally, let us consider the question – so emotionally argued about for so long – of the relationship between cannabis and crime. From experience in England of a great many smokers the impression has been that there seems hardly any connection at all. The risk with the hashish smokers seen by the author was certainly not of aggressiveness or undue activity, but rather, on the contrary, of too much lethargy, indifference and apathy. However, in the past, e.g. in the USA, the taking of cannabis was held responsible for all types of crimes, including murder. In fact, the name hashish stems from 'hashishins', a gang of assassins employed by an ambitious leader to attack and kill neighbouring tribes [42] (see Section 5.3). Allegedly they were given hashish and so went berserk, ran riot and attacked and killed the people they were meant to go for. A comment in a recent review states that the hashishins were in fact not given the drug to enable them to commit crimes but as a reward after they had carried out their murders. This question and all others concerning cannabis, is complicated by the fact that the term cannabis in the past has been used to describe quite different concoctions of substances, taken in varying strengths at varying intervals by different groups of people in quite different socio-cultural conditions (see Section 5.3). Not unnaturally, therefore, reports about the effects of cannabis coming from different sources varied a great deal. However, a sober, rational appraisal has recently come from a WHO Scientific Group Report (1971) [16].

Three types of argument have in the past been used with respect to the connection between cannabis and crime. These are (a) that loss of control during cannabis intoxication might result in impulsive and violent behaviour, (b) that lethargy due to cannabis may affect the earning capacity and lead to petty thieving, and (c) that persons predisposed to criminality may obtain sufficient 'Dutch courage' from cannabis to commit antisocial acts. Clearly a great deal of research in this field is required, a task which should be made easier and more revealing as future research will be able to use active principles of known chemical content (see Section 5.3).

Meanwhile the WHO Report concludes that at present perhaps a suitable method of assessing the contribution made by cannabis to crime and violence, is by a comparison with alcohol. On this basis, most authors regard alcohol to be much more closely associated with aggression and violence than is cannabis – a conclusion with which the author would fully concur.

Traffic accidents [11]
Recent studies have shown that alcoholics contribute much more than their fair share to traffic accidents, in particular to the more serious and fatal ones. Of 200 male alcoholics, among whom 60 % were car drivers, one quarter admitted in answer to a questionnaire to having got into trouble in the past because of drunken driving, i.e. every third male and every second female car driver respectively. Not until an average of 39 years were these men first seen by a doctor for some other manifestation of alcoholism, and not until an age of 41 did they admit to themselves that they were indeed alcoholics. It became evident that the better one got to know an alcoholic or his relatives, the less likely was one to find an alcoholic car driver who had not been driving regularly for several years in a state where his performance must have been seriously impaired by heavy drinking. Minor scrapes and accidents were very common, and such drivers often admitted to having taken appalling or fantastic risks for years, or to having driven in a state of alcoholic blackout [43].

The alcoholic car driver, therefore, must be considered a menace on the road particularly since he usually starts his alcoholic-impaired driving very early in his alcoholic career. In our view, recurrent driving whilst in an alcoholic-impaired state must be regarded in basically non-psychopathic personalities as a common and important prodromal symptom of alcoholism [11, 43]. Alcoholic-impaired car driving is of course a problem of alcohol as well as a problem of alcoholism, the latter because many serious and fatal accidents occur in car drivers with relatively high blood alcohol values such as are likely to be achieved in the main by alcoholics and not by 'casual roisterers'. However even fairly low amounts of alcohol have also been shown to affect judgment and driving performance. The British legal limit of 80 mg of alcohol per 100 ml of blood is higher than the limits of certain countries, lower than those of others. According to Dr J. D. Havard [44] who has taken a special interest in this subject for many years, the probability of being involved in an accident was, at a blood level of 80 mg per 100 ml, increased by a factor of approximately five.

So far little research has been carried out on the effect on driving of drugs other than alcohol. A review published in 1970 has estimated that between two-thirds and one-half of the general population in technically developed countries at least once a year drive after taking psychotropic drugs. Seven per cent of these drivers take alcohol as well as drugs.

In a recent review of the problem, Havard [45] refers to possible dangers arising from the unpredictable and possibly marked changes in behaviour and mood brought about by stimulant drugs, such as amphetamines, phenmetrazines and methylphenidates. An example of this is over-confidence possibly leading to unnecessary risk taking, followed by fatigue when the effect begins to wear off. Psychomotor and perceptual skills are impaired even by therapeutic doses of barbiturates. The evidence on the effect of tranquillisers which may reduce attention and wakefulness and lead, in larger doses, to drowsiness is conflicting. In trials, carried out with police drivers in Basle, Kielholz, Goldberg and co-workers found no significant impairment of driving performance from the use of relatively small doses of meprobamate (400 mg) and chlordiazepoxide (10 mg). In contrast, there was marked impairment from alcohol use [46]. There is little evidence of opiate users causing traffic accidents possibly because such addicts are unlikely to drive. It might be interesting however, to inquire about the effects of such drugs in car driving, by professional addicts. There is no evidence of increased risk of accident involvement from taking commercial preparations of the minor analgesics such as salicylates. The depressant side effects and unpredictable effect of antihistamines could be dangerous for car drivers, as could be the drugs likely to alter perception, such as cannabis, LSD, STP, etc. Heavy goods vehicle and public service drivers are warned not to drive at all whilst they are on medication with barbiturates, tranquillisers, stimulants, thymoleptics, antihistamines, hypotensives, and hypoglycaemic agents. As regards the use by long distance drivers of amphetamines in order to combat fatigue, the BMA Working Party on Amphetamines in 1968 came out strongly against this dangerous practice [47].

Many young drug abusers when closely questioned by the author about their driving exploits whilst on drugs have spoken freely of risks they took when in a drug-affected state (in the main due to amphetamines but occasionally also to cannabis). They claimed that in a drug-free state they would never have dreamed of driving in such a reckless and irresponsible fashion. Often the risks were increased because in a drugged condition some such youngsters may steal cars with which they may be unfamiliar. In the case of cannabis, a number referred to problems arising out of the perceptual distortion of sense of time and distance. I have also known cases where a combination of even moderate amounts of alcohol and other drugs has led to hazardous situations on the road.

Measures such as the introduction of the legal blood alcohol limit, and of the 'breathalyser' for detecting alcohol, have probably greatly contributed to the lessening of the dangerous impact of alcohol-impaired driving. Matters as regards drugs in this respect are much more difficult, because only certain types of drugs can be readily detected in the urine (opiates, amphetamines, sedative–hypnotics) and even these cannot be quantitatively determined as can alcohol. No reliable method exists as yet for the detection of cannabis. The Road Safety Act of 1967, which authorised the use of breath tests for proof of consumption of alcohol, resulted from a BMA Report in 1965 on 'The Drinking Driver'. Last year the BMA convened a Working Party to prepare some notes which might be of help in dealing with the problems caused by the drug taking driver.

Financial cost to the community
Though outweighed in importance by the vast amount of human misery and waste of human lives brought about by alcoholism and other forms of drug dependence, the economic loss to the community must not be forgotten. This includes such items as the upkeep of the unemployed or sick, alcoholic and drug abuser and (mainly in the case of alcoholics) their families. Also involved are maintenance costs in hospitals or prisons, the loss due to the lowering of industrial efficiency, the cost of accidents and, in the case of notified drug addicts, the supply (often over many years) of expensive drugs by the Treatment Centres etc. In the USA it has been estimated that excessive drinking costs the community well over a billion dollars each year.

3.5 MORBIDITY AND MORTALITY

Risks to health in alcoholism and drug abuse
Brief reference has already been made to the physical complications of alcoholism. Chiefly affected are the gastro-intestinal tract and the nervous system. To what extent such complications are due directly to the toxic action of alcohol itself and to what extent they are 'deficiency

diseases' following the neglect of nutrition, defective absorption etc., is not yet clear.

It is interesting to note that at present the pendulum has swung back towards the notion that the toxic action of alcohol contributes greatly to the development of alcoholic cirrhosis of the liver. In recent years this has been held to be a consequence of protein deficiency. Incidentally, the common liver affection in alcoholics is the reversible fatty infiltration, perhaps occurring in about 80% of alcoholics, not the much rarer, irreversible liver cirrhosis (occurring in about 8% of alcoholics). However, the relative contribution of alcoholism to liver cirrhosis cases varies greatly in different countries, being considerably higher, for example, in France (over 90%) than in the UK (about one third) [48]. The most common alcoholic affection of the nervous system is polyneuropathy, occurring in roughly 20% of alcoholics. More rarely affected are the cardiovascular system (e.g. alcoholic cardiomyopathy) and the blood (e.g. anaemia, leucopenia, which is perhaps responsible for the lack of resistance to intercurrent affections, and thrombocytopenia, which may contribute to the tendency to bleed readily).

A recent Australian survey [49] on the frequency of physical diseases in alcoholism among 1000 patients (825 men, 175 women) seen between 1964 and 1969, showed the commonest acute complications to be acute alcoholic liver disease (25·1%), peripheral neuropathy (19%), hypertension (16·9%) and alcoholic gastritis (13·3%). The commonest chronic diseases were chronic bronchitis (17·3%), cirrhosis (9·8%), chronic brain syndrome (8·5%), epilepsy (7·5%) and peptic ulcer disease (7·2%). Major traumatic injuries, mainly resulting from road traffic accidents, had occurred at some time in 11·6% of the patients.

A recent Canadian study investigated the causes of death among 738 Canadian patients out of a total of 6500 treated at the Toronto Clinic of the Addiction Research Foundation between 1951 and 1963 [50]. The Canadian investigators found a greatly increased risk from alcoholism (or, from the life style of alcoholics) in cancers of the upper digestive and respiratory organs, pneumonia, cirrhosis of the liver, heart diseases, ulcers, accidents, suicides and homicides. In theory, the deaths caused by cancer of the lung, pharynx, larynx, and oesophagus occurring in alcoholics could have been ascribed to heavy cigarette smoking, as alcoholics are usually heavy smokers. However, the investigators concluded that it was the excessive drinking that effected the development of cancers in pharynx, larynx, and oesophagus. Suicide was found to be six times higher than normal, attributed by the authors to predisposing social and personality factors, social isolation, and alcohol-induced depressive states. Alcoholics are also very vulnerable to accidents, arising from poisoning, falls and fires and to traffic accidents.

Of great interest is the point made by the authors, W. Schmidt and J. de Lint that, 'The characteristics of alcoholics – their drinking behaviour, smoking habits, emotional state and life style – are uniquely expressed in their mode of dying' [50]. Acute effects of alcohol are seen in poisoning, falls, fires, pneumonia, and probably suicide. The chronic effects are seen in cancers, cirrhosis and heart disease. Smoking of cigarettes added to the risk of accidents such as fires, pneumonia, cancer and heart trouble. Moreover, malnutrition, personal neglect and poor living conditions may add to the hazards possibly contributing to deaths, e.g. from pneumonia, accidents and liver cirrhosis.

As regards the relationship between alcoholism and misuse and dependence on other drugs, it is again of interest to point out how the common association between heavy drinking and heavy cigarette smoking and the not unusual association between abuse of alcohol and drugs, in particular barbiturates, greatly adds to the risks of health and life of alcoholics. For example, whilst in a depressed and befuddled state from alcohol intoxication and looking for a good night's rest, it is all too easy to take a handful of barbiturate tablets when they are at hand anyway – if the drinker is also a habitual barbiturate misuser – and then to forget that one has taken them already and to repeat the performance (automatism). Likewise it happens all too commonly that alcoholics who smoke in bed whilst in a befuddled state fall asleep and the cigarette then drops onto the bedclothes.

How many of such risks to health and life apply not only to alcoholics but also to people dependent on 'other drugs'? It is true that a number of the illnesses common to alcoholics are much less common in drug addicts. Also, these illnesses, such as cancer, ulcers, heart disease* and liver cirrhosis, are often not a direct consequence (pharmacologically) of their drug abuse. Nevertheless, V. Marks and Chapple [52] found a relatively high incidence of liver function abnormalities (80%) in i.v. 'H-C' abusers. The risks arising out of all kinds of accidents – accidental or intentional overdosage, falls, fires – and from intercurrent infections (such as pneumonia) suicide and homicide, seem at least as high in other

---

* Very recently, transient electrocardiographic abnormalities have been described in approximately one-fifth out of 104 young Canadian poly-drug abusers [51]. These findings have as yet not been confirmed elsewhere

forms of drug dependence as in alcoholism. Indeed, the hazards arising out of life style factors such as malnutrition, personal neglect and exposure to poor living conditions are probably higher in young drug abusers, who often come from a poor, underprivileged background, or have turned their back on their family and ordinary society.

Patterns of drug transfer
Alcohol and other drugs may often be taken by an individual at the same time. For example, in England over recent years, many youngsters have combined drinking with the consumption of the highly psychological and physical dependence-producing hypnotic mandrax containing the non-barbiturate methaqualone. In this way, they achieve a state of intoxication more rapidly and more cheaply. The 1966 WHO Expert Committee [5], which recommended the combining of services for alcoholics and other drug addicts, listed three general patterns of drug transfer. These were:

(a) transfer from one drug to another in the same group with a particular type of dependence, e.g. from opium to morphine or heroin. More common in England nowadays is the shift from heroin to methadone, brought about by the Treatment Centres prescribing policy,

(b) transfer from one drug to a closely related one, e.g. the all too familiar switch from alcohol to barbiturates, and finally

(c) transfer from one type of drug to another of substantially quite a different kind, e.g. transfer from barbiturates to amphetamines.

In recent years London drug abusers have been switching around quite indiscriminately between drugs that are quite different from each other and often combine them. David Archibald refers also to North American reports of the use of quite different drugs in sequence. For example, the use of barbiturates for a limited period, followed by alcohol for a few days, then by amphetamines, marihuana, LSD etc. [53]. At the present time (1973) some American methadone maintenance programmes find that one-third or more of their patients receiving methadone have also become excessive drinkers or alcoholics.

In the author's experience over a period of 20 years, the use by the same individual of similar or dissimilar drugs at the same time or at different periods, has been quite common. For example, at Warlingham Park Hospital in the 1950s it was found that as many as 30% of (mainly middle-aged) alcoholics had also at times prior to admission taken other drugs to excess. These were mainly barbiturates, but also taken were amphetamines, paraldehyde etc. and at a somewhat later stage, the stimulant phenmetrazine, sometimes combined with the sedatives carbromal or methylpentynol [54]. Another quite different sample is that of several hundreds of young drug-dependent men, in their late teens or early twenties, observed over the past ten years in a London prison. Here the most common pattern was that having started on alcohol and cigarettes in their early teens, this was followed shortly afterwards by the various types of soft drugs and often somewhat later by hard drugs. After starting on drugs, they had as a rule practically given up alcohol, though not cigarettes, because they found drugs much better for a variety of reasons.

According to a Chinese tradition, drinking, along with womanising, gambling and narcotics, is one of the four disasters [55]. The present chapter has touched on certain relationships between all of them, but it would seem that in present-day Western society excessive drinking may be the worst of these 'disasters'. Like the other socially and legally approved Western tranquilliser, tobacco, alcohol is responsible for a much greater hazard to health and life than all other dependence-producing drugs. However, it is the latter which steal the limelight through their presentation by the mass-media. The mass-media has a grave responsibility. A recent report of the Ontario Addiction Research Foundation [56] has shown that youngsters rate the news media as most influential sources of information – above family, friends, church, and school, and far above their own experiences. Twenty-three million, i.e. more than one in two adults in the UK smoke tobacco and an even higher proportion – three in four – take alcoholic drinks. Suggesting that addiction to tobacco, alcohol and drugs should be regarded as one whole problem, a 1971 report on 'Drink, Drugs and the Family' by the National Society for the Prevention of Cruelty to Children [57] drew up a ranking list of drugs according to their order of danger. Tobacco topped the list followed by alcohol and cocaine. Cigarette smoking has been blamed for 50 000 deaths per year in the UK. Alcohol has been estimated to enslave 300 000–400 000 people, with the number probably increasing [11]. This is indicated by a gradual but steady rise of most of the indirect indices, such as drunkenness offences, offences for driving under the unfluence, deaths from alcohol cirrhosis and alcoholism [29] and admission rates to psychiatric hospitals. Alcoholics apart, a much greater number of people occasionally or habitually drink 'heavily'. The overall cost, therefore, caused by over-indulgence in alcohol, in terms of human suffering and health and in the cost to the community must be enormous. Whatever reason there may have been in the past for the relative neglect by the mass-media of the two drugs, which although legal, cause much more danger to health and life than the more newsworthy illicit drug abuse, one must hope that in future these problems will receive the coverage which their importance and their dangers deserve.

In summary, it is clear that drugs and alcohol share risks to the individual (due to constant preoccupation with the drug to the exclusion of other vital interests, or due directly to the effects of the drug) and to society. However, through their vastly greater numbers, alcoholics are responsible for much greater social damage than addicts to other drugs.

3.6 YOUNG ALCOHOLICS [58]

Among the young nowadays there is a more insistent demand for involvement and a tendency towards direct action. This springs to a large extent from disillusionment with, and a more critical awareness of, the shortcomings of the Establishment. However, disillusion and disenchantment with the ideas and the ways of their elders by no means immunises the young against repeating their elders' follies and maladaptive behaviour.

Drinking patterns among the young

What are the differences between the drinking patterns of normal adolescents and those who become dependent at an early age? Basically, 'normals' do not drink for 'kicks'. They drink as an aid to social acceptance. For example, in a small study among nurses in a London general hospital, we heard such comments as, 'I do not like it at all but if you are out with a boy who asks you to have a drink, you do not want to look a right nut and say orange juice; I drink gin even if I do nearly choke,' or, 'When you are at school you tend to follow the crowd and you drink even if you feel that it nearly kills you'. Another girl said, 'It was my father who offered me my first drink and I felt proud and grown up'. According to Menzies, 'The difficulty as regards alcohol and relations with the opposite sex could be expressed as the inability to say 'no'. At this age to be different from others is to be alone and lonely, and it is clear that many boys and girls would accept alcohol rather than to be the odd one out' [59].

Amongst young alcoholics, on the other hand, there is definite evidence that the alcohol was used at a very early stage for the effect it gave and sometimes it was taken in solitude. A young male alcoholic, aged 25, stated, 'Drink has been a problem since I was nineteen. I would drink at night after work until I was on the floor and quickly built up to the point where I was drinking $1\frac{1}{2}$ bottles of spirits on each occasion, two or three times a week.' It is more the rule rather than the exception that young alcoholics will ascribe their early heavy drinking to a need for warmth, freedom from worry, a need to forget or to sleep. It would seem that drinking behaviour amongst young people largely depends on the way in which they view their own situation. If they look upon themselves as teenagers, then drinking is not a part of their everyday life although they may drink on occasions to relieve their feelings of hostility towards adults (parents). On the other hand, if they view themselves as adults, then drinking is accepted as a normal social function. An adolescent does not have to invent the idea of drinking, he learns it whilst growing up in a society in which most adults drink [60]. Often the development of abnormal drinking patterns seems to be an attempt at a short cut to an adult role, supplying a false feeling of omnipotence to the disturbed personality acting out his inadequacy.

Aetiology of adolescent alcoholism
Certain factors deemed to be significant in the histories of our young alcoholics:
  (a) Many show early emotional deprivation and have commonly experienced both physical and psychological trauma in childhood.
  (b) There is often evidence of heavy drinking by one parent and dominance by the other.
  (c) Unsatisfactory sexual adjustment.
  (d) Over-identification with a parent of the opposite sex.
  (e) Overcompensation for feelings of inadequacy by antisocial behaviour and withdrawal from society.
  (f) Difficulty in accepting an adult role with a confused attitude to their own children. They are often unable to relate to their children responsibly.
As regards the personality characteristics of young alcoholics, it would seem that by and large young alcoholics, although naturally a heterogeneous group comprising many types of personalities who may have started drinking for a variety of psychological and social reasons,

are emotionally much more disturbed than the hypothetical average adult alcoholic. Often they seem to have been more insecure from the beginning, not infrequently emotionally deprived, and to have started drinking in order to reduce anxiety, tension, feelings of inadequacy, etc. Initially, alcohol may have been helpful by providing the missing feelings of adequacy and acceptability. However, as dependence on alcohol develops, which happens very rapidly in these youngsters, the alcohol releases (a) hostility directed against themselves (suicide attempts) or others, (b) a need for self-punishment or revenge on others and (c) an explosion of anger directed against themselves or others. In this situation, these young alcoholics are often unable to cope.

However, the above study concerns young alcoholics who were observed six to ten years ago. Meanwhile heavy drinking among younger age groups has become increasingly common. Under such circumstances it could perhaps be expected that a higher proportion of young alcoholics in the future may show less evidence of pre-alcoholic personality disturbance, than the sample described in the foregoing paragraph. In addition, because of the wider acceptance of heavy social drinking among the young as the norm, 'average' youngsters may become exposed to the risk of becoming alcoholics, due to the combination of such social factors and the pharmacological action of alcohol itself.

REFERENCES

1. Jellinek, E. M. (1960). *The Disease Concept of Alcoholism* (New Haven, Conn.: Hillhouse Press).
2. Glatt, M. M. (1967). *WHO Chronicle*, **21,** 293.
3. Glatt, M. M. and Leong Hon Koon (1961). *Psychiat. Quart.*, **35,** 1.
4. Glatt, M. M. (1970). *A World Dialogue on Alcohol and Drug Dependence*, **311** (E. Whitney, editor) (Beacon Press)
5. WHO Expert Committee on Mental Health (1967). *WHO Tech. Rep. Ser.*, **363.**
6. Pittman, D. J. (1967). *Brit. J. Addict.*, **22,** 337.
7. WHO Alcoholism Subcommittee (1952). *WHO Tech. Rep. Ser.*, **48.**
8. WHO Expert Committee (1954). *WHO Tech. Rep. Ser.*, **84.**
9. WHO Expert Committee (1955). *ibid.*, **94.**
10. Laurence, D. R. (1966). *Clinical Pharmacology*, 3rd ed. (London: Churchill).

92 A guide to addiction and its treatment

11. Glatt, M. M. (1972). *The Alcoholic and the Help He Needs*, 2nd ed. (London: Priory Press).
12. Salzman, L. (1972). *Psychiatry in Medicine*, **3**, 29.
13. Jellinek, E. M. (1952). *WHO Tech. Rep. Ser.*, **48**.
14. Glatt, M. M. (1961). *Acta Psychiat.*, **37** (1), 88.
15. Carlini, E. A. *et al.* (1972). *Cannabis and its Derivatives*, 154 (W. D. M. Paton and J. Crown, editors) (London: Oxford Univ. Press).
16. WHO Working Party on Cannabis (1971). *WHO Tech. Rep. Ser.*, **418**.
17. Wikler, A. (1972). *2nd Int. Symp. Drug Abuse, Jerusalem* (Abstracts), 27.
18. Glatt, M. M. (1973). *1st Int. Med. Conf. Alcoholism, London*.
19. Wilkins, L. (1965). *Narcotics*, 140 (D. Wilner and G. Kassebaum, editors) (New York: McGraw-Hill).
20. Young, J. (1971). *The Drugtakers* (London: McGibbon and Kee).
21. Keller, M. (1972). *Brit. J. Addict.*, **67**, 153.
22. Merry, J. (1966). *Lancet*, **i**, 1257.
23. Interdepartmental Committee on Drug Addiction (1961). *1st Report* (London: H.M.S.O.).
24. Glatt, M. M., Pittman, D. J., Gillespie, D. G. and Hills, D. R. (1969). *The Drug Scene in Great Britain*, Revised Reprint (London: Edward Arnold).
25. Walton, K. J. (1968). *Brit. J. Psychiat.*, **117**, 761.
26. Cameron, D. (1971). *WHO Tech. Rep. Ser.*, **448**, 34.
27. Glatt, M. M. (1967). *Brit. J. Addict.*, **62**, 35.
28. Gomersall, J. (1972). *Drugs and Society*, 12 (May).
29. Zacune, J. and Hensman, C. (1971). *Drugs, Alcohol and Tobacco in Britain*, 89 (London: Heinemann Books).
30. Hewetson, J. and Ollendorf, R. (1964). *Brit. J. Addict.*, **60**, 110.
31. *Brit. Med. J.* (1972) (Annot.) **2**, 63.
32. Trocchi, A. (1966). *Cain's Book*, 95 (London: Calder and Boyars, Jupiter Books).
33. Trico, H. M. and Roman, P. M. (1972). *Spirits and Demons at Work: Alcohol and Other Drugs on the Job* (N.Y. State School Indust. and Labour Relations: Cornell Univ.).
34. Glatt, M. M. and Whiteley, J. S. (1956). *Mschr. Psychiat. Neurol.*, **132**, 1.
35. Edwards, G. *et al.* (1972). *Psychol. Med.*, **1** (5), 388.
36. Glatt, M. M. (1962). *Bull. Narcot.*, **14** (2), 19.
37. James, P. I. (1969). Quoted from *The Drug Scene in Great Britain*,

by M. M. Glatt *et al.* 93 (revised edition) (London: Edward Arnold).
38. Camps, F. E. (1968). *Int. Conf. Drug Dependence*, Optat, Quebeck.
39. Glatt, M. M. (1968). *Gradwohl's Legal Medicine*, 2nd ed., 584 (F. E. Camps, editor) (Bristol: John Wright and Sons).
40. Hawks, D. V. (1970). *Bull. Narcot.*, **22** (3), 15.
41. James, I. P. (1969). *Brit. J. Criminol.*, **9**, 108.
42. Glatt, M. M. (1969). *Brit. J. Addict.*, **67**, 99.
43. Glatt, M. M. (1964). Lancet **i**, 16,1.
44. Havard, J. D. (1972). *Drugs and Society* (March).
45. Havard, J. D. *Medical Aspects of Fitness to Drive*, 42 (A. Raffle, editor (London: Medical Commission on Accident Prevention).
46. Kielholz, P., Goldberg, L. *et al.* (1967). *Dtsch. Med. Wschr.*, **92**, 525.
47. Brit. Med. Assoc. Working Party on Amphetamines (1970). *Brit. Med. J.* (Suppl.), **3**, 48.
48. Stone, W. D. (1973). *Pract.*, **210**, 612.
49. Wilkinson, P., Kornaczewski, A., Rankin, J. G. and Santamaria, J. N. (1971). *Med. J. Australia*, **1**, 1217.
50. Schmidt, W. and De Lint, J. (1972). *Quart. J. Study of Alcoholism*, **33**, 171.
51. Vogelsang, A. (1973). *Lancet*, **i**, 1248.
52. Marks, V. and Chapple, P. A. L. (1967). *Brit. J. Addict*, **62**, 189.
53. Archibald, H. D. (1970). *A World Dialogue on Alcohol and Drug Dependence*, 297 (E. D. Whitney, editor) (Boston: Beacon Press).
54. Glatt, M. M. (1959). *Lancet*, **i**, 887.
55. Singer, K. (1972). *Brit. J. Addict.*, **67**, 3.
56. *Addictions* (Summer 1972).
57. *Drugs and Society* (Nov. 1971) 2.
58. Glatt, M. M. and Hills, D. R. (1968). *Brit. J. Addict.*, **63**, 183.
59. Quoted from Ref. 58.
60. Maddox, G. L. and McCall, B. C. (1964). *Drinking among Teenagers* (New Brunswick, N.J.: Rutgers Centre of Alcohol Studies).
61. Eddy, N. B. *et al.* (1965). *Bull. WHO*, **32**, 721.

Part 4

RELATED TYPES OF DEPENDENCE

Although not directly included in our brief, it may be of some interest to take a look at the subjects which are more or less closely related to drug dependence.

4.1 TOBACCO*

The preoccupation of the general public – to a certain extent aided and abetted by the mass-media – with the problem of young narcotic abusers whose known numbers throughout the past decade have never exceeded 3000, has helped to conceal the sobering fact that the two drugs causing most social, physical and mental damage in contemporary society are those two most beloved by adults, legitimate in the eyes of the law and sanctioned and encouraged by tradition and custom. More than half the adult population in Britain are smokers, consuming between them approximately 350 million cigarettes per day.

Hazards to health and life

As in the case of alcohol and most other drugs (barbiturates being the main exception) smoking is relatively less common among women (two-fifths of whom are smokers) than among men (7 in 10 men smoke). Giving up smoking might raise the average life expectancy for men by two years, as indicated by the Medical Officer of the Department of Health and Social Security in his 1971 Annual Report. That few men (apart from doctors) do give up smoking, indicates the strength of the psychic (and probably also physical) dependence on the drug, as now-

* Certain aspects of tobacco (nicotine) dependence were discussed in Part 2 and Part 3

adays nearly everyone knows of its hazards to health and life. According to the Report, cigarette smoking is the single largest avoidable cause of death in Britain at the present time, the three main causes of such deaths being lung cancer, bronchitis and coronary heart disease. Smoking may be responsible for as many as 9 out of 10 lung cancer deaths, 3 out of 4 bronchitic deaths, and 1 in 4 deaths due to heart attacks. Other reports have indicated that continued smoking reduces the life span of a young man by an average of 4 years; and by 7 years if he smokes more than 40 cigarettes per day [1]. Such figures amply explain the great importance given to the subject by the Royal College of Physicians, whose Second Report (1971) estimates the number of premature deaths a year caused by cigarette smoking in men aged 35 to 64 as between 20 000 and 24 000 [2].

Parallel to the mortality there is of course the greatly increased morbidity risk in heavy smokers, seeing that some of the illnesses involved are chronic and often very disabling (e.g. chronic bronchitis). Harm to the family is naturally not as severe as in the case of alcoholics, although other family members may find the continual smoking irritating and resent it. However, there seems to be an almost double chance of women smokers' pregnancies terminating in spontaneous abortion, stillbirth or neonatal death [1]. Whilst other people's smoking has not been found to be dangerous to healthy non-smokers, it may distress such individuals who are allergic or suffer from heart or lung disorders. The carbon-monoxide level produced by smoking in rooms that are overcrowded and ill-ventilated or in enclosed spaces can reach a level (50 p.p.m. or more) surpassing that permitted in industry [3].

Mortality and morbidity apart, smoking imposes an enormous economic strain on the community. The number of working days lost annually through illness directly attributable to smoking has been estimated to be more than 20 times the number lost through industrial disputes [1]; the number of hospital beds occupied each day by people needing hospitalisation solely because of their smoking has been estimated as between 5000 and 8000.

Nicotine dependence

Regarding the causation of smoking (see Part 2), a number of factors seem to be involved, in the main probably psychological and social ones. Social factors are probably most important in initiating the habit. Once the process has started, pharmacological factors probably help to maintain it later on. Russell [4] has described physical withdrawal symptoms when smoking is stopped which include sleep disturbances, changes in brain wave patterns, a fall in pulse rate and blood pressure and impaired driving. Nicotine can thus apparently lead to physical dependence as well as to psychic dependence, the latter manifested by such symptoms as depression, anxiety, tension and craving for cigarettes, following sudden withdrawal. Such symptoms are characteristically relieved – as in the alcoholic's hangover – by a 'hair of the dog', so that pharmacological reinforcement helps to maintain the habit. Naturally there is also strong social reinforcement arising from the widespread social habit of smoking. As is the case with alcohol many youngsters seem to start to smoke because they want to feel adult, i.e. to behave like their parents, whereas starting other drugs clearly denotes a turning away from the parental habits.

The development of dependence in the case of cigarette smoking proceeds much more quickly than in the case of alcohol and most other drugs. It has been stated that the adolescent who has smoked twice has a 70% chance of smoking for the rest of his life [5]. Intensity of dependence on smoking in general seems strong: 3 out of 4 smokers wish to or have tried in the past to give up cigarettes but less than 1 in 4 ever succeed [1]. Therefore, it is important to try to induce the young not to take up the habit in the first place, by health education that must start in school; many youngsters have taken up the habit by the time they leave school. In order to succeed, such health education should be less concerned with horror stories but rather emphasise the advantages arising out of non-smoking [5]. It should be non-smoking which is regarded as normal practice and not, as unfortunately is still the case today, smoking. As in the case of other forms of drug dependence it seems to be less difficult to give up smoking altogether than to reduce the amount. Some little progress has in fact been made since the 1971 publication of the Royal College of Physicians, as there has been a slight reduction in cigarette consumption in this country.

Alcoholism and excessive smoking

As regards the connection between excessive smoking and alcoholism, it would seem that the great majority of alcoholics are heavy smokers, and that often, whilst under inpatient treatment for alcoholism their cigarette consumption may go up even further. On the other hand, a study carried out in the late 1950s by the present author on a sample of 100 alcoholic ex-patients of Warlingham Park Hospital – whose drinking habits had been greatly improved – showed that there was no consistent smoking pattern involved: one-third smoked less than before, one-third smoked more than before and one-third about the same as before. On the other hand, it is well known that smokers who give up the habit have to be careful not to start eating too much. To some extent this corresponds to the great appetite alcoholics often develop as soon as they give up drinking. This may last for a short period only, though quite a few alcoholics after giving up alcohol seem to be left with a strong desire to eat sweets (which previously they may have abhorred) and often for non-alcoholic drinks such as tea, coffee etc.

It might also be of interest to note that in our experience the great majority of young drug abusers had started to take alcohol and smoke cigarettes before first experimenting with other drugs. As a rule, once they began to take other drugs they practically cut out drinking, except on special occasions, but persisted in often very heavy smoking of cigarettes.

'Action on Smoking and Health'

Much valuable, up-to-date information has just been published [3] by an Expert Group of the organisation Action on Smoking and Health. ASH was set up by the Royal College of Physicians following its report on 'Smoking and Health Now' in 1971, in order to coordinate and stimulate voluntary efforts in this field. The new report of this expert group confirms (despite certain contrary reports from Switzerland) that the smoking of pipes and cigars is much less dangerous than smoking cigarettes, although with pipe and cigar smokers, too, the risk of developing cancer of the mouth, throat, oesophagus and lung is higher than in non-smokers. However, the increased risk of developing lung cancer is much less for long-standing pipe and/or cigar smokers than for cigarette smokers. To give up smoking is the only way in which tobacco smokers can avoid the danger to their health. However, those cigarette smokers who find it impossible to give up the habit, can reduce the risks if they switch over to pipe or cigar, taking care to smoke less tobacco and not to inhale. Those heavy pipe or cigar smokers who smoke 10 or more cigars or 20 or more pipes daily and inhale, take on a similar risk to life as light smokers of cigarettes.

The new report also suggests important public health measures.

(a) Higher priority should be given in public places to the right to be free from smoke than to the right to smoke, with certain areas to be set aside for smokers.

(b) Before starting to smoke at work or at meetings, smokers should ascertain whether their habit would upset non-smokers.

(c) Ample provision should always be made at home, in public transport, at work, etc. enabling non-smokers 'to breath air free from pollution by tobacco smoke' [3].

4.2 COMPULSIVE OVEREATING*

'Moral attitudes die hard in medicine' read the opening sentence of a recent editorial in a medical magazine [6]. Health education is the doctor's concern and, 'It is part of the doctor's job to inform patients of the dangers of overeating or excessive drinking, to counsel against smoking, and spell out the risks of unwanted pregnancy and venereal disease. . . . (But) doctors are not there to read moral lectures. . . . (Nevertheless) there is no question that patients suffering from diseases of indulgence . . . are conscious of attitudes of censure when attending for treatment.' Thus embarrassment and fear of medical disapproval may often inhibit girls from going to a doctor or a family planning clinic for contraceptive advice.

In spite of some progress, this statement often also applies to the conditions discussed in this book. For example, rightly or wrongly one is often told, when alcoholics or their families apply for help and one advises them, first to go to their family doctor, that this was useless as he would just adopt a moralistic attitude, tell them to use will power and cut down on their overindulgent habits. Similarly, overeating has in the past attracted much moral and social censure. 'For a long time . . . the compulsion of overeating was considered the consequence of weakness, sinfulness, or inadequate self-control, rather than a medical condition', writes Dr L. Salzman. 'Like drug or alcohol addicts, severe cases of excessive eaters are compulsively driven to eat, not through taste or hunger – for they often stuff and gorge without any enjoyment to the point of illness – but by inner drives that they can neither understand nor control' [7]. Of course, not all overeaters or grossly obese persons are compulsive eaters or food addicts. Many factors, often working in interaction, may be responsible, such as physiological (metabolic or, rarely, genetic), socio-cultural and psychological ones. Malnutrition, though less prevalent nowadays than in former times, is unfortunately still all too common in many parts of the world. A

* Certain aspects of compulsive overeating were discussed in Part 2 and Part 3.

well-fed, well-nourished state has often been regarded as representing health, happiness and security.

Risks to health
It is probably only in fairly recent years that increasing attention has been given to the risks accompanying overeating (i.e. ingestion of more calories than physiologically required) and obesity, and the latter is now considered probably the most common nutritional disorder in Great Britain. American insurance statistics have indicated that men who are overweight by 20% or more for their age and height have a 33% greater probability of mortality than men of normal weight. To be overweight by 10% has been said to constitute a greater health risk than smoking 25 cigarettes per day [8]. Among the physical complications ascribed to obesity are those affecting the cardiovascular, renal, respiratory, alimentary and skeletal system. They include disorders such as atheroma, hypertension, coronary thrombosis, chronic bronchitis, osteoarthritis, etc. Metabolic disorders include diabetes mellitus, chronic lopaemia, raised blood cholesterol etc.

Thus as regards physical complications excessive eating may have at least as many serious consequences as alcoholism and drug dependence. As to psychological and socio-cultural consequences, obesity is less destructive than alcohol and drug dependence but it nevertheless seriously affects and undermines the psychological well-being of the sufferer, his domestic and interpersonal relationships, and his performance at work. He or she may feel unattractive and repulsive and the butt of ridicule, may become miserable and depressed, and may tend to withdraw increasingly from social contacts, becoming more and more isolated and lonely. This reduction of physical activity and mobility may lead to impaired work performance. Fortunately as in the case of habitual smoking there are none of the antisocial activities which so often follow in the wake of dependence of alcohol, other drugs, or gambling.

Relief eating
By looking at the Chart of Alcohol Dependence (Figure 1, in Appendix), it is possible to compare the case of the compulsive eater or food addict with that of the alcoholic. (The food addict differs from the social overeater who suffers from simple obesity). Thus a predisposed, inadequate or anxious personality, may drive him to complement his ordinary food intake (and the 'feasting' encouraged on socio-cultural

or festive occasions), by occasional relief eating when feeling in need of a comforter during moods of depression, tension, or when feeling lonely or bored. The choice of food rather than, say, alcohol may perhaps be more common when such an individual belongs to a community where for cultural or religious reasons the consumption of alcoholic drink may be frowned upon. Occasional relief eating may gradually lead to eating whenever such an individual finds himself under mental strain and stress and when the occasion presents itself – a process of conditioning helping to bring about such development. Gradually he eats more and more frequently but, like the alcoholic, the overeater is good at rationalising and denying to himself the full extent of his food intake. He (or she) may nevertheless feel guilty and avoid overeating in front of wife, husband or children, often storing his food supplies in places unknown to the family, and making sure to gulp food in short 'eating binges' when on his own. Sometimes he may try to make himself vomit immediately after such a 'binge' in order to avoid excessive weight again. Thus the family is often unaware of the degree of overeating, and may be more sympathetic to the eater's theory of a glandular origin of the obesity [7]. The 'eating binge' may increase the guilt feelings, and these, as the eater at this stage cannot see any way out, lead to increased anxiety and tension, requiring relief by further overeating. Promises and resolutions to refrain from excessive eating usually fail again and again, and if dietary restrictions are imposed, such an individual is deprived of his customary means of obtaining relief from anxiety through food intake. Moreover, under these dietary restrictions, the compulsive eater will exhibit psychological-dependence symptoms, such as irritability, tension, anxiety and fatigue (although, at this juncture, one cannot say to what extent withdrawal of foodstuff is directly responsible for symptoms which would parallel those following withdrawal of alcohol, other drugs and tobacco).

Management of compulsive overeating

Personal vanity, fear of physical complications, pressure and pleas by the family may finally encourage the compulsive eater to seek help. However, like the compulsive drinker or drug taker, he may tend to look for 'magical help', such as a pill which may help him to slim in spite of continued overeating rather than having to stick to a diet and psychotherapeutic help. Like alcoholism and drug dependence, the so-called food addiction (food dependence seems to be a more suitable term) is a relapsing disorder. Only too often, rather than refraining from overeating, 'all that such obese individuals lose is the sheet with the carefully calculated diet' [9]. This is analogous in some way to the tendency of alcoholics to forget to take the alcohol-deterrent disulfiram, thereby giving themselves the chance to resume drinking.* Unfortunately, as we shall see later (see Section 5.1), most drugs so popular a few years ago in the treatment of overeating, such as the amphetamines, can themselves lead to dependence, although other, allegedly non-addictive substances have been introduced in their place as adjuncts in the overall management of the problem of overeating.

Since emotional factors often play an important role in the problem of compulsive overeating, a psychological approach may often be required apart from dietary control, encouragement of exercise and pharmacological adjuvants. In Dr Salzman's view [7] compulsive eaters, '... like compulsive drinkers, gamblers, drug-takers and masturbators' have an obsessive − compulsive personality structure, with a '... manifest goal to control everything: (but) the illness consists of a total inability to control (their) addictive behaviour. . . . Some compulsions may be bizarre and unusual while others may be exaggerations of commonplace activities, like eating, drinking or washing'. The compulsive addict continues to take drugs clearly because he gets something from such drugs which he feels do something for him [10]; but as Matussek [11] has pointed out, in a compulsive neurosis, the impulse experienced is more foreign to the personality than that experienced in drug dependence. The compulsive neurotic's act cannot be enjoyed in the same way as the drug addict enjoys his drugs, even though such enjoyment may be marred by guilt feelings and fears of unwanted side- and after-effects. Whereas the compulsive neurotic fights against his obsessions and comfort sessions, the drug addict (though he may have ambivalent feelings about drug taking) fights for his drugs − defending its merits against the therapist who attempts to withdraw the drugs, and playing down the extent of the harmful effect of his drug taking [10]. Therefore by no means everybody would thus share Selzman's view that the majority of addicts have such a pre-addictive personality

---

* An interesting comment on the similarities between alcoholism and compulsive eating was recently given to the author by the wife of an alcoholic who for years had refused to admit that he had a drinking problem. Although his excessive drinking had produced difficulties at home as well as at work, his wife had been able to take it all rather well. Her own craving for food (under stress)—which she indulged in, mainly when by herself and which she felt very guilty about but which she had been unable to overcome—had provided her with an understanding of her alcoholic husband's behaviour and of his problems in admitting it

structure and exhibit the obsessive – compulsive syndrome ('. . . a disorder in which the individual is compelled to behave in certain ways which are beyond his control') even before the outset of their addictive illness. However, many would agree with his proposition that '. . . in the long run, the treatment of obesity must use the same modalities as the treatment of other addictive disorders' [7]. At any rate, largely influenced by the success of the group approach of Alcoholics Anonymous 30 years earlier, techniques based on similar principles and introduced a few years ago have also proved very helpful in the management of compulsive eating (Weight Watchers) and of compulsive gambling (Gamblers Anonymous) – although proving so far, somewhat less effective in the treatment of dependence on other drugs and apparently also of the excessive smoker.

The aetiology of obesity

The last few paragraphs have reviewed certain problems involved in food dependence and have illustrated some similarities and a few dissimilarities between compulsive overeating and alcoholism. Additional comment on this theme is contained in Diagram 1 (see Appendix) which presents a scheme depicting the roles of host, agent and environment in the causation of obesity [12].

As regards the host factor, the search and need of the inadequate, immature, neurotic personality for relief, security and affection should not be overlooked. These needs may lead to attempts to assuage such hunger symbolically by the intake of food. Again, just as alcoholics sometimes substitute other drugs in the place of alcohol, so some alcoholics, when giving up alcohol and trying to maintain abstinence, may occasionally substitute food – in particular sweet foodstuffs – in the place of alcohol (see case history below). Many alcoholics, after giving up alcohol begin to drink large amounts of (usually sweetened) tea or coffee etc. and to eat chocolates and sweets which often they had actually disliked as long as they were practising alcoholics. Such substitution may be partly based on the need to replace the high intake of carbohydrates in the past (in the form of alcohol) by other foodstuffs containing as much carbohydrate, but this is unlikely to be the whole explanation.

In a recent interesting article, G. D. Campbell [13] described the marked rise in sugar consumption over the past 150 years as a consequence of demand as well as of availability. He refers to the 'sugar orgy' of the Pondo cane cutters who eat an enormous amount of raw sugar in a very short space of time; to Charles Darwin's description of two groups of primitive people becoming immediately hooked as soon as they had tasted sugar (tobacco following sugar in immediate popularity); and to the finding that certain mammals (e.g. dogs) may become rapidly addicted to sucrose, whereas others (e.g. cats) do not. He mentions the hypothesis of sugar having a sedative effect, e.g. when sweetened tea is drunk by obese, overworked housewives. This is also reflected in the high sugar intake of smokers. The addictive effect of sugar – as Campbell points out – may consist in the addiction to a sweet taste and not to sucrose itself. (In view of its probably psychological rather than physical origin it would seem preferable to use the term 'dependence producing' rather than 'addictive'). Campbell feels that, 'Sugar probably is in fact addictive but that the addiction may easily be modified by substitutes', especially when the addictive agent is not readily available. But he also stresses (as we have seen so often in questions pertaining to problems of dependence), that the verdict on the question as to whether sugar is really addictive at present must remain that of 'Not Proven'; and quite rightly he points out that, 'The actual dividing line between a liking and an addiction is not easy to delineate'. Here the term should certainly be 'dependence', as there seems little evidence in the case of compulsive eaters of a loss-of-control and of a physical abstinence syndrome (see case history below).

Mention has already been made of the risk that addicts giving up alcohol or tobacco may turn to substitute-gratification by stepping up their food intake. It has also been pointed out that one effect of recent antismoking campaigns has been the increase in the consumption of sweets. The risk of replacing one form of habitual abuse (tobacco) by another (sweet food) reminds one of the danger of one addictive drug being replaced by another more readily available drug when the first one is suddenly prohibited – as has often been demonstrated in the history of drug abuse. Further to the role of the agent in the development of obesity it is obvious that, apart from the quantity of food taken, its type is of crucial importance: it is carbohydrate-containing foodstuffs, such as chocolates, cakes etc., which provide large amounts of calories. Similarly, alcohol contains large amounts of calories. For example, half a pint of bitter contains 90 kcal and a tot of whisky contains 50 kcal [8]. This explains to a large extent why alcoholics, who so often restrict their food intake to alcoholic drinks for weeks or months, may suffer from protein and vitamin deficiency and malnutrition but at the same time may put on weight (quite apart from the oedema which accompanies certain forms of nutritional deficiency).

Finally, to illustrate some of the points made in the foregoing, here is the brief case history of a female compulsive eater, first seen a few years ago for alcoholism and again a few months ago, when she had given up alcohol and developed an eating compulsion:

Case history

Mrs. A.B., a middle-aged divorced, intelligent but neurotic, loss-of-control (gamma) alcoholic, had managed, despite considerable domestic stress, to get over her alcoholic problem, and to abstain from alcohol altogether for a period of several years – largely with the help of Alcoholics Anonymous. She was also somewhat overweight. Fifteen years earlier she had tried to cut down on her food intake by taking phenmetrazine (Preludin), but feeling so good on the prescribed doses of phenmetrazine she had soon started to take this drug by the handful, having managed to obtain it by devious means. Shortly after giving up alcohol she joined the Weight Watchers, taking a keen interest in their programme which she understood well because of its similarity with the AA philosophy. She lost a little weight but nevertheless was unable to refrain from having regular 'eating binges'–varying from one to three per day. During these binges she was consuming – always on her own – '. . . enormous amounts of food-stuffs such as cakes and buns'. In order not to put on more weight she took care always to follow up these 'binges' by drinking enormous amounts of coffee to bring the food up. This worked on all occasions. (A similar method was adopted by another female over-eater, seen recently, who incidentally was also a neurotic who had (at least temporarily) recovered from alcoholism.) Apart from these deliberately planned and prepared 'binges' she sometimes went on eating too much after her usual meals, stating, '. . . When I begin to eat I eat too much. I don't seem to be able to stop. When I have anything in the stomach it seems to send wrong messages, as it seems to want more.'

She was very worried and felt guilty, and in an attempt to find a solution she consulted a hypnotist. Subsequently for one week she was able to cut down on her food intake but soon increased it again. When seen she was about 15 pounds overweight.

She explained that whilst drinking in the past, she did not have any 'food binges'. (Feeling very guilty and tense she had had two short-lived drinking bouts after four years of sobriety.) Her

compulsive eating started with slight 'binges' of overeating at meal
times and these made her feel very guilty because of her association
with the Weight Watchers. However, she went on overeating.
'It is the comfort I derive from it: that is why I choose soft and
usually sweet things. But once when I thought I should not spend
so much money I bought a lot of bread and marmalade, toasted it
and ate the whole lot.' This reminds one somewhat of alcoholics
who – when no longer able to afford spirits – may take to the drinking of cheap wine or surgical spirit. She tried to keep the 'binges' –
and her supply of cakes etc. – hidden from her children who were
out most of the day, and had the 'binges' only when the children
were not at home. She herself stressed the connection between her
state of mind and the frequency of her 'food binges'. 'When happy
I don't eat so much,' she declared. To a certain extent this behaviour
reminds one of statements occasionally heard from LoC alcoholics
who claim that they are sometimes able to cut down their drinking
when in a cheerful or relaxed frame of mind but not when
depressed or worried (see Part 3). Whilst having a satisfactory
relationship with a man friend for eighteen months, her 'binges'
became infrequent; they occurred mainly when problems arose in
this relationship – the 'binges' provided escape from thinking.
Again, an attempt to escape from 'having to think' may also seem
to be a plausible reason for some drinking bouts of alcoholics.

   She was very worried, depressed and disgusted with herself
about her dependence on food and was very anxious to force
herself off it but despite her previous failure with hypnosis (and
though she showed considerable insight) she still hoped for a
magical, relatively painless solution, requiring little effort on
behalf of herself.

4.3 COMPULSIVE (PATHOLOGICAL) GAMBLING*

The types of dependence discussed in this book may initially have
started with activities approved by family and society and experienced
by the individual as pleasurable. In the course of time however such
activities become an intolerable burden and develop into obsessions,
which are defined in a recent 'Encyclopaedia of Psychiatry' [14] as
'... contents of consciousness which are associated with a subjective

* Certain aspects of compulsive gambling were discussed in Part 2 and Part 3

feeling of compulsion together with a desire to resist', and which
'... may ... be recurrent and pathological in that they may substantially interfere with adequate performance and mental activity'.
Alcoholics, for example, may originally have liked the taste and
certainly the effect of alcohol, but later on they usually come to a
point, where, as Seldon Bacon has expressed it, they '... hate liquor,
hate drinking, hate the taste, hate the results, hate themselves for suc-
cumbing but they cannot stop' [15]. Compulsive eaters, as we have seen,
do not embark on their 'eating binges' because they enjoy the taste and
the flavour of the meal or because they want to satisfy an ordinary
hunger or appetite. Similarly, the compulsive (or as Moran [16] prefers
to call him the pathological) gambler does not gamble mainly for
material gain. 'The main point', wrote Dostoievski – himself a pathological gambler, 'is the game itself. I swear it is not greed for money,
although I am sorely in need of money' [17]. One young gambler
whose dependence had landed him in prison started each morning with
looking at the sports column of the newspaper and picking out likely
winners although of course he was unable to bet on them, and he
waited anxiously all day long to learn the result. To a lesser extent a
similar principle may be involved in the case of the man who day by
day places small bets and who sometimes may indeed have developed a
degree of mild psychological dependence. 'Such a man', wrote the
French philosopher and mathematician Blaise Pascal, 'spends all his life
playing every day for small stakes. Give him every morning the
money that he may gain during the day, on condition that he does not
play and you will make him unhappy. It could perhaps be said that
what he seeks is the amusement of play, not gain. However, let him
play then for nothing and he will lose interest and be wearied' [18].

At the times when not actually involved in drinking, drug taking,
overeating and gambling, such addicts are only too well aware of the
irrationality and the dangers arising out of their behaviour. As Carstairs
[19] put it in the case of the gambler, 'Many gamblers are keenly aware,
in the intervals of their gambling, of their own folly and culpability ...
(and may) beg for help in mastering an uncontrollable urge – as may
be the case with alcoholics, sexual deviants, and even the obese ....'.
But if such people at the start of their career which leads ultimately to
complete dependence, proceed from occasional to habitual drinking,
drug-taking and gambling, it seems likely that there is some emotional
reward or gratification involved that drives them to continue such
risky activities. In some such cases there may indeed be a self-destructive

and self-punitive urge at work as postulated by some analysts. K. Menninger has spoken of the 'gradual suicide' and of the 'Man Against Himself' [20]. Alternatively, one might feel that in such individuals, who are often very ambivalent in their attitude towards their addiction, the hankering after the emotional gratification may prove stronger than their fear of the bill presented the next day in the form of personal suffering, remorse, intense guilt feeling and rebuke by the family. Gamblers Anonymous talks of the compulsive gambler as a compulsive loser [21] – and the same may be said of the ultimate fate of those who have become dependent on drink, drugs etc. Nevertheless, like these fellow addicts and gluttons for punishment, the pathological gambler comes back again and again. What he seeks and enjoys, according to Bergler [17], is '. . . an enigmatic thrill . . . compounded of as much pain as pleasure'. This pleasurable–painful tension is derived from uncertainty of the outcome of his gamble. 'The normal person does his best to avoid painful uncertainty, but uncertainty is precisely what the gambler seeks.' The gambler looks forward to the interval between placing his bet and hearing the result and to the accompanying tension, and 'the craving for this strange thrill frequently overshadows the desire to win'. The gambler may have no end of conscious reasons or rationalisations for his gambling, but he '. . . doesn't gamble because he consciously decides to gamble; he is propelled by unconscious forces over which he has no control'.

Thus in the case of the pathological gambler the personality factor (host) is often of decisive importance. As with other forms of dependence, other factors being equal, inadequate, immature, insecure, neurotic and psychopathic personalities may tend to escape into the gambler's dream world more often than the more stable individual, provided that the facilities and opportunities for gambling are within reach. Therefore the environment (but not the agent) factor also plays a role in the development of dependence on gambling; and in social or occupational groups where gambling is widely accepted, and in areas where facilities and opportunities for gambling are plentiful, environmental influences may become relatively more important than personality. Environmental factors probably also explain (e.g. money, opportunity etc.) the predominance of men among pathological gamblers. These differences in the proportions of men and women becoming dependent on gambling which seem to arise mainly on the basis of environmental factors, can also be seen in cases of alcoholics and addicts to other drugs.

To a certain extent, the host factor is reflected in the finding that gambling and excessive drinking often go hand in hand. Possibly about 5% of our alcoholic patients were also excessive gamblers. As Moran [16] remarks, where pathological gambling and heavy drinking occur in the same person, sometimes the gambling is primary, the heavy drinking providing the individual with 'Dutch courage' for his gambling; in other cases, the alcoholism is primary, as the drinker hopes to win money enabling him to continue drinking. Older men, mostly with a history of alcohol or drug abuse and broken marriages, were one of two groups of gamblers observed by a probation officer among recidivists in a London prison, the second group consisting of gamblers whose criminal career had started with juvenile offences [22].

Types of gambling
Moran [16] divides pathological gambling into five types:
  (a) *Subcultural gambling*, arising mainly on the basis of the individual's family and social background.
  (b) *Neurotic gambling*, which is a reaction to some stressful situation or emotional problem. Possibly, 'reactive gambling' might be a more appropriate term for this variety.
  (c) *Impulsive gambling*, associated with loss of control. In these cases gambling has become irresistible and is simultaneously longed for and feared. Possibly, 'compulsive gambling' might be a more appropriate term, bringing the condition more in line with Jellinek's classification of addictive alcoholism and its associated loss of control [23]. The compulsive gambler, like the gamma alcoholic, apparently can not be certain of being able to stop his gambling activity whenever he wants to once having resumed his gambling, possibly after a period of total abstinence (see the first case history below). This loss of control in the compulsive gambler may be the consequence of psychological and possibly social factors. In the case of the loss-of-control (gamma) alcoholic it would seem that, apart from psychological and social factors, physiological (biochemical) factors may also be involved (see Part 3).
  (d) *Psychopathic gambling*, which is part of a generalised psychopathic personality disturbance. (Clearly, there are many pathological gamblers who exhibit features simulating psychopathy only getting 'hooked': such people are *not* psychopaths).
  (e) *Symptomatic gambling*, which occurs in the context of mental

illness, such as depression. Apart from psychotic gambling, neurotic and psychopathic gambling might also be classified as symptomatic in nature, similar to Jellinek's classification of alpha (symptomatic) alcoholism (see Section 3.1).

One could also attempt to give a classification of pathological gambling in terms of Jellinek's classification of the various alcoholisms (see Section 3.1). Thus 'alpha gambling' would comprise the types of gambling which are symptomatic of an underlying personality disturbance, which may be mild (neurotic) or more serious (psychopathic, or in other cases psychotic) in nature. 'Beta gambling' would roughly correspond to Moran's subcultural type, i.e. the gambling arises mainly on the basis of environmental and socio-cultural influences in the absence of marked primary psychological disturbances and of marked psychological dependence. Nevertheless, it could lead to marked economic, social or secondary psychological complications, although not to the severe physical complications which may occur in beta alcoholism. Gamma (and possibly also delta) gambling corresponds to Moran's impulsive type, with the loss of control superimposed upon and added to the original psychological or social reasons which started the gambler on his gambling career in the first place. As a result of his (psychological) loss of control he usually goes on gambling once he starts; moreover he becomes preoccupied with thinking about gambling all day long and may be unable to abstain from it (similar to Jellinek's delta alcoholism). Unlike Jellinek's gamma and delta alcoholisms, there are, however, no physiological factors involved in the corresponding gambling varieties. Finally, in analogy to Jellinek's epsilon alcoholism, there is the periodic (epsilon) gambler who has no difficulty in refraining from gambling for long periods, only to plunge once more into a gambling 'binge' for the most trivial reasons, or for no reason at all. In the experience of Gamblers Anonymous such periodic gamblers are not free from abnormal symptoms even in their gambling-free intervals, when they often suffer from irritability, frustration, nervousness etc.

Developmental progress of gambling

There are also many similarities in the developmental paths of alcohol and gambling dependence, as seen from a quick glance at the Chart of Alcohol Dependence (Figure 1 in Appendix). The individual gradually proceeds from occasional to habitual gambling, in spite of the uncertainty of material rewards. Unpredictable, intermittent reinforcement may, however, lead to operant conditioning [24] which is '. . . the learning process resulting from the selective reinforcement (rewarding) of certain emitted responses or rewards. This reinforcement increases the probability of the same response occurring on subsequent exposure to the same stimulus situation' [14] (see Part 2). At any rate, as financial reward is not the most important reason but rather the craving for the painful–pleasurable tension derived from the uncertainty of the result, whether he wins or loses the gambler will have received his reward or reinforcement. He gambles more and more frequently, risking higher and higher stakes and becomes increasingly preoccupied with it, to the neglect of other interests and sometimes also of his work. Losing money, feeling guilty and fearing reproach by his family, he may try to keep his gambling secret; he rationalises it and plays its extent and importance down. From time to time he may refrain from gambling altogether but in the long run all his well-meant resolutions and promises fail. He loses control, and once having started he goes on gambling whether he wins or loses, till the place closes for the day, or he has no money left. In order to afford gambling and to pay his debts he may take recourse to unlawful activities (larceny, fraud, embezzlement etc.) and land in prison. It has been estimated that gambling, alcohol abuse and drug abuse account for over half of Britain's prison population [25]. Occasionally, such a gambler – forsaken by family and friends, having gambled away all his money and laving lost his job, left with neither money nor interest to look after himself and his nutrition, may also go downhill physically. Having remained overoptimistic and living in a grandiose dream world for a surpsisingly long time, remorse and guilt feelings coupled with worry about his hopeless financial situation may lead to serious depression, heavy drinking or suicide attempts. Finally he may ask for help, though more often it will be his wife who does so on his behalf.

With increasing recognition of the pathological gambler's need for assistance and treatment, one might hope that in future gamblers too may come forward at earlier phases of their downward path than in the past. Treatment includes psychological (individual and group), physical (e.g. aversion [26]) and social (e.g. hostel) methods and, last but not least, there is the fellowship of Gamblers Anonymous [21], which started in California in 1957 and came to England in 1964. It has modelled its approach very much on the lines of Alcoholics Anonymous. 'Compulsive gambling is an illness, progressive in its nature, which can never be cured, but can be arrested. . . . The compulsive gambler is a very

sick person who can recover if he will follow a simple programme. . . .
The first small bet to a problem gambler is like the first small drink to
an alcoholic. . . . The first bet is the one to avoid . . .'. Spiritual and
group (sharing of experiences) factors are as important in GA as in AA.
Like other forms of dependence, pathological gambling is essentially a
relapsing disorder. Therefore continuing support is as necessary for
those afflicted with it as in the case of other addictions.

Some of the points discussed above will be briefly illustrated by
abstracts from two case histories of men whose pathological gambling
led to prison sentences:

Case history 1

An intelligent, elderly man from a good family background,
described by his (second) wife as a good husband and father
and a conscientious worker, had spent most of his adult life in
prison, all his offences arising from his extreme dependence on
gambling. His gambling started forty years ago when he was in his
early twenties (clubs, car and dog racing), and even then he was in
trouble with the law for receiving and selling stolen goods as
he needed the proceeds for gambling, i.e. backing horses. His
whole life, then and later, was centred on gambling, such as at
dog- and horse-racing meetings. The reasons he gave for embarking on his gambling habit in the first place were first, the
'thrill' he obtained from attempting to win, and second, that he
just followed the local trend since most of his friends attended
local clubs and gambled to some extent. Moreover, on the
occasion of his first attempt at real gambling in a West End club
he won £20, playing chemin-de-fer: 'I then thought how easy
it was to win.' (The importance of a large win early on in one's
gambling career has been stressed by many authors.)

His first marriage broke up mainly as a result of his gambling.
He liked going to the horses because of the thrill he obtained from
watching them and from 'beating the bookie'. He managed to
abstain from gambling for a year but as soon as a friend had asked
him to take him to a race meeting, he . . . was at it again, until he
was again convicted for receiving. 'Whether I won or lost, I always
stayed to the last race', and similarly at gambling clubs, 'I stayed
until I couldn't win any more, or until I was broke'. Being preoccupied with dog races, horses, clubs etc., he ran into trouble
repeatedly, for offences mainly consisting in obtaining credit by

fraud – although by then he had remarried and his marriage was happy apart from the continual problems arising from his gambling. For a brief period he again managed to abstain from gambling, apart from putting a few shillings on the pools. However, he then entered a newly established betting shop, mainly from curiosity, and started to gamble again, losing £40 in one bet. The next day, he '. . . had to go back – you think about it all the time . . . you want your money back', and from then on he attended the betting shop practically every day and obtained credit; he also began going to Casinos which fascinated him. Although he realised that there were grave risks involved and that he would lose as he had so often done through the years, he thought that he would get goods on credit, play a gamble, win and then be able to pay the money back, adding spontaneously, 'Of course, this never happens but I keep on thinking it must happen some time'.

During frequent interviews he reiterated, 'I do not believe I will ever gamble again' – having promised his wife he wouldn't. 'I cannot understand my behaviour . . . I come from a highly respectable family . . . I behave like a madman . . . I am normal apart from gambling . . . I have never exactly stolen anything in my life'.

Case history 2

A 25-year-old waiter, who had never before been in trouble, found himself in prison after forging cheques. 'I had become so compulsive a gambler that I needed more and more money in order to be able to go on gambling. By then I had sold my car and lost all my savings.'

He had been a manager at a restaurant for 2 years, a conscientious, hard worker who had saved money because of constant overwork, although he gave all his money to the mother with whom he lived. He did not smoke and drank very little. He had started to gamble eighteen months before and was initially attracted by noticing.

   (a) the occasional win, and

   (b) the excitement of some relatives when he was watching their modest, weekend gambling on horse racing.

On the first occasion he put a few shillings on a horse and was very excited, but then very disappointed when getting up early next morning he saw he had lost. In order to get his money back, he gambled again the next day; this time with a few pounds which he took from his savings. He began to gamble two or three days a week, as he could not leave his shop more often to go to the book-maker. After six months he started doing more overtime in order to earn more money for gambling purposes. Occasionally he won up to £300 per day, and this led him to forego selection and bet on each race. ('Sometimes I had bad dreams then, like someone strangling me; dreams which I had never had before'.) He felt depressed (but not guilty) when losing, but elated when winning: 'I didn't feel I was doing anything wrong, as I was losing my own money.' Initially I didn't feel it was getting out of hand, but after nine months all my savings had gone (£600) and I had run into debt. . . Even after nine months when I had to sell my car I hoped I would win the money to buy it back.'

'Even in prison I still use a method given to me earlier in my betting career of betting on favourites, naturally now without putting money on. Whenever I get the papers I look at the races, so I stopped the paper, but since then I have borrowed a paper. The thing is still inside me – I'd need a few shocks to get it out of me.'

'I can't get out of the betting shop till the last race (i.e. loss of control). When I'm satisfied that the races are over, I can then go home or to work.' In his case LoC apparently set in after a few months of gambling.

He looked forward to gambling in all his spare time. He often arranged nightshift work with the object of being able to go into betting shops the next day. At the same time he was afraid of gambling, '. . . because I can't resist or avoid it' (ambivalence). He felt certain that he'd not have gambled anywhere else if there had been no betting shops.

He showed no asocial or antisocial tendencies prior to the onset of his gambling dependence. In Moran's terminology he would seem to be an impulsive gambler with loss of control, the gambling dependence apparently having arisen in a somewhat immature but certainly not psychopathic personality, mainly because of availability and opportunity.

REFERENCES

1. Russell, M. A. H. (1971). (quoted from *Drug, Alcohol and Tobacco in Britain*, 221 (J. Zacune and C. Hensman, editors)).

2. Royal College of Physicians (1971). *Smoking and Health Now*, 2nd Report.
3. Action on Smoking and Health, Expert Group (1973). *Practit.*, **210**, 645.
4. Russell, M. A. H. (1972). *Drugs and Society* (April), **2**, 15 (August), **2**, 17.
5. *Drugs and Society* (1972). (August) **2**, 15.
6. *World Medicine, Editorial* (1972). No. 20, **7**, 7.
7. Salzman, L. (1972). *Psychiatry in Medicine*, **3**, 29.
8. Office of Health Economics (1969). *Obesity and Disease* (London).
9. Bruch, H. (1957). *The Importance of Overweight* (New York: Norton).
10. Glatt, M. M. (1970). *Brit. J. Addict.*, **65**, 51.
11. Matussek, F. (1958). *Nervenarzt*, **29**, 252.
12. Mayer, J. (1959). *Postgrad. Med.*, **25**, 623.
13. Campbell, J. D. (1971). *Acceptable Addictions*, 7 (Documenta Geigy).
14. *Encyclopaedia of Psychiatry* (1972). 297 (D. Leigh, C. M. B. Pare and J. Marks, editors) (London: Roche Products Ltd.).
15. Bacon, S. (1952). Quoted from L. Williams, *The Sober Truth*, 13 (London).
16. Moran, E. (1970). *Brit. J. Addict.*, **64**, 419.
17. Bergler, E. (1967). *The Psychology of Gambling* (Hill and Wang) (Reprinted from *Gambling*. (1957). 113 (R. D. Herman, editor) (New York, London: Harper and Row)).
18. Pascal, B. (1971). Quoted from, N. Polsky, *Hustlers, Beats and Others*, 43 (London: Penguin Books).
19. Carstairs, G. M. (1968). *Brit. Med. J.*, **1**, 239.
20. Menninger, K. (1938). *Man Against Himself* (N.Y.: Harcourt)
21. *Questions and Answers about the problem of Compulsive Gambling and the G.A. Recovery Programme, London.*
22. Ball, R. (1969). Conf. Churches' Council on Gambling, London. *Lancet*, **i**, 619.
23. Jellinek, E. M. (1960). *The Disease Concept of Alcoholism* (Connect.: Hillhouse Press).
24. Skinner, B. F. (1953). *Science and Human Behaviour* (New York: Macmillan).
25. *Drugs and Society* (1971) (Dec.), **1**, 6.
26. Seager, C. P. (1969). Conf. Churches' Council on Gambling, London. *Lancet*, **i**, 619.

Part 5

DEPENDENCE ON OTHER* DRUGS

5.1 STIMULANTS

Whereas dependence on such drugs as morphine and cocaine has for long been a condition of which both the professional as well as the lay public have been well aware, the same cannot be said for the recognition of states of dependence on hypnotics and stimulating drugs, often wrongly described as minor addictions. In many ways the problems caused by these substances are more important, not only because so many people even today are not fully aware of the possible dangers of taking such drugs to excess, but also because of the much greater number of abusers involved. Second to alcohol (and nicotine), barbiturates and amphetamines are responsible for the bulk of all problems of drug dependence in this country.

THE AMPHETAMINES

The amphetamines belong to a number of compounds called sympathomimetic amines and adrenergic drugs which are similar in structure and place of action to adrenaline (epinephrine) and noradrenaline (norepinephrine USA). The latter are described as catecholamines, i.e. compounds in which the phenyl ring of catechol (1-4,dihydroxybenzene) has a side chain attached which bears the amine (NH_2) group. Adrenaline and noradrenaline are hormones secreted by the medulla of the suprarenal gland, and released on stimulation of adrenergic

* Certain aspects of dependence on 'drugs other than alcohol' were discussed in Parts 2 and 3

(sympathetic) nerve fibres. The main effect of noredrenaline is to constrict the blood vessels thus leading to a rise in systolic and diastolic blood pressure. The sympathomimetic amines (which apart from the amphetamines also include ephedrine and isoprenaline (drugs used in asthma) probably act by stimulating the release of adrenalines from their store. The adrenalines are destroyed by several enzymes, among them monoamine-oxidase, whereas the amphetamines are not broken down by this enzyme. The amphetamines are powerful mental stimulants. They lessen fatigue, make for liveliness and talkativeness, stimulate wakefulness and excite the mood. However, among their unpleasant effects are nervousness, excitability, irritability, restlessness, agitation, insomnia and anorexia.

Classification of CNS stimulants and antidepressants
Although the amphetamines in the past have been employed in the treatment of depressive conditions their use for this purpose has now been abandoned, but several other groups of antidepressant drugs have more recently been introduced [1]. Under the classification central nervous system stimulants and antidepressants we may list the following four groups:

(a) *Amphetamines and pharmacologically related compounds*
    e.g. phenmetrazine
        methyl phenidate
        pipradol
        pemoline
    Of the amphetamines the first one to be used clinically (1937) was 'Benzedrine'; others are dextro-amphetamine and methylamphetamine.

(b) *Amphetamine–barbiturate and other combinations*
In this group is the mixture of dextro-amphetamine and amylobarbitone, known under its proprietary name of 'Drinamyl', which a few years ago, acquired fame and notoriety as 'purple hearts', due to the colour and tablet shape.

(c) *Monoamine-oxidase inhibitors*
    among them hydrazine derivatives (e.g. phenelzine
                                      nialamine)
    and non-hydrazine derivatives, e.g. trancylpromine

These MAO inhibitors block the action of the enzyme monoamine-oxidase which normally assists in the clearing of some mood-elevating amines, such as tryptamine and noradrenaline. MAO blockage leads in animals to accumulation of such amines in the brain. The therapeutic effect of MAO inhibitors may be due to MAO inhibition but this has not yet been definitely proven.

(d) *Thymoleptics* (iminodibenzyl derivatives)
    e.g. imipramine
        amytryptiline
        nortriptyline

This group of drugs has an antidepressant effect like the MAO group, but does not inhibit monoamine-oxidase.

These modern antidepressants have found a very useful place in the psychiatrist's armamentarium in treating depression. They obviously have their dangers too. For example, MAO inhibitors may potentiate morphine, pethidine and imipramine, or may produce agitation, and have occasionally been responsible for attacks of extremely painful headache, rise of blood pressure, or even subarachnoid haemorrhage. This occurred sometimes in patients who had been eating cheese before the attack. Cheeses are rich in tyrosine which normally is not converted into tyramine, because the liver contains monoamine-oxidase. In the presence of an MAO inhibitor, however, the tyramine level may rise and, as tyramine is a pressor amine, cheese ingestion in an MAO-treated patient may give rise to hypertensive attacks. This has been reported most often in the case of the combination preparation Parstelin (Parnate plus Stelazine). As a result of this, the use of this substance – which proved very useful in the treatment of minor depressive conditions in general practice – has been markedly reduced.

Amphetamine abuse and dependence

The risk of development of dependence is considerable in amphetamines and related substances, and in the amphetamine–barbiturate combinations. Occasional cases have been described with MAOI-type agents, but so far this has not been shown to be a problem with the other antidepressant drugs. Caffeine is another mild cerebral stimulant which is occasionally taken to excess by unstable personalities.

The amphetamines and the related stimulant drugs with similar properties (such as phenmetrazine) have enjoyed great popularity. Ten years ago in the UK they accounted for $2\frac{1}{2}\%$ of all National Health Prescriptions. Recently voluntary restriction of prescribing exercised by doctors on the advice of the British Medical Association, and a greater awareness of their hazards, has dramatically reduced use and availability of amphetamines. Nevertheless, there is still considerable illicit consumption since small-scale peddlers still manage to obtain a surplus from their own doctor or from different doctors under some pretext or other, or by forging prescriptions and theft. Where overprescribing is involved, the blame may be placed partly on patients, but mainly on certain doctors for their too ready and uncritical prescribing, though this frequently happens under strong pressure from patients – as in the case of barbiturates.

Ten to twenty years ago, the present author found that the amphetamines, second to barbiturates, were the drugs most commonly misused by alcoholics either concurrently or, usually in an unsuccessful bid to get off alcohol. Cases of abuse of and dependence on amphetamines [2] as well as on phenmetrazine were also seen among harassed, overworked housewives and others. Over the past decade there has been a great deal of evidence of world-wide widespread use, abuse and dependence on amphetamines amongst teenagers [3]. Scott and Wilcox found in a London Remand Home, through urine testing, that of all the male delinquent teenagers, 18% were taking amphetamines [4]. Apart from the epidemic of amphetamine abuse after the last war in Japan (chiefly affecting young men from low socio-economic backgrounds) other cases of abuse have been reported. For example, in Europe from East Germany (mainly methylamphetamine users, developing a toxic psychosis), Austria, Czechoslovakia and Sweden, where youngsters assumed the dangerous habit of giving themselves intravenous injections of phenmetrazine with the frequent result of toxic paranoid psychosis. The abuse of these drugs in Canada and USA may also be more widespread than generally realised. Amphetamine psychosis, moreover, closely simulates schizophrenia, so much so that O. J. Kalant [5] suggests the administration of routine chemical urinary tests for amphetamines in schizophrenic patients. For twenty years following their introduction in the mid-thirties, amphetamines were the only drug competitors to the electroconvulsive treatment in the therapy of depressive conditions, and their risks were hardly appreciated. Of course it is not only the psychopath who runs the risk of misusing the amphetamines. Kalant's [5] comprehensive review (1966) of 201 cases reported in the literature of psychotic reactions associated with chronic consumption of amphetamines show that most of them were adults aged 20 to 50 years. Whereas in earlier years most patients were men, in the following years the proportion of women increased a great deal. Among them were certainly many psychopathic personalities, psychoneurotics and personality defects; and in some cases of amphetamine psychosis, the condition was merely a precipitation of a schizophrenic state in patients with latent psychotic traits. Likewise, states of dependence were seen in 'normal' as well as in inadequate, neurotic and psychopathic individuals. There is, therefore, no characteristic mental or emotional picture by which a high risk patient can be identified in advance.

The most numerous groups represented in the literature among individuals developing an amphetamine psychosis were found to be people in the medical and paramedical professions, and obese housewives. The most common reasons for starting the use of the drug were attempts to improve mood and performance and to inhibit the appetite. Another point emerging from Kalant's review is that at least 50% of these people had at some time or other taken alcohol or other drugs to excess. In this country, fifteen years ago, the type of amphetamine- (or phenmetrazine-) dependent person most commonly seen was the middle-aged woman, often an overanxious, overworked or lonely housewife [3]. (Apparently a similar type of person in Switzerland may tend to abuse the minor analgesic drugs.) Having initially taken amphetamines on a doctor's prescription in order to help her slim, or alternatively, having been told by a friend that these drugs would give her zest and energy to go on with her housework, the housewife becomes so satisfied with the results – the increased energy, enthusiasm and the feeling of well being and euphoria – that she tends to increase the dose and to continue to do so even if by that time the doctor has become suspicious and attempts to cut down her supplies. Another type of patient commonly seen was the alcoholic who also habitually took amphetamines or more frequently barbiturates and amphetamines to excess, or who became dependent on amphetamines when trying to abstain from alcohol with the help of such medication prescribed by his practitioner. In other cases amphetamines were taken by addicts to other drugs as an additional stimulating 'fare'.

These types of patients, usually middle-aged, are quite different from the youngsters seen frequently in the early 1960s in this country – also in North America, Japan, Sweden and Western Europe – taking amphetamines for their 'thrilling' effects. Such youngsters often begin to take the drug during the weekend to give them sufficient 'pep' and 'staying power', and to help them to remain active and awake, before returning on Monday morning to their parental home [3]. Among such youngsters – who initially certainly did not take the drug compulsively but quite deliberately – one comes across many cases of drug dependence and of psychotic reactions (sometimes only after a few exposures).

The consequences of amphetamine abuse

(a) *Acute amphetamine poisoning*
Compared to the high incidence of acute barbiturate overdose, acute amphetamine poisoning is seen relatively rarely by doctors and reported cases of a fatal outcome are few and far between. By comparison to the much greater risks stemming from chronic abuse (psychosis and dependence) of amphetamines and of acute and chronic abuse of barbiturates, acute amphetamine poisoning thus constitutes a relatively minor risk.

(b) *Amphetamine psychosis* [2, 5]
Some individuals can take amphetamines for long periods without ill effects, and apparently also without developing a state of dependence. On the other hand, others may suffer from a psychotic state clinically indistinguishable from a paranoid schizophrenia. Amphetamine psychosis may supervene whether the individual originally started taking the drug on medical prescription as an anorexiant, or took it quassi-medically himself to profit by its euphoriant and energy-giving properties, or whether he started off by taking it for 'kicks', thrills or for curiosity. Nor does short duration of administration necessarily protect from the development of psychotic reactions.

The comprehensive review of the features of amphetamine psychosis by Kalant [5], showed that the daily dose used had ranged from 20 mg of d-amphetamine sulphate to 985 mg of amphetamine base (equivalent to 1687 mg of amphetamine sulphate). The characteristic clinical picture of amphetamine psychosis emerging from the study of the world literature is one of paranoid delusions as the most common feature, with hallucinations of various kinds. These are most commonly visual and auditory, tactile and olfactory ones being rare. Ideas of reference occur frequently. An important feature is the relative rarity of disorientation, which was only noted in 7%. This setting of a clear consciousness is remarkable as it is usually regarded as being characteristic of a toxic state. Other common mental features include excessive activity, excitability, anxiety, aggressiveness, agitation and depression. Physical signs in this condition are much less conspicuous than the mental features and may be absent altogether, but in many cases signs such as anorexia and weight loss, increased postural tone, and mydriasis are present and should be of help in the diagnosis. Occasionally insomnia, tremors of limbs and tongue, facial twitching etc. have also been noted.

The description of cases of psychotic reactions occurring on withdrawal of amphetamines is rare in the literature. The evidence does not permit any conclusions about the authenticity of psychotic episodes as amphetamine withdrawal phenomena. On the other hand, withdrawal of amphetamines in patients suffering from an amphetamine psychosis usually rapidly leads to disappearance, or at least to a marked improvement of the acute mental symptoms without any special treatment. Therapy must naturally be directed afterwards towards improvement of any underlying or precipitating conditions.

Some cases of amphetamine psychosis will turn out to be true schizophrenics. This condition should be suspected when, on withdrawal of the drug the picture does not clear up. However, it is possible that the patient may surreptitiously continue with the amphetamines; in such cases urinary tests should be carried out. Otherwise there should be rapid improvement, the only common mental withdrawal sympton being depression, occasionally with the danger of suicide. Physical withdrawal features are rare. Prognosis, however, is not good as many of these patients tend to resume their drug habit again and are then likely to suffer from a recurrence of the psychotic state.

Common reasons given for having originally started the drug are the control of obesity, depression, and as a substitute for alcohol and other dependence-producing drugs. Among other reasons given are fatigue and the necessity to perform extra work or study, and finally one 'legitimate' indication, narcolepsy. In the great majority of cases (80%) drug taking started without a doctor's initial prescription. All drugs of the amphetamine type may lead to an amphetamine psychosis, and care must be taken not to be misled by the great variety of names under which they are known in the various countries.

In the great majority of Kalant's cases the drug had been taken orally, in a small number by intravenous injection. An interesting and

10

dangerous development took place in London during 1967 and 1968. A few doctors started to prescribe methylamphetamine ampoules – a custom which soon became very popular, widespread and dangerous [6, 7]. The names of two London practitioners who were foremost in doing this, were well-known among young drug abusers, and at the time it was rare to meet young London drug abusers who were not mainlining methylamphetamine (methedrine). Many became severely psychologically dependent on it, and quite a few presented with the clinical picture of a (temporary) paranoid psychosis.

Though the danger became well-known (in fact, a number of cases of serious methylamphetamine dependence had been noted about ten years earlier among middle-aged neurotic patients who had been treated by their psychiatrists with repeated intravenous methedrine abreaction), it took some time before active steps were taken. However, the epidemic stopped practically overnight, after the British Medical Association, the Government and the pharmacists agreed to a voluntary ban on the prescribing of methderine ampoules by General Practitioners. From then onwards (i.e. mid-1969) there have been very few new cases of intravenous methylamphetamine abuse in the UK. The sudden termination of this minor epidemic throws an interesting sidelight as to how in certain situations quasi-legal steps can be effective.

(c) *Drug dependence of the amphetamine type*
Drug dependence of the amphetamine type is a state arising from repeated administration of amphetamine or an agent with amphetamine-like effects on a periodic or continuous basis. The characteristics can perhaps be best discussed here under the headings given by the WHO Expert Committees on Dependence Producing Drugs.
(i) An overpowering desire or need (compulsion) to continue taking the drug and to obtain it by any means.

There is no doubt—from the cases reported in the literature and from our own experience—that this condition is fulfilled by many cases of amphetamine-dependent individuals. Cases of forgery of prescriptions and theft have occurred, sometimes with the object of selling, but very often also in order to satisfy the abuser's own overwhelming desire.

One typical example is that of an intelligent middle-aged housewife, whose General Practitioner prescribed Drinamyl, as a substitute for alcohol. (Although this preparation contains both an amphetamine and a barbiturate, it seems from the way such patients talk about the effect of the drug that the amphetamine action is the predominant one, at least with respect to the patient's desire to continue taking the drug, but see paragraph below.) She managed to keep off alcohol but developed an irresistible desire to continue taking the Drinamyl, gradually increasing the dosage. The patient's doctor noticed this and stopped the drug after having been warned of the patient's drug taking by her husband, but she managed to turn up regularly at the surgery when he was absent and to forge the prescription.

(ii) A tendency to increase the dose.

Amphetamine abusers often take large doses in one day. A unique feature of the amphetamines is their capacity to induce tolerance – a quality possessed by few CNS stimulants. The wish to obtain even greater euphoria and energy may be additional reasons for increasing the dose. The ingestion of such high doses may often produce a psychotic state, accompanied by such amphetamide side-effects as agitation, restlessness and insomnia (all of which may be reasons for the preference shown by some abusers towards amphetamine–barbiturate mixture as against attraction to the pure amphetamine).

(iii) A psychic (psychological) dependence on the effects of drugs. (As described in the following discussion there is no clinical evidence of physical dependence in the case of amphetamines.)

As these drugs initially improve mood and provide energy and a feeling of well-being, individuals may well develop a psychological dependence on the effect of the drug which may become very intense. On sudden discontinuation, psychological withdrawal symptoms are seen in varying degrees, of which the main one is depression. This depressed state in itself may act as an added motivation to continue taking the drug, or to resume taking, possibly in increased dosage. Certainly withdrawal from large doses of amphetamines is *not* symptomless [8]. Amphetamine abusers often complain of and are afraid of the intense 'come-down', and features such as depression, sleepiness and lethargy might well be regarded as characteristic symptoms of the withdrawal of any stimulant drug [5]. One possible reason for the relative medical neglect of amphetamine withdrawal symptoms is that because of their low rate of excretion withdrawal symptoms develop more gradually.

Apart from suicide attempts which may occur during the depressive state following withdrawal from amphetamines, such withdrawal is never life-threatening. Incidentally, as Wilson and Beacon [9] demonstrated in a 'double-blind' trial, among individuals dependent on amphetamines, a certain proportion stated that they could not do without pills; they had become dependent on the taking of pills rather than on the substance as a drug, being unable to distinguish placebo tablets from active tablets in the trial.*

Clinically a physical abstinence syndrome has never been seen in the case of amphetamine withdrawal, and these drugs are generally described as not producing physical dependence, as measured by the criterion of a characteristic and reproducible abstinence syndrome. However, Oswald and Thacore in 1963, found that withdrawal of amphetamine or phenmetrazine in women abusers produced physical abnormalities of nocturnal sleep patterns which disappeared either on readministration of the drugs or (more slowly within weeks) if these drugs were not given again. The nocturnal sleep patterns were studied by recording the electroencephalograms and eye movements during sleep, and the authors concluded that these patients were patients physically dependent on the drugs [12].

(iv) Detrimental effect on the individual and on society.

To the chronic abuser the drug may bring unpleasant side-effects, such as anorexia, restlessness and agitation. Behaviour becomes more drug-centred, and he or she may become more selfish in outlook and attitude, with a progressive deterioration of character. Not infrequently the abuser may develop a state of paranoid psychosis. Some symptoms – psychomotor involvement, fatigue, carelessness and overconfidence – may lead to accidents. Detrimental consequences to society may arise from preoccupation with acquiring the drug if not by legal then by illegal and antisocial actions. Criminal behaviour has been described by some authors and more definite behaviour changes and antisocial actions may be a serious risk in cases of intravenous administration. The individual's change of attitude at home may lead to a deterioration of the domestic emotional climate to the detriment of family relation-

---

* To a certain extent these findings remind one of the 'needle addict' to whom the psychological effect of 'gear' is more important than the pharmacological effect of the drug and who gets his main 'kick' from the act of 'fixing'. Another illustration of the great importance of psychological factors in the spread of drug abuse is provided by the stories emanating a few years ago from the USA and for a short period enjoying popularity in London, of alleged hallucinogenic effects of bananas. The white fibre scraped from inside the banana peel was smoked in a pipe. An American underground paper described the effect as a mild 'high' resembling '. . a psilocybin (rather) than a marihuana high'. However a study of 50 banana smokers in Greenwich Village failed to give convincing evidence of true psychosomimetic action. The effects appear to be psychological rather than pharmacologic. The baked skins do produce mild autonomic effects which are secondarily given psychologic elaboration and experienced as 'high' [10]. The 'Practitioner' sees this story as evidence that, 'There is apparently no limit to the ingenuity shown by the human race in finding, or at least attempting to find, means of escaping from reality' [11]

ships. Deterioration of working habits may involve the family or individual in debts and antisocial actions. The costs for imprisonment, hospital stay, and looking after dependents, may put a considerable financial burden on the community.

Diagnosis of amphetamine abuse
Among the variety of symptoms, there may be periods of euphoria, extreme talkativeness and overactivity followed by depression, lethargy and fatigue. There may be tension, agitation, irritability, aggressive and uninhibited behaviour. Insomnia and roaming around at night may be followed by difficulty in getting up in the mornings and sleepiness during the day (leading to deterioration of performance in school or at work, failure to get up in the mornings, truancy and loss of jobs). Loss of appetite may be followed by loss of weight. Dryness of lips and mouth may lead to licking of lips by the tongue. There may be tachycardia, brisk reflexes, dilated pupils and 'cocaine bugs' (tactile hallucinations, a feeling that insects are crawling under one's skin).

Thus, if a stable, well-behaved, tidy, punctual youth begins to be slovenly, shows marked mood changes or a deterioration in dress, school or work performance, roams around at night and sleeps during the day etc., it is reasonable to consider amphetamine misuse as a possible cause of such a change in behaviour. There are of course many other reasons for such changes of attitudes and often a clinical diagnosis of amphetamine taking is not possible on symptomatology and physical examination alone. However, diagnosis can be established by urine testing for the presence of the drug.

DRUGS WITH AMPHETAMINE-LIKE EFFECTS

There are a number of newer drugs with amphetamine-like effects on the market. Whilst the origin of the alleged appetite-reducing action of these drugs is still obscure it is often held to be related to their stimulating effect on the CNS and this brings with it the risk of chronic abuse or dependence. The risk of abuse of such tablets obviously is greatest in the case of individuals who formerly abused amphetamines. Some drug abusers seem more particular than others in the choice of their drugs. For example, some seem to concentrate entirely on stimulants and tend to use to excess any new stimulant drug put on the market, even if occasionally they may combine it with sedatives to counteract its excessive stimulative and exciting effect. Others concentrate mainly on sedative-hypnotics, and some abuse all these varying types. Alcoholics, although essentially dependent on a CNS depressant also abuse stimulants occasionally, although by and large sedative-hypnotic drugs seemto be more popular with them. Of interest in this connection may be the experimental findings obtained by Eysenck [13]. Different personality types may react to drugs in a different way. Thus individuals who score high on extraversion on the introversion-extraversion continuum (e.g. hysterics), tend to respond to small doses of depressants by marked alterations of behaviour but are little affected by stimulant drugs. Introverted (dysthymic) patients on the other hand react in the opposite way to these different types of drugs; being centrally inhibited they are more easily influenced by stimulants but large doses of depressant drugs tend to leave them rather 'cold'.

It is an old rule in the history of drug dependence that drugs which have been widely used and abused for a longer period are at a great disadvantage if their undesirable side-effects are compared to newer drugs with similar properties, in particular if such newer drugs are initially claimed to be 'not habit forming'. It often takes some years before dependence-producing characteristics are brought into light and the initially put forward claims to the contrary proved wrong.

In practice most reports on drug abuse and dependence among amphetamine-like agents refer to phenmetrazine – probably reflecting its greater popularity than that of other such drugs. Phenmetrazine use rapidly became popular in Great Britain in the mid-1950s after amphetamine preparations had been put under restrictions (Schedule IV). It was not long before one saw quite a number of cases of phenmetrazine abuse, psychosis and dependence closely resembling the corresponding conditions previously described in cases of amphetamine abuse [14]. Similarly the previously popular abuse of a combination of amphetamines and barbiturates was for a period replaced by combining phenmetrazine with non-barbiturates, in particular carbromal [15]. Most of the cases of phenmetrazine abuse seen by us at the time concerned middle-aged women, which confirms Kalant's findings of 43 women among 45 cases described in the world literature [5].

It is of some interest that in recent years despite widespread misuse of amphetamines by the young in this country, phenmetrazine never seems to have had much following. This is particularly surprising in view of the large-scale intravenous abuse of this drug over years by youngsters in Sweden [16]. This is one of various examples illustrating the importance of local fashion on the choice of drugs of abuse. However, another amphetamine-like drug, has, over the past few years, become very popular with young British poly-drug abusers. This is methyl phenidate which is often taken in the form of intravenous injection. It was synthesised in 1954 and has sometimes in the past been employed by psychiatrists during treatment of patients with LSD. At least twelve cases of dependence on this relatively mild CNS stimulant – when taken orally – had been reported by 1963. A few cases were also reported of dependence on another amphetamine-like drug, diethylpropion [17].

It would therefore seem not unlikely that all such appetite-reducing drugs with even mild central stimulating properties, carry risks of abuse and dependence, particularly if taken by unstable, immature and inadequate individuals. As a rule such danger seems greater when control of such drugs is lax, e.g. where such drugs are available without medical prescription or where doctors seem to be careless or unduly generous with their prescribing habits. The BMA Working Party on Amphetamines (1968) felt at that time that among appetite-reducing substances, fenfluramine was the safest – though recently this drug too has been described by a group of authors as a drug of dependence though not of abuse (see Part 2) [18].

KHAT [19]

In certain districts in East Africa and the Arabian peninsula the habitual chewing of leaves of the khat plant may produce psychological and physical effects similar to those following ingestion of some of the less potent amphetamine preparations. It is the feeling of euphoria and the lessening of fatigue which is sought after – as is the case with amphetamine abusers – and is responsible for the development of a state of psychological dependence. Another amphetamine-like effect of khat is lessening of hunger. Thus supplies are procured without consideration for other more vital needs, such as food. As a result of this and different geographical and social circumstances, khat abuse leads to socio-economic complications different from those associated with the amphetamines. These include loss of working hours and income, financial impoverishment, malnutrition and lack of resistance to disease. Unlike amphetamine abuse, khat abuse also leads to gastrointestinal complaints which result from the presence in khat of a non-amphetamine-like substance, i.e. tannin, in considerable amounts. However, two amphetamine-like active principles have been found in khat-norpseudoephedrine (cathine) and a closely related substance. Their presence is responsible for the development of a moderate degree of psychological dependence in cases of habitual and excessive chewing. As with ordinary amphetamine dependence, physical dependence does not develop. Perhaps because only limited amounts of khat are absorbed by the user, tolerance does not develop (unlike the case of ordinary amphetamine dependence) and there are no withdrawal symptoms and no psychotic complications.

COCAINE

Cocaine is one of the alkaloids contained in the coca leaves of the plant erythroxylon coca. The stimulating effects of coca leaves have been well-known among the natives of South America for many years, and when Francesco Pizarro entered Peru in the 16th century he found its inhabitants chewing the leaves in order to overcome fatigue and to feel happy. Cocaine was the first local anaesthetic that was discovered and used as such in 1884 in Vienna. Koller Siegmund Freud just missed the fame, before starting on his psychoanalytic studies, of being the first to use cocaine in this way in ophthalmology, having been the first one to suggest its use. Shortly afterwards he suggested the use of cocaine as a treatment to a fellow scientist who was a chronic morphine addict and suffered a great deal. Cocaine did indeed cure this condition of dependence on morphine but only at the price of substituting for it a condition of dependence on cocaine, to which this man finally succumbed. Cocaine may be injected, swallowed, chewed (chewing the coca leaves is the method used in South America), and inhaled as snuff or 'snow' – the latter method gradually leading to ulceration of the nasal mucosa and perforation of the nasal septum.

The effects of cocaine are very transient as it is rapidly destroyed in the body. Thus the feeling of the 'flash' passes off so quickly that the addict is for ever trying to keep it going by repeating the drug again and again at short intervals and very large amounts may be taken throughout the day. For example, 30 g per day (1800 mg) were injected by heroin-cocaine addicts during the 'heyday' of this form of combined addiction in London in the mid-1960s [3].

In contrast to morphine which produces solitary introverts who like to be left alone with their visions, cocaine temporarily changes the individual into a social extrovert, who is charming, superficially witty and full of apparently brilliant ideas. Acting as a cerebral stimulant cocaine helps the user to make up his mind quicker and to talk more rapidly. It raises confidence, relieves fatigue, dilates pupils and accelerates the heart beat. However, if stimulation becomes too strong the user will become overexcited and thereafter may require a CNS depressant as a kind of antidote to the restlessness and delirium. This is one of the reasons why those using cocaine in high doses as a rule combine the drug with heroin, a combination recalling the habits of many drug abusers who combine the use of other stimulants with that of sedatives (e.g. amphetamines and barbiturates, phenmetrazine and carbromal, etc.). The addict who habitually takes large doses of cocaine, in an attempt to recapture for longer periods the ecstatic 'flash', may find it produces a delirious state plagued with paranoid delusions and hallucinations – visual, auditory and the characteristic tactile (haptic) ones. The latter may feel like insects crawling beneath the skin ('cocaine bugs'). The cocaine addict is often basically a psychopathic individual and such a person, experiencing hallucinations and paranoid delusions may become dangerous.

In England in the early and mid-1960s heroin addiction was so regularly associated with dependence on cocaine ('H' and 'C') that the layman may have got the idea that these two drugs bear a close chemical and functional relationship to each other. In reality not only are these drugs chemically quite different but their effects are also diametrically opposite to each other, heroin being a depressant of the central nervous system, cocaine a stimulant. It is however precisely the fact that the central nervous system effects of cocaine and heroin are opposed to each other that leads to them being taken so often simultaneously. 'Skinpopped' or 'mainlined' – often in the same dirty syringe – the young addict has the intention of counterbalancing the unpleasant effects of each agent, overcoming for example the extreme slowing down and depressive effects of heroin by the excitant, stimulating effect of cocaine (or a few years later, methylamphetamine [3]). However, very soon addicts realised that cocaine is much more dangerous and much more destructive to them than heroin, although it is not pharmacologically addictive. The following case history is typical of a great many English young 'H–C' addicts of the mid-1960s.

Case history

A 21-year-old boy of fairly high intelligence had started to smoke marihuana at the age of 16, soon changing to hashish. He found that 'hash' was too much of a stimulant of the mind. 'It made me think too much, and thoughts went round in circles in my mind. I wanted something to sedate me and after about a year I began to buy heroin from addicts, starting with $\frac{1}{6}$ g (10 mg) but gradually getting up to 4 g (240 mg) per day.' At that time he was registered with a doctor as he could no longer afford to buy heroin from addicts. He obtained 5 g from the doctor. He was smoking hashish and mainlining heroin at the same time although he gradually cut down the hashish and increased the heroin (reducing the amount of cannabis taken is common in those smokers who have progressed to the hard drugs). He developed a severe hepatitis with jaundice and went abroad in an attempt to get off drugs but resumed them immediately on returning to this country six months later. Having occasionally had a little cocaine he registered again with another practitioner who immediately gave him 5 g heroin and 5 g cocaine after having been told that this was the amount the patient had taken all along. Whereas this boy had been able to work on and off whilst on cannabis and heroin, he left work for good almost immediately after starting on cocaine. 'I got a mental craving for more and more, buying additional "Coke" from other addicts and occasionally exchanging "H" for extra "C". I could use all my supply of "C" (5 g) within four hours and I had none left in the afternoon. . . . I kept shooting it up. . . . Many people gave themselves overdoses of "C" . . . I once nearly killed myself through such an overdose: I felt a terrible explosion in my head and my heart beat violently. On that occasion the "C" crystals were damp so I didn't know how much I was using. . . . the effects were much stronger than usual. Ordinarily after mainlining "C" the "flash" came within seconds: my heart started beating fast, there was a nervous excitement which usually scared me. . . . The first time when I took "C" I got the "flash", although I only took very little, perhaps $\frac{1}{3}$ g, but later on I needed more to get the "flash". I liked the stimulation but every time I took "C" I had a fear of overdosing myself. . . .'

'When I started on heroin I felt fine but later on after becoming addicted to it I didn't feel anything nice any more though I took larger amounts, and I no longer got the mental explosion in the head from heroin. I felt low and depressed but taking "C" gave me the sudden "flash". . . . Five grains of "H" was a necessity for me because of the withdrawal symptoms and because I didn't want to come down to earth, but five grains of "C" were a luxury because they gave me the sudden "flash".'

However, this addict paid a high price for his luxury. 'My whole personality began to change, I became very aggressive, I used to think people were persecuting me and I used to insult them. . . . I almost became violent when I accidentally bumped into people . . . I had to give up work; my existence was just between home, the doctor and the chemists: there was nothing else, apart from occasional stealing to get money to buy extra "C" – I had never stolen before . . . I was getting in a very untidy state. I stopped washing, shaving, bathing . . .'.

Cocaine does not lead to physical dependence and thus would not be classified as addictive if strict pharmacological criteria were to be applied – yet clearly adopting other criteria, for example social criteria, the drug is at least as dangerous as (or more so than) any other physically dependent-producing drug. Psychological dependence to cocaine is very pronounced and the addicts need to continue its use though there is little evidence of development of tolerance. Occasionally one hears of jazz musicians and others who have apparently managed to stick to sniffing cocaine rather than taking it by injection. They have done this at irregular intervals for long periods and have apparently come to no great harm. However, these individuals must be regarded as exceptions. As a rule habitual cocaine abusers exhibit changes of personality with increasing emotional and ethical deterioration, loss of self-control and increasing unreliability and untruthfulness, sometimes accompanied by physical impairment. Following the introduction of the Treatment Centres prescribing of cocaine has been greatly cut down and as a consequence cocaine dependence in England – prevalent only a few years ago – has practically disappeared from the British drug scene*. This is certainly an important (and perhaps not sufficiently appreciated) success of the changed British System. It constitutes an advance, even though temporarily (in 1967/8) the H–C combination was replaced by the heroin-methylamphetamine epidemic [3] and despite the fact that nowadays many young British poly-drug abusers mainline the stimulant methyl-phenidate alongside the CNS depressants, Chinese heroin, methadone and the barbiturates.

---

* Over the past few months some drug users have mentioned that cocaine has once more become available on the illicit market.

CAFFEINE AND THEOPHYLLINE

The world over, even more popular and widespread than the CNS-depressant drug alcohol, are the stimulant beverages coffee and tea which owe their popularity to the presence of certain purine bases, the Xanthines, i.e. caffeine and theophylline. Coffee contains 1–1·5% caffeine, tea about 3·5% caffeine and theophylline. Caffeine is also responsible for the activity of the Cola Nut which contains about 2% caffeine, apart from the weaker alkaloid theobromine. Cocoa also contains theobromine apart from small quantities of caffeine.

The widespread use of coffee and tea in Europe goes back a few centuries only. Coffee first cultivated in Arabia conquered Europe in the 16th and 17th centuries. Tea widely consumed by the Chinese in the 15th century likewise reached the rest of the world not until the end of the 16th century [20]. As with other drugs affecting the CNS, approval and acceptance of tea and coffee was by no means unanimous. In 17th century Paris for example, coffee was '. . . proved to shorten life'; in 18th century Germany coffee drinkers were threatened with caning. King Frederick II of Prussia attempted to wean his citizens off coffee in order to get them to drink beer which he regarded as far healthier. The method he employed was the modern one of imposing high taxes (on coffee). Similarly in the case of tea – described by one 16th century author as – '. . . a medium for ensuring health and long life', history frequently witnessed '. . . a repetition of the conflict between praise and condemnation . . . like that found in the history of other excitants'. But in spite of many objections over the years to coffee and tea – in Lewin's words, 'Substances which act on the brain mock at all obstacles which oppose their extension. Their attraction grows slowly, silently, but surely' [20]. (Silently would not be quite the appropriate term to be used in the case of some of today's popular CNS-affecting drugs.)

There is no evidence of chemical dependence on caffeine but there must be many people who are mildly emotionally dependent on the drug. 'Many of us would find it difficult to make it through a day without one or more analeptics' [21]. Habitual tea drinkers were described by a doctor member of the House of Commons in 1952 as the 'truest types of addicts'. Tea consumption in England amounts to over 10 lb per head annually. A cup of tea contains 90 mg of caffeine [21]. Most of the world's supply of coffee now comes from Brazil: 40 million bags (of 132 lb each) supply the world's annual requirements.

Americans prefer coffee beans, consuming 17 lb annually on a *per capita* basis [21]. Malcolm [22] quotes an estimate that one person in four relies on coffee to get him functioning in the morning.

Caffeine and the less strong theophylline are stimulants of the CNS which may provide a feeling of well-being, stimulate activity and delay the onset of fatigue. Effects vary greatly from person to person. 'In general, caffeine and amphetamine induce feelings of alertness and well-being, euphoria or exhilaration and postpone onset of boredom, fatigue, inattentiveness and sleepiness' [23]. Excessive intake of caffeine may lead to symptoms such as tension, insomnia, '... an excessive state of brain excitation showing itself by a remarkable loquacity with accelerated associations' [20].

Caffeine is a constituent of some analgesic powders and tablets which occasionally have been taken to excess in continental countries such as Switzerland. In London a few years ago one occasionally came across cases of habitual abuse of pills containing caffeine (Pro Plus) in unstable youngsters who, encouraged by advertisements, believed these tablets could give them as much pep as amphetamines without their associated dangers. Caffeine is also a fairly regular constituent (averaging about 20 %) of the Chinese heroin powders nowadays peddled in London's West End.

Caffeine is thus a weakly-stimulating drug that can lead to mild emotional dependence. The fact that the beverages containing this substance (coffee, tea, cocoa, the 'cola' drinks) have been enjoyed for hundreds of years by millions with relative impunity probably testifies to its general safety (though the example of nicotine with the very delayed recognition of its dangers must be kept in mind). It is however interesting to note that quite recently articles in the medical press have taken up this subject. For example, an apparent relationship between heavy consumption and myocardial infarction has been noted by the Boston Collaborative Drug Surveillance Program [24]; and a strong correlation has been shown between annual *per capita* consumption and fatal ischaemic heart disease in 24 countries, comparing different countries' coffee consumption and their death rates from ischaemic heart disease [25]. In such cases the matter is made more complicated by the finding that coffee drinkers are frequently heavy smokers, a point to be kept in mind in the desirable prospective clinical trials designed to study coffee consumption as a risk factor in the pathogenesis of atherosclerosis [25] and other conditions.

5.2 SEDATIVE–HYPNOTICS, TRANQUILLISERS AND NON-NARCOTIC ANALGESICS

SEDATIVE–HYPNOTICS

The barbiturates

For many hundreds of years the only CNS depressants known to mankind were ethyl alcohol and opium. The modern era of the therapeutic use of hypnotics dates back less than a hundred years. At that time the bromides* were employed as sedatives, and in 1869 Liebreich introduced chloral hydrate.† Ever since, the pharmaceutical industry has worked overtime to make available more and better hypnotic drugs. Chloral was followed by paraldehyde,‡ sulphonal and urethane§ and about a hundred years ago barbituric acid (malonyl urea) was synthesised. In 1903 Fischer and von Mering [26] introduced the first barbituric acid derivative into clinical practice – barbitone or Veronal. Since then, a large number of barbiturates have been prepared and used therapeutically, usually classified into a very short-acting (e.g. thiopentone), a short-acting (e.g. pentobarbitone), an intermediate (e.g. amylobarbitone) and a long-acting (e.g. barbitone) group.

Often barbiturate intoxication is not recognised as it may not be suspected and so it is often associated with abuse of alcohol or other drugs. Frequently the clinical picture is mistaken for a chronic neurological condition. However, the fact that barbiturates may give rise not only to psychological but also to physical dependence and may cause mental and physical complications has been known for many years. The serious risks involved in indiscriminate barbiturate prescribing were first stressed by the Home Office Pathologist, William Willcox [27, 28]. The fact that the barbiturates were true drugs of addiction was proved beyond any doubt by the experiment of Isbell and his associates

---

* Bromide poisoning and bromide dependence were (until the late 1930s) once quiet common. Though probably rare nowadays, the possibility of such an occurrence should still be kept in mind. The psychic dependence which is produced is mild and there is no physical dependence. Symptoms of bromide intoxication include drowsiness, confusion, restlessness, ideas of persecution and hallucinations [29].

† Second, to opium and alcohol, chloral hydrate is the oldest of the CNS depressants. It enjoyed great popularity in the second half of the 19th century; but like the bromides many years later, chloral hydrate use was largely abandoned in favour of the barbiturates. Chloral hydrate can produce psychological and physical dependence (withdrawal delirium), causing dependence of the barbiturate–alcohol type [30]. (A similar risk may exist in the case of some of its more recently introduced derivatives.)

‡ Paraldehyde is rarely used today. It can cause psychic and physical dependence of the barbiturate–alcohol type. Such cases are occasionally seen in alcoholics.

§ Urethane, a mild hypnotic, belongs to the group of monoureides (see footnote on page 154)

[31] at Lexington in 1950. In this experiment a number of morphine addicts who had been off morphine for some time were regularly given barbiturates for periods ranging from three to nearly five months. On sudden withdrawal, convulsions were seen in some patients and delirium (or convulsions and delirium) in others. None of these patients exhibited these symptoms whilst taking the drug. Clinically, the same syndrome of convulsions and delirium was observed by us in 1952–1955 in a number of alcoholic patients (at Warlingham Park Hospital) who had not divulged their barbiturate habit when admitted to hospital. Although it soon became clear that a very similar picture might supervene on sudden withdrawal of alcohol from long-standing heavy drinkers, in some individuals such an abstinence syndrome undoubtedly followed the sudden discontinuation of barbiturates [32, 33]. It was not surprising that in 1954 the *Lancet* in a leader entitled 'Shadow over the Barbiturates' [34] named the barbiturates '. . . true drugs of addiction (a risk which was) . . . the least appreciated and . . . most sinister'. Further, a *British Medical Journal* editorial (1954) – after a remark that '. . . the sinister potentialities of the barbiturate hypnotics have been a perennial subject of debate in the medical press for the past 30 years . . .' – agreed that apart from the relatively slight tendency to increase the dosage compared with the behaviour of morphine addicts, '. . . barbiturates otherwise fulfil all the criteria for drugs of addiction' [35].

Yet even these denunciations and warnings failed at the time to stem the rising tide of barbiturate misuse. More than 60 years after the introduction of the first barbituric acid derivative into therapeutics and over 30 years after the 'Battle of the Barbiturates' [36] was at its height, in the mid-1960s barbiturates still enjoyed great popularity among the medical profession and the lay public. This was evident at the time from the rise in annual consumption rates, suicide attempts, suicides, fatal accidents due to barbiturates [36], and very likely also a rising incidence of emotional and physical dependence on these drugs (36, 37).

Barbiturate consumption
The percentage of National Health Service prescriptions for barbiturates rose from $1 \cdot 1 \%$ in 1934 to $4 \cdot 6 \%$ in 1947. Between 1957 and 1960 the percentage of NHS barbiturate prescriptions in England and Wales rose to approximately 7%. Also at this time non-barbiturate hypnotic–sedatives (excluding the 'tranquillisers') accounted for $2 \cdot 5$–$3 \cdot 2 \%$ of all NHS prescriptions. However, since then there has been a gradual increase in prescriptions for non-barbiturate hypnotics and an even

greater rise for prescriptions for tranquillisers. There has also been a rise of antidepressant prescriptions and a fall of prescriptions for stimulants and appetite suppressants (see Table 2 in Appendix). It seems clear that the campaign during the 1960s against the well-known, dependency-producing barbiturates and amphetamines seems to have contributed indirectly to the relative increase in popularity of the newer non-barbiturates, tranquillisers and antidepressants, which, on the whole, carry somewhat lesser dependence risks.

The number of barbiturate prescriptions between 1961 and 1968 remained constant at just over 15 million; however in relation to total drug prescriptions this amounted to a fall from 7·4%–5·7%. The dependence-producing stimulants and appetite suppressants fared even worse, the number of prescriptions falling from 6 million in 1961 to under 4 million in 1968. In contrast, non-barbiturate hypnotic prescriptions in the same period increased from 3·4 million–5·8 million, or from 1·6%–2·2%, tranquillisers from 6·2 million (1961) or 3·0% to 16·0 million or 5·9% (and the non-dependence producing antidepressants from 1·4 million prescriptions in 1961 (0·6%) to 5·3 million or 2·0%). The total prescriptions in England and Wales between 1961 and 1968 increased by about one third; the number of prescriptions for barbiturates, non-barbiturate hypnotics, tranquillisers and antidepressants rose from just over 26 million in 1961 (or 12·6% of total prescriptions) to 42·4 million (or 15·8%) in 1968 [38]. The same trend in prescribing habits has continued over recent years, i.e. diminishing popularity of barbiturates and amphetamines and rising prescription of non-barbiturate hypnotics, tranquillisers and antidepressants (see Table 2 in Appendix). Thus barbiturate prescriptions fell from 13·1 million in 1969 to 10·9 million in 1971 and amphetamine prescriptions (and related stimulants) fell from 3·3 million to 2·7 million. On the other hand the number of prescriptions for non-barbiturate hypnotics increased from 5·9 million in 1969 to 7·1 million in 1971. Similarly, the number of prescriptions for tranquillisers increased from 15·4 million to 17·1 million and for antidepressants increased from 5·4 million to 6·6 million.

It seems very difficult to accept that the vast amounts of barbiturates, non-barbiturate sedatives, tranquillisers and analgesics prescribed nowadays (50 million prescriptions per year) are really necessary for the treatment of patients. Confronted with a large number of patients with functional troubles (these may form more than one-third of people asking for the General Practitioner's help) and insomnia (estimated to be the main or only symptom in at least one-third of patients in general practice), all clamouring for rapid relief, the harassed practitioner, lacking time (and psychiatric education) to inquire more fully into the patient's history often can do little else but give drugs to sedate, in spite of all warnings that sedatives and stimulants are not placebos. The family doctor could argue that many of his neurotic patients referred to a psychiatric in-patient or out-patient department are probably referred back to him sooner or later with the suggestion to continue treatment with (in the past) barbiturates or (nowadays) tranquillisers. The doctor may further argue that patients having heard of new 'wonder drugs' insist that they should be given them.

There is, of course, no doubt that CNS-affecting drugs are necessary and valuable in the case of many people suffering from emotional ill-health, e.g. anxiety or depression. However, referring to the possible reasons for the modern use of CNS-affecting drugs, the 1961 Report of the First Interdepartmental Committee on Drug Addiction [39] regarded their alleged role in modern society as very doubtful. Intensive advertising was seen as one possibly important factor together with a materialistic attitude 'towards therapeutics leading to a search for, and application of, a specific chemical corrective aimed not only at eradicating major and minor ills, but also if possible at positively enhancing health'. The hazards of the widespread use of psychotropic drugs must be recognized and balanced against any accepted, alleged or apparent benefits.

Non-medical use of barbiturates

In spite of the fall in prescriptions for barbiturates, their abuse – in particular by middle-aged women – still seems very widespread. This is a problem of many years standing [9]. However, a new development regarding the non-medical use of barbiturates in the late 1960s was the emergence of the young barbiturate abuser [40]. Youngsters in this country – prior to this period – had as a rule kept away from the barbiturates. Their claim was that they left the use of 'sleepers' and alcohol to the middle-aged, whilst they (the young) preferred being 'pepped up' by stimulant amphetamines or obtaining consciousness-expansion by 'hash' or 'acid'. Whereas the middle-aged therapeutic and non-medical users of barbiturates take them orally, the modern young British poly-drug abusers inject the powdered and dissolved tablets intravenously (usually nembutal – pentobarbitone or tuinal – quinal-barbitone and amylobarbitone). At one time, 1968—1970, the habit of mainlining barbiturates became quite common among young British poly-drug abusers, the fashion superseding and following the methyl-amphetamine epidemic of 1968. Whereas previously the methyl-amphetamine-dependent youngsters had been very restless and moved around a great deal, after the advent of intravenous barbiturate abuse such intoxicated youngsters on the Piccadilly 'scene' became sleepy and staggered and fell about a great deal. They also risked acute overdosage (often fatal), local abscesses and gangrenous ulcers at the injection sites, and generalised complications, such as septicaemia and viral hepatitis. These youngsters claimed that they were driven to the use of barbiturates as a consequence of the Treatment Centres' approach which did not provide them with as much narcotic 'stuff' as they needed (or as often perhaps as they wanted). They therefore took to increased black market oral use of the non-barbiturate hypnotic mandrax and the intravenous injection of Chinese heroin and of barbiturates. They obtained the latter on the illicit market, or by attending various GPs as temporary patients. Few medical practitioners at the time were aware of this new fashion among the young, so that the latter had little difficulty in obtaining large amounts from doctors. However, doctors became gradually aware of this new barbiturate risk among the young. Drug abusers themselves grew frightened of the many dangers attached to the mainlining of barbiturates – although for a period they sometimes used such well-known risks as a kind of blackmail to induce Treatment Centre doctors to prescribe more narcotics for them in order to keep them away from the 'sleepers'. Today one still meets many young poly-drug abusers who also 'fix' barbiturates and are often in a state of sub-acute or chronic barbiturate intoxication, but fortunately this extremely dangerous intravenous barbiturate abuse by youngsters seems to be declining.

Acute barbiturate poisoning (suicides, accidental deaths and attempted suicides – self-poisoning)

During the past decade this country has witnessed a remarkable steady fall in the suicide rate, among men and women alike (see Table 3 in Appendix). The number of suicides fell from 3261 among men and 2378 among women in 1963 (a combined rate per 100 000 of 12·0), to 2263 among men and 1682 among women (a combined rate of 8·1 in 1971.The only other countries in which a decline in suicide rates has been reported, are Israel and Japan. In the view of Dr R. Fox, the 34% drop in suicide in England and Wales from 1963 to 1970 is '... associated with the growth of the largest suicide prevention organisation in the world' – the *Samaritans* [41].

Ten years ago when the present author reviewed 'The Abuse of Barbiturates in the UK' [36], the barbiturates were '. . . surpassed only by coal gas in the frequency of causing suicidal and accidental death'. Barbiturates among drugs, and carbon monoxide among non-medicinal cases, still remain today the two major agents in deaths due to poisoning [42]. However, coal gas has lost its position as the most common cause of suicide as it is gradually being replaced by non-toxic natural gas. The number of domestic gas suicides – amounting in 1962 to 1392 among men, 1069 among women (a combined rate per 100 000 of 5·3) – had fallen by 1971 to 215 among men and 131 among women (a combined rate of 0·7). On the other hand, poisoning by solid and liquid substances rose from 459 males and 660 females (a combined rate of 2·4) in 1961 to 750 males and 1097 females (a combined rate of 3·8).

Barbiturates remain by far the main cause of suicidal deaths by drug poisoning. Deaths from suicidal and accidental poisoning in England and Wales in 1970 totalled 2909, of which 1895 were due to barbiturates. In 1968, out of nearly 4600 suicides, 1926 (42%) were caused by drugs. The great majority of these deaths – over 1400 – were a result of taking barbiturates; 210 deaths were a result of taking aspirin and 74 deaths were a result of taking mandrax [43].

In contrast to the overall decline of suicide rates in this country, the number of attempted suicides has continued to rise. As at the time of our previous review ten years ago [36] drugs, and in particular the barbiturates, remain the most popular agent chosen by individuals attempting suicide. Ten years ago coal gas was the method responsible for most actual suicides, being a more lethal weapon than the barbiturates. However, today, the readily available barbiturates are far more frequently used for actual suicide and suicide attempts, than is coal gas.

There are no reliable official statistics available about the number of attempted suicides. The number of annual hospital admissions for attempted suicide has been estimated to exceed 50 000, and to be rising each year by 10% [44]. From our review of certain official figures for this country in the 1950s [37] and from an American estimate quoted by Stengel *et al.* [45] in 1958 the ratio of attempted to fatal suicides at the time was thought to be in the region of six to one. The increase in suicide attempts in the 1960s in contrast to the fall in actual suicides seems to support Stengel's hypothesis that different motives may often be at work. In Stengel's view the failed suicide bid has not been bungled but was from the beginning often meant as an appeal for help; the individual attempting suicide may often be quite a different type of person from the one who actually commits suicide.

The preponderance of barbiturates among the causes of hypnotic self-poisoning is also borne out by Scottish statistics. Over 70% of cases of poisoning by hypnotics admitted to the Edinburgh Regional Poisoning Treatment Centre between 1968 and 1970 [46] were due to barbiturates (706 patients); followed in order of frequency by the two non-barbiturates mandrax (about 300) and nitrazepam (about 100). Other hypnotics together amounted to no more than 80 cases. The relatively high representation of mandrax and nitrazepam among cases of hypnotic poisoning probably reflects the high rate of prescribing of these drugs, which together account for the bulk of increase of prescriptions of non-barbiturate hypnotics (see Table 2 in Appendix).

The rise of non-barbiturate prescriptions as we have seen has accompanied a decline in the prescribing of barbiturates in recent years. The total number of annual hospital admissions for barbiturate poisoning – according to Locket – is nowadays about 14 000, compared to 16 500 in 1963 (with a constant mortality rate of about 2%) [29]. These figures are still high, but Locket makes the point that 'Hospital admissions for poisoning have shown a steady fall in percentage due to barbiturate poisoning . . . paralleled by a fall in NHS prescriptions for barbiturates'. Thus barbiturate prescriptions in 1970 made up approximately 29% of all psychotropic drug prescriptions and less than 5% of all prescriptions. Corresponding to this, in 1971 no more than 16% of all poison admissions to Dr Locket's North-East Metropolitan Regional Poisoning Centre were due to barbiturates.

This parallelism between prescribing habits and the risk of self-poisoning had also been apparent in our earlier review ten years ago [36] when it seemed that, 'The continual increase of suicidal and accidental deaths caused by the barbiturates proceeds in some respects parallel to their rate of consumption'. Thus barbiturate output in Great Britain increased four-fold between 1938 and 1950, whilst deaths from barbiturate poisoning multiplied by $4\frac{1}{2}$ times from 1938 to 1948. Barbiturate suicides have increased twelve-fold in the past 20 years (i.e. the 1940s and 1950s) and accidental (barbiturate) deaths have increased about ten-fold [36].

Prescribing habits of doctors thus seem to exert some influence on the type of drug chosen for acts of self-poisoning. Therefore, a

Matthew *et al.* [46] point out, the relative safety in overdosage should influence the choice of hypnotic by the doctor. They feel that, 'Despite the mounting incidence of self-poisoning, the prescribing habits of doctors seem hardly to have changed' – though clearly the (by-and-large safer) benzodiazepines (and also methaqualone which is probably as dangerous as the barbiturates) have in recent years pushed down the prescribing rates of the barbiturates.

Overdosage is one major risk with the barbiturates, the development of dependence is another danger. The incidence of overdosage seems considerably higher in those taking the drug habitually to excess than among the general population. This reminds one of the much more frequent occurrence of episodes of acute drunkenness among alcoholics compared to other drinkers though the latter also may occasionally imbibe too much. A high rate of barbiturate poisoning points to the likelihood that a state of (at least emotional) dependence on these drugs may not be uncommon. Indeed, fifteen years ago–some 4–6 % of attempted suicides were estimated to be '. . . barbiturate addicts accidentally taking overdoses or attempting suicide' [42]. Drugs, and in particular the barbiturates, are clearly the most popular agent chosen by individuals attempting suicide, and because of their ready availability in many households the barbiturates and similar drugs take a heavy toll of human lives.

Barbiturate dependence
60 years ago, Willcox [27] reading a paper on the 'Veronal Habit' at the 17th International Congress of Medicine described how this drug taken in repeated small doses could lead to chronic veronal poisoning characterised by features such as tremor, ataxia etc., an abnormal mental state and disorganisation of the moral sense. 'Tolerance', he stated, 'undoubtedly occurs in some cases', though is only slight in degree. He repeatedly stressed the risk of – sometimes fatal – overdosage especially in those taking the drug habitually: 'Persons who have been taking the barbituric acid derivatives daily for a long period very commonly take a large overdose when they are faced with mental stress and worry and often death results thereby.'

It is impossible to estimate how prevalent the state of emotional dependence to the barbiturates is and how often physical dependence develops among those who over a certain period take higher than therapeutic doses (i.e. at least 0·4 g daily [47].) A certain proportion of those admitted to hospital following an acute overdosage are discovered to have taken the drug habitually and often excessively over a considerable period. The event that leads to hospital admission in such cases is no more than one episode in, and an acute exacerbation of, a chronic though often unrecognised condition. Not infrequently the state of affairs is at first not even recognised in hospital when the patient, as occurs so often, gives a misleading history and the state of physical dependence comes to light only when physical abstinence symptoms supervene (and are recognised as such!).

Chronic barbiturate intoxication though probably not uncommon – in particular among middle-aged women – often may go unrecognised. As long as the addict is able to satisfy his demand and need for drugs he may feel tolerably well in spite of his symptoms. If such symptoms persist and the patient keeps coming back to the doctor asking for drugs and insisting it is only some special type of drug that is any good for him, the possibility of drug dependence should be kept in mind. If this demand is not met the addict may suffer from symptoms such as anxiety, depression, insomnia, i.e. withdrawal symptoms which may easily be mistaken for a recurrence of the condition for which these drugs were originally prescribed: more barbiturates may thus be prescribed in higher doses [48]. Occasionally, persisting chronic tension states may be caused by an underlying state of chronic barbiturate dependence. As one might expect, most cases of barbiturate dependence are caused by the intermediate and short-acting preparations though more rarely they may also occur with the long-acting ones. According to Eddy *et al.* (1965), 'There is no evidence that physical dependence develops to a detectable degree with continuation of the therapeutic doses usual for the production of sedation or hypnosis; the daily dose must be appreciably above the usual therapeutic level before abstinence symptoms will appear on abrupt withdrawal' [8].

Psychic dependence, on the other hand, may occur even with therapeutic doses. Some degree of tolerance may rapidly develop in the case of the barbiturates. This, combined with the underlying emotionally disturbed and tense state and the interference with proper judgement produced by the drugs, may lead to a stepping up of the dosage into the levels needed to produce physical dependence. Rapid increase of dosage may also occur when barbiturate consumption is combined with that of amphetamines. In the 1950s this combination was quite popular among unstable personalities, alcoholics, etc., long before its properties were discovered by the modern teenager. In such cases the 'primary' dependency may be on either type of drug, amphetamine or barbiturate.

For example, barbiturates taken in fairly high doses for some time may lead to a state of depression. In an attempt to counteract this effect, the barbiturate-dependent individual may take amphetamines. A few years ago, when the risks accompanying the indiscriminate use of barbiturates became more widely appreciated and when the amphetamines were subjected to stricter legal precautions, the previously popular barbiturates–amphetamine combination was followed for a time by the misuse of another similar combination, i.e. that of the sedative carbromal preparations with the stimulant phenmetrazine (see Section 5.1). Simultaneous consumption of alcohol may occur alongside habitual overdosage of barbiturates and amphetamines. Recovered alcoholics as well as those who still practise their alcoholism are very prone to also take other drugs to excess – chiefly barbiturates [49].

Apart from causing depression by a direct pharmacological effect, habitual excessive consumption of barbiturates, like any other form of dependence, may interfere with the individual's relationships at home and in society and may produce deterioration and difficulties at work. Domestic friction, loss of employment, financial problems etc., may all indirectly heighten his depressive state. As barbiturates are readily available, the frequent occurrence of suicidal attempts by means of these drugs is easily explained. Forty years ago Willcox went as far as to say that in his experience, 'Most of the fatalities from poisoning by the barbiturates occur in people who have been taking the drugs in repeated daily doses': they were '. . . hardly ever used as a means of suicide except by persons accustomed to their daily use and effect' [50]. This certainly must be an oversimplification and an exaggeration but an important aspect in regard to the barbiturates is the extent to which their widespread medical use has made them socially respectable. Many people who would not dream of taking opiates or of drinking regularly to excess, see nothing wrong or risky in habitually taking sedatives or hypnotics and occasionally repeating the doses if the required effect is not obtained very rapidly. The higher incidence of suicide attempts by means of barbiturates in the case of women than among men may be due to several reasons, such as a preference for the less lethal method of drug overdose as compared with the more lethal coal gas, but it may also point to the relatively greater prevalence of the barbiturate habit among women. One explanation for this may lie in the fact that unstable men feeling in need of psychological relief at times of strain and stress may turn to heavy drinking with the tacit consent of or even encouragement by society. This escape route, even today, is still con-

sidered taboo in the case of women in similar circumstances. The
woman who feels in need of emotional relief may thus be more inclined
to turn to drugs than to alcohol. Substantial quantities can be obtained
legitimately and will arouse less suspicion than regular purchase of
wine, gin, or vodka; tablets are more easily carried in a handbag, they
are cheaper [36], and there is no smell to give her away.

Drug dependence of the barbiturate type has been described by
Eddy *et al.* [8] as '. . . a state arising from repeated administration of a
barbiturate on a continuous basis, generally in amounts that exceed
the usual therapeutic dose levels'. Desire or the need to continue taking
the drug is strong. 'There is a psychic dependence . . . related to subjective and individual appreciation of the effects of the drug, and there is
physical dependence requiring the presence of the drug for maintenance
of homeostasis and resulting in a characteristic and self-limited syndrome . . . on sudden cessation of drug intake, or . . . on reduction of
intake below a critical level.' Barbiturate-type dependence is detrimental to the individual because of the user's preoccupation with the
drug, but even more so because of the effects of the drug on his mental
and physical health (as described above). The detrimental effect on
society is related to the user's preoccupation with the drug, the neglect
of his obligations to family and society at large and the effects of the
drug on his mental and physical functions and interpersonal relationships etc.

One often encounters patients who have been taking barbiturates in
small doses for years without increasing the dose and who swear that
they could not possibly sleep without their night-time dose. Nevertheless because of its prevalence, the danger of a supervening state of
physical dependence and of chronic intoxication and the risks of
accidental and deliberate self-poisoning, barbiturate dependence is a
problem of considerable importance.

Many people who misuse these drugs are emotionally unstable. The
view has been repeatedly expressed that barbiturate addiction is rare
except in fundamentally very disturbed individuals, such as psychopaths and severe hysterics. If that were so the prognosis would naturally
be very poor. But, on the other hand, the habit of taking a hypnotic at
night-time is so prevalent (it is often regarded as being harmless,
medically sanctioned and prescribed), that also psychologically relatively 'normal' individuals (i.e. with no more emotional unbalance than
the average person) may embark on it and for reasons already briefly
discussed may persist with it, thus developing tolerance. Once an

individual has started on the pill-taking habit it may easily grow. It seems therefore by no means certain that the majority of barbiturate-dependent individuals are psychologically very abnormal. There are many among them, in particular perhaps professional addicts, who may prove very amenable to treatment.

Chronic intoxication

The picture of chronic barbiturate intoxication has been already touched upon. Mentally, such an individual may be confused, slow, forgetful; judgement, attention, concentration and memory may be poor, he may be unreliable, emotionally labile, irritable etc. All such symptoms depend to some extent on the underlying personality characteristics. Physical (neurological) features may include ataxia, slurred speech (dysarthria), giddiness, nystagmus, tremor etc. The abdominal reflexes may be decreased, and ankle clonus and the Babinski sign may be present. In contrast to the alcoholic, nutrition in the barbiturate addict is said to be usually well-maintained, though in our experience he may often be in a poor nutritional and generally neglected state.

Withdrawal symptoms begin to appear within the first 24 hours of discontinuation of the drug and rise in intensity within two to three days before gradually fading away. They include anxiety, agitation, disorientation in time and place, nausea, tremor and dizziness, insomnia and a fall of blood pressure on standing. In severe cases, with marked physical dependence, the abstinence syndrome may include convulsions, and a picture resembling alcoholic delirium tremens with restlessness and frightening visual hallucinations. Psychotic episodes with paranoid, schizophrenic and other types of reaction have also been noticed.

Barbiturate abstinence symptoms in infants

The special features of young abusers of barbiturates who inject these drugs intravenously have been described above. Recently, moreover, cases have been reported of infants showing features of physical dependence shortly after birth [51, 52]. In such cases the mothers were either barbiturate addicts or had been prescribed the drug throughout pregnancy or during its last few months.

The phenomenon of physical barbiturate dependency in infancy reminds one of the better known neonatal abstinence syndrome supervening in infants of the heroin-addicted mother. Unlike the infants of heroin-addicted mothers, those born to barbiturate-addicted mothers were fully-grown and showed no respiratory depression. They were restless, jittery, tremulous, or febrile etc. Such symptoms first started in most cases a few days after birth. Most infants required the administration of sedatives or tranquillisers.

As barbituates have been widely used and abused for more than half a century it seems strange that the phenomenon of barbiturate-dependent infants was not recognised long ago. One answer given in a recent editorial in the British Medical Journal [52] is that observation of newborn infants frequently ends after 4-6 days, whereas symptoms of barbiturate-dependent infants often only start later on. Probably now that the syndrome has been described, more cases may come to light.

Non-barbiturate sedative–hypnotics

In view of the risk attached to the misuse of barbiturates, particularly in the case of emotionally vulnerable personalities, non-barbiturate sedatives seem preferable. In accordance with a dictum of a World Health Organising Sub-Committee on Addiction-Producing Drugs some years ago that any drug which can adequately replace another addictive drug may itself lead to dependence, it may be expected that such non-barbiturate sedatives too may not be free from such a risk. With many such drugs, both those used before the advent of the barbiturates and the new products introduced in recent years, this has indeed proved to be the case. However, in our own experience, whilst as a group the newer non-barbiturate sedative–hypnotics are possibly somewhat less effective than the barbiturates, by-and-large the risk of addiction also seems slightly less than with the barbiturates. For example, we have been using several newly-introduced hypnotics in successive years as a routine in alcoholics (who temporarily required an hypnotic). The use of these non-barbiturate sedatives and tranquillisers has enabled us to dispense altogether with barbiturates (and paraldehyde) in the case of alcoholics for 20 years. Certain alcoholics – even those who have received treatment or have found sobriety with the help of Alcoholics Anonymous – seem for ever on the search for new drugs as alcohol-substitutes to bring them immediate relief, and tend to abuse practically any new CNS-affecting drug as soon as it has been put on the market.

Cases where such abuse of non-barbiturate hypnotics has led to psychological and – even less so – physical dependence, have been in our experience much rarer than in the case of barbiturates. However, probably no non-barbiturate sedative can be regarded as completely free from the danger of dependence. We have come successively (not long after their having become available) across cases of psychological dependence on methylpentynol – which enjoyed a high degree of temporary popularity in the mid-1950s – glutethimide, methylprylone, dichlorphenazone, methaqualone (especially in the form of mandrax) and ethchlorvynol, apart from cases of dependence on older non-barbiturates, such as paraldehyde, chloral hydrate and carbromal preparations. Probably because we have always been careful to 'taper off' such drugs in those who had taken them to excess over a certain period – having learnt from our bitter experience with the barbiturate abstinence in the early 1950s – we have not seen cases of a physical abstinence syndrome with any of these drugs. However, this is well-documented in the clinical literature, for example in the case of glutethimide, methylprylone, ethchlorvynol and ethinamate metha-qualone [53]. All these drugs can therefore produce dependence of the barbiturate–alcohol type. With such non-barbiturate substitutes, as with the barbiturates, the continuing search for relief from anxiety, tension, emotional strain and stresses etc. may lead to a rise in tolerance and increase of the dose and establishment of psychic dependence, higher doses continued for a certain period (at least with certain of the newer drugs) also producing physical dependence.

An interesting phenomenon in our experience was that cases of psychological dependence on drugs such as methylpentynol and methylprylone tended to occur much more frequently at a time when there was no restriction on their sale. Thus we saw quite a number of cases of dependence on methylpentynol in the early days after it had come on the market and had attracted a great deal of favourable publicity in the national press. At this time it could be bought freely without prescription over the counter and some of these patients also suffered from episodes of acute accidental or deliberate self-poisoning, chronic intoxication and psychotic periods etc. [54]. Similarly, the two cases of methylprylone seen by us fifteen years ago occurred in former residents of South Africa where apparently (as in Western Germany) this type of dependence was then not uncommon and where the drug could at the time be bought without prescription. Australia is another area where dependence on the various non-barbiturate sedatives has been reported as being not uncommon and as giving rise to diagnostic problems, similar to those arising with the barbiturates. Thus Bartholo-mew [30] found within a period of six months, no less than 38 cases of intoxication with glutethimide in a selected population of alcoholics, psychopaths, neurotics and inadequate and immature personalities. The majority of these individuals had also taken other drugs such as carbromal preparations, barbiturates and tranquillisers. James[55] found among patients admitted to an acute psychiatric ward that 12 % had for years been consuming grossly excessive doses of barbiturates, bromureides,* or glutethimide. All these patients had been admitted in a state of chronic intoxication – a condition which had remained undiagnosed in more than half of them while they had been treated elsewhere for symptoms ascribed to a number of psychiatric illnesses.

Glutethimide was one of the main drugs widely abused by American adolescents. According to Nyswander in 1965, heroin, glutethimide, and amphetamine were the predominant dependence-producing drugs taken by North American adolescent drug addicts. The effect of heroin and glutethimide is synergistic and in East Harlem this combination of drugs at one time constituted, 'the major cause of death from overdose' [56]. In this country the abuse of glutethimide by heroin addicts seems virtually unknown (at least in our experience) and seems to have very little black market status. This is another example of how local fashion, customs of a drug-subcult and similar factors may influence the choice of a given drug by an unstable segment of the population.

A non-barbiturate sedative–hypnotic drug used successfully in cases of alcoholism in recent years is chlormethiazole [57]. Compared with the long history of barbiturates, all these newer non-barbiturates have so far a much shorter observation period which gives them an unfair advantage as regards the observation of possible side-effects, dependence etc. This is a point which of course must always be kept in mind when comparing the merits and risks of old established and recently introduced drugs.

In the case of chlormethiazole, since starting its use, we have rarely come across patients who ask their GPs for further supplies of the drug and who keep on increasing the dosage. Such patients may maintain that chlormethiazole is the only drug that helps them to feel less tense. (In general, where a patient claims that it is just one given CNS-affecting sedative or stimulating drug that provides him with the

---

* These drugs are derivations of urea, monoureide form – '... a group of very weak, slowly acting sedatives, some of which act by releasing bromine' [53]. They are not known to cause physical dependence. Carbromal is the best known example; urethane is another. A combination tablet of carbromal with the barbiturate pentobarbituratone (Carbrital) is occasionally abused in this country, leading to psychic and physical dependence (Incidentally, the barbiturates are derivatives of barbituric acid which is malonyl urea. In contrast to the monoureides which are weak hypnotics, the barbiturates or diureides are of course strong hypnotics)

desired effect and that no other drug will do, the question of a possible or at least threatening state of drug-dependence should be seriously kept in mind.) Such cases of abuse of this drug seem to occur more commonly in areas where practitioners use it for prolonged daytime sedative medication in emotionally unstable personalities. There have been reports of a physical abstinence syndrome, so that chlormethiazole seems to belong to the barbiturate–alcohol dependence-producing-type of drugs. Therefore, except in DT this drug should not be given to vulnerable personalities such as alcoholics for the treatment of withdrawal symptoms for longer than six to seven days (see Section 6.4).

New drugs may have their own special dangers and it may take a long time before they come to light, a danger which was brought home a few years ago by the thalidomide disaster. This potent sedative-hypnotic soon became widely used even when it was found to lead to peripheral neuritis until in 1961 it was discovered that its consumption by women in their early months of pregnancy was fraught with the danger of producing malformed babies. Fortunately nothing similar has as yet been reported with any other newly-introduced non-barbiturate sedatives but they are all likely to have their share of undesirable side-effects and disadvantages. They may vary from case to case but in general the picture of chronic intoxication with these newer drugs resembles that seen in chronic barbiturate poisoning, and a separate, detailed description is unnecessary. Likewise, as stated by the 1964 WHO Expert Committee on Addiction-Producing Drugs [58], 'The characteristics of dependence of the non-barbiturate sedative type are essentially identical with the characteristics of dependence of the barbiturate type . . .'. A great deal of what has been said above in the discussion of problems encountered in the case of barbituric acid derivatives applies equally well to the non-barbiturate substitutes. In certain unstable, immature and inadequate personality types practically any drug with sedative or stimulating effects will sooner or later be discovered to lead to psychological dependence and in the case of the sedatives also physical dependence. The only exceptions to this rule known so far are among the hypnotic drugs, nitrazepam (a benzodiazepine) and among the tranquillisers, the phenothiazines. Though obviously the observation period is much shorter in the case of nitrazepam than, say, with the barbiturates, it is remarkable that over the past ten years there has been no definite report of cases of dependence. In our experience, alcoholics can be relied upon to misuse practically any CNS-affecting drug as soon as they can lay their hands on it. We saw cases of abuse and dependence, for example, as soon as methylpentynol, glutethimide, methylprylone, meprobamate, methaqualone, mandrax, or the stimulants phenmetrazine and methylphenidate became available [59, 60]. The finding that among alcoholic patients (requiring a hypnotic) we have not seen a case of abuse of nitrazepam [61] – despite its use as our routine hypnotic with such patients over the past six or seven years – seems certainly to indicate that any tendency of causing dependence must be very low.

In contrast to nitrazepam, the misuse of, and dependence on, the other popular non-barbiturate hypnotic mandrax (by youngsters even more than by alcoholics) is quite common. Youngsters who are poly-drug abusers often ask for mandrax whilst rejecting nitrazepam. Next to the barbiturates, these two non-barbiturates are probably the hypnotics most commonly taken in suicide attempts [46]. Matthew et al. [46] regard nitrazepam as, '. . . the hypnotic of choice for all patients who are at risk from overdosage', because of its relative lack of toxicity. The common choice of nitrazepam and mandrax as agents of self-poisoning, reflects their high prescribing rates. Parish [62] has calculated that during the six year period 1965 to 1970 the prescriptions of psychotropic drugs (in England and Wales) rose by 19% (from just below 40 million to over 47 million. During the same period prescriptions of non-barbiturate hypnotics increased by 145%, although the annual prescribing rate for all hypnotics remained fairly stable at roughly 20 million. The rise of prescriptions of non-barbiturate hypnotics was caused by the increasing popularity of two drugs, mandrax and nitrazepam. Introduced in the mid-1960s, by 1970 mandrax (2·5 million) and nitrazepam (2·6 million) together accounted for one in four of all prescriptions for hypnotics. There seems little doubt however, that on the illicit market, mandrax is one of the great favourites, nitrazepam, on the other hand is hardly used at all.

TRANQUILLISERS

Since the advent of chlorpromazine, which was synthesised more than 20 years ago, a great many tranquillisers have been marketed and have enjoyed widespread popularity, both in psychiatric hospitals – where they revolutionised the treatment of certain conditions such as schizophrenia and led to a complete change of the therapeutic climate even in the most old fashioned institutions – and in general practice. Some tranquillisers are phenothiazine derivatives like chlorpromazine. Such *major tranquillisers* are often employed in high doses for the treatment of psychotic conditions. Others have quite a different chemical composition, e.g. meprobamate and the benzodiazepines such as chlordiazepoxide and diazepam. The latter drugs – sometimes called the *minor tranquillisers* – are used more often for the treatment of excitable, restless, agitated, tense and anxious states and of neurotics in general practice and in general hospitals. Both types of tranquillisers are also used in the acute withdrawal stage of alcoholism and sometimes of other forms of drug dependence. Although unfortunately such drugs sometimes seem to be used as a convenient, rapid substitute for the proper investigation of the patient's problems, many tranquillisers have proved of the greatest value in the treatment of many minor and major psychiatric conditions and their use over the past twenty years has become more and more widespread. Their field of employment covers to a large extent just those personality types whom one would regard as especially vulnerable to the risk of drug dependence. Under these circumstances the relative rarity of reports of cases of dependence on tranquillisers is striking. The only common exception is meprobamate, and it is interesting to note that pharmacologically it is related much more to the sedatives than to the major tranquillisers such as phenothiazines. Most cases not only of psychological but also of physical dependence (with a physical abstinence syndrome on sudden withdrawal) including major epileptiform convulsions and delirium, have been reported from the USA [53] where the use of the drug is very widespread. During one decade it became '. . . as popular in its way as aspirin', being taken by '. . . about 80 million people, including millions of businessmen, women at home, adolescents facing school examinations and generally anyone reluctant to face the stresses of contemporary life'.

However, cases of meprobamate abuse and dependence have also been seen outside the USA, as for example in Austria, Czechoslovakia, Norway and in this country. In England meprobamate though less popular than in the USA accounted ten years ago for 15% of all tranquilliser preparations. The patients seen by us with psychological dependence on meprobamate were usually unstable personalities who previously had also abused other drugs—such as intelligent but very neurotic alcoholics.

Although in the UK the use of meprobamate was never as popular as in the USA, the other type of minor tranquillisers, the benzodiazepines, have been favourites on both sides of the Atlantic ever since the introduction of chlordiazepoxide in 1960 and of diazepam in 1963. In fact, a recent editorial in the *Lancet* [63] comments that, 'Nothing has equalled the extent to which the benzodiazepines have been used . . .' since their first appearance; and it raises the question as to what extent this large consumption represents '. . . correct use, overuse, misuse, or even abuse, and to what extent do physicians, patients, and the pharmaceutical industry contribute?' to the problem. Occasional cases of psychological and physical dependence – usually following the prolonged intake of rather high dosage – have been described, mainly in USA [1, 53] but also in European countries, such as Austria [64] and Germany [65]. The excessive use of any of these minor tranquillisers may lead to drowsiness, difficulty in thinking, ataxia etc. and may be responsible for traffic accidents, falls, impairment at work and aggressive behaviour. Withdrawal may produce psychological and physical symptoms, including, in severe cases, generalised convulsions, delirium, delusions and hallucinations.

In our own experience with chlordiazepoxide with a great number of unstable personalities, including hundreds of alcoholics during the withdrawal phase, we saw only rare cases where such patients requested the continuation of the drug after it had been stopped by the doctor, or where such patients tried to increase the dose after discharge from hospital. Occasionally one comes across unstable personalities who – having in the past swallowed habitually any CNS-affecting drug to excess at one time or another – had also tried some such tranquilliser as chlorpromazine or chlordiazepoxide in high doses for a day or two, only to declare disgustedly that these had failed completely to give them whatever they were looking for. Similar replies are often given with an air of righteous indignation by individuals (including many modern young drug abusers) dependent on other drugs. These people may profess a willingness to give up their drugs provided they could be supplied with a satisfactory substitute, but they usually declare that these tranquillisers '. . . don't do anything for me; they are no good whatsoever!' This experience is certainly quite different from the one we had in the past in the withdrawal treatment of alcoholics with drugs such as barbiturates, meprobamate and, in the rare early cases, even paraldehyde, all of which were found extremely pleasant (or 'rewarding') to the patients who were very reluctant to discontinue them when asked to do so.

Such experiences seem to show that compared with these other drugs, the risk of psychological and physical dependence certainly seems to be much smaller in the case of the major tranquillisers. To a somewhat lesser extent, this may hold good also for the benzodiazepines, although if used in lighter dosage over prolonged periods psychological and physical dependence may occur. Phenothiazines used by us among the dependence-prone alcoholic population without (so far) producing any definite case of dependence include, apart from chlorpromazine, promazine, perphenazine, trifluoperazine and thioridazine. We came across a few cases of psychological dependence on the proprietary preparation parstelin (which includes trifluoperazine) but the dependence-producing component was probably the stimulant tranylcypromine. Responsibility for the lack of dependence-producing qualities of tranquillisers such as phenothiazines may perhaps be partly due to the fact that they do not lead to an improvement in the feeling of relative well-being or euphoria. From the description of features observed in cases of dependence on the benzodiazepines and meprobamate the similarity to barbiturate dependence – and to some extent also to alcoholism – seems clear. These minor tranquillisers therefore belong to the group of drugs producing dependence of the barbiturate-alcohol type [53].

NON-NARCOTIC ANALGESICS

Among this group of weak pain-killers are drugs such as the salicylates (e.g. aspirin), aniline derivatives (e.g. phenacetin – acetophenetidin – and paracetamol, the substance into which phenacetin is converted after absorption) and pyrazolone derivatives such as phenazone. Aspirin poisoning frequently occurs among young people (self-poisoning) and very young children. However, habitual misuse must be rare, apart from where it occurs as a constituent of the compound codein tablet (which contains aspirin 250 mg, phenacetin 250 mg and codein 8 mg. (Codein is methylmorphine and has a slight analgesic and narcotic action.) Phenacetin is a constituent of several popular proprietary analgesic compounds which sometimes also contains the mildly-stimulating caffeine, e.g. the preparation containing aspirin, phenacetin and caffeine.

Most of the reports of habitual misuse of the minor analgesics come from abroad. As the abuse usually concerns analgesic mixtures it must often be difficult to decide which of the various constituents is the main culprit. In Switzerland such abuse and mild dependence seems quite common and fashionable [66, 67]. The analgesic mixtures there contain mainly phenacetin as well as hypnotic and caffeine; the widespread use

1 2

is indicated by the fact that in 1955, 30 single doses of analgesic tablets or powders were sold per head. The regular users of such drugs in Switzerland are women who belong to an age group in which they are able to follow a gainful occupation, and who are often overworked, tired and harassed, or lonely individuals. Abuse of analgesic mixtures has also been reported from Sweden. Thus in a Swedish town some years ago a high proportion of the population felt unable to start the day without taking a powder consisting of a mixture of phenacetin, phenazone and caffeine; and there was a relatively high number of deaths from renal insufficiency in this area [23]. (Incidentally phenazone is also a constitutent of the non-barbiturate hypnotic compound dichloralphenazone, the other constituent being chloral. We have seen a few cases of habitual excessive use of this preparation.)

Other parts of the world in which analgesic abuse has been reported to be common are Australia and Japan. In a study in Brisbane, second to barbiturates, the non-narcotic analgesics were found to make the greatest contribution to the drug problem. Female abusers, as with barbiturates, were more common than males. Personality instability and alcoholism was found frequently and pain was the reason most often given for starting analgesics [68]. In Japan, from 1964 onwards, abuse of hypnotics began to decrease, whilst abuse of analgesics started to rise following the introduction of stricter control measures for the hypnotic drugs. This indicates that under certain conditions analgesic abuse can form a substitute for abuse of hypnotics. The most commonly abused proprietary analgesic compound in Japan contains allopyrabital, phenacetin, caffeine and benactyzine [69].

The symptomatology of habitual self-medication with such analgesic mixtures – as described by Prof. R. Battegay [70] who has seen many such cases in Switzerland – often resembles the picture of chronic barbiturate intoxication (in particular of course when the compound also includes a barbiturate). Often patients start taking such tablets because of a state of emotional tension and psychosomatic complaints. A vicious circle may arise because compounds containing phenacetin, when taken frequently in high dosage, may themselves lead to headache, inducing the patient to take an even higher dose.

Not much has been written about the misuse of analgesic tablets in this country, although it is probably much more common than generally suspected. Unless patients are specifically questioned about this point they are unlikely to volunteer any information. One occasionally comes across abusers of analgesic compounds (though more frequently those containing codein preparations) among alcoholics and other unstable personalities.

The two most commonly used mild analgesics in this country are aspirin and paracetamol, and although the latter is a metabolite of phenacetin, it seems very much safer. One of the major complications of prolonged consumption of high doses of analgesic mixtures containing phenacetin is renal damage (interstitial nephritis and papillary necrosis) and much has been learned about the danger of phenacetin abuse from observation of patients suffering from analgesic nephropathy [71]. Thus a report from Newcastle [72] describing 14 patients with analgesic nephropathy found that almost all (12 patients) were middle-aged or elderly women, occasionally with a propensity for addiction to tobacco, alcohol and other drugs, who during initial interviews had not referred to their intake of analgesics, probably, '... because they regarded analgesics as harmless domestic remedies unworthy of special mention'. The history often indicated a cycle 'headache-analgesic – withdrawal headache – more analgesic', and these patients had consumed several kilograms of phenacetin, in analgesic or sedative mixtures, over many years. Newcastle workers stress the need for early, life-saving diagnosis. They draw attention to the diagnostic value of sterile pyuria but they go on to say that the best screening test for the condition is careful interrogation of all patients with chronic renal disease of unknown aetiology. However, in view of the improvement of renal function in the majority of these patients it is emphasised that, '... analgesic withdrawal is ... worth achieving even in the presence of advanced renal failure'.

It has been estimated that there is a minimum of 500 new cases of analgesic nephropathy in England and Wales, and even more in Scotland [73]. The number of people in Britain taking five or more analgesic tablets daily without doctor's advice, has been estimated as about a quarter of a million (putting the sales of 'across-the-counter' analgesics as more than £15 million). The total annual number of NHS prescriptions of analgesics in England and Wales between 1965 and 1968 was about 20 million.

Phenacetin has no different therapeutic properties from those of aspirin and paracetamol, and thus there seems no need for its continued use. But aspirin may be responsible for a quarter of the 28 000 annual hospital admissions with gastrointestinal bleeding. R. M. Murray [73], referring to these statistics and literature findings, concludes that the habitual abusers of analgesics are '... extremely vulnerable people who become dependent on the only drugs freely available to them'. He believes that such dependence is encouraged by advertisements for proprietary analgesics stressing their benefits in relieving nerve pains and tense, depressed headaches. He therefore urges doctors to take action in an area of preventable disease by pressing for stricter statutory control of the advertising and sales of 'across the counter' analgesics.

Clearly the wide availability of the minor analgesics favours their abuse, in particular by emotionally-vulnerable personalities, with possible development of psychological dependence and dangerous complications, especially in the case of phenacetin. However, similar to the findings that the non-barbiturate substitutes of the barbiturate-hypnotics are themselves not free from risks, paracetamol – a more recent arrival on the therapeutical scene – has already produced its own problems. Gradually becoming more popular and a constituent of more than fifty compounds sold over the counter, its rising abuse is reflected in the increasing use for intentional self-poisoning. Five years ago there were 150 cases of attempted suicide, now the annual figure has reached 2000. Whereas normal therapeutic doses are said to be safe, any dose over 30 g will damage the liver. However, as recent experiences at MRC Liver Research Unit at King's College Hospital, London have shown, patients stand a good chance of recovery if they are treated within 24 hours of paracetamol overdosage.

One group in whom drug taking should obviously be reduced to a minimum are pregnant women. Recent reports however, have indicated that many pregnant women take CNS-affecting drugs even without a doctor's prescription. Nearly 50% – according to a recent study carried out by Professor John Forfar in Edinburgh – had taken analgesics as self-medication – usually aspirin [74].

Interesting in this connection is Forfar's comment that, '... two other forms of self-administered drug medications were common among these pregnant women, of whom two thirds (including those taking them on prescription) took analgesics: 57% smoked, 88% drank alcohol at least occasionally'.

5.3 CANNABIS AND HALLUCINOGENS

About half a century ago the pharmacologist Louis Lewin employed the term 'Phantastica' to describe drugs giving rise to sense illusion [20]. This is a much better term than the now commonly used name

'hallucinogens', since most of these drugs do not give rise to true hallucinations but to distortions of perception [75]. Hallucinations are false
sensory perceptions which arise on their own in the absence of an
outside objective stimulus, whilst most of the false perceptions arising
out of the taking of these drugs do not occur 'in the absence of an
outside stimulus'. They are usually based on the distortion of something
that is actually there, that is seen or heard [76]. Thus one usually deals not
with hallucinations but with 'illusions', i.e. false perceptions as a
consequence of distortion of real sensory perceptions. In practice it is
often very difficult to know, after listening to an individual's description
of his experiences, whether they were illusions or hallucinations. Other
terms employed for these drugs are *psychotomimetic* (a mimicker of
psychosis, in that their effects resemble brief, temporary states of
schizophrenia), and *psychedelic* (mind-expanding or mind-revealing)
as they are claimed to reveal possibilities of experience which the drug
taker was not aware of before.

Among this group of drugs many have been used for thousands of
years. Some are relatively mild, and others like the most famous
example, LSD 25, are extremely potent. Among them are substances
originating from plants, such as mescaline from a cactus (peyotl),
psilocybin from a mushroom, nutmeg from the nutmeg tree and the
seeds of several varieties of morning glory. The more modern drugs
have been synthesised by the chemist, e.g., LSD, DMT (dimethyl-
tryptamine) and STP, which may stand for 'serenity, tranquillity and
peace', but which chemically is dimethoxy-methyl-amphetamine, or
DOM.

Volatile solvent type. Occasionally a mild hallucinatory state may be produced by
a group of substances, described as volatile solvents, organic solvents,
inhalants or deliriants. However, their main effect is usually a state of
intoxication, with mild euphoria, excitement and mild delirium, at times
ending in unconsciousness. The forerunners of these modern sniffers of the
commercial solvents were, in previous times, substances such as nitrous
oxide, ether, and chloroform, which were inhaled in order to produce a
pleasurable state of intoxication, even before these drugs became officially
used anaesthetic agents. Anaesthetic agents are still today abused by unstable
people, although rarely, and, in isolated cases, abuse by anaesthetists has been
reported. The solvents inhaled by today's sniffers include airplane glue,
gasoline, paint thinners, cleaning fluids, nail-polish removers etc. Glue
sniffing apparently started in California in the late 1950s [77], and enjoyed
much greater popularity in the USA [78], [79] and Canada [77] – chiefly
among underprivileged and unstable youngsters – than in the UK. The

active ingredients of these substances are usually toluene trichloroethylene, aectone etc. (The dependence produced by substances such as toluene, acetone and carbon tetrachloride etc. has been described by a recent WHO Study Group as being of a separate volatile solvent type.) In this country only isolated cases or pockets of glue sniffing in certain localities were reported. The only patients seen by the author were three young, emotionally very unstable and inadequate male glue sniffers, and a fair number of young poly-drug abusers were observed in prison who occasionally inhaled paint thinners. (*Thinner addiction* has previously been reported, e.g. in Sweden [56]. They were not at all enthusiastic about their newly-detected fad, and they used it only – they said – because in prison they could not get hold of anything better, They certainly 'ranked' it far below any other drug which they had abused in the past. Occasionally one comes across heroin and other addicts who give a history of having used such substances in passing and finding them a very unsatisfactory means of obtaining a 'high'. Occasionally mild states of psychological dependence develop in predisposed, unstable people. Often such abuse has unpleasant side-reactions (headaches, nausea, vomiting etc.), and many of the solvents used in industry and at home can be highly toxic.

Chemically the hallucinogens belong in the main to three main sub-groups [53], i.e. indoles, phenylalkylamines, and tetrahydrocannabinols. Among the indoles are LSD, DMT (a short-acting hallucinogen effective when smoked or injected), and psilocybin (effective both by mouth and injection). To the phenylalkylamines belong mescaline (chemically very similar to amphetamine) and STP (which has mescaline-like effects). The tetrahydrocannabinols are '... all hallucinogens if taken in a sufficient dose'; more than 100 have been synthesised. (The whole subject is well documented in a WHO monograph written by H. Isbell and T. L. Chrusciel [53], who list a large number of substances with minor hallucinogenic effects when taken in high dosage). As Dr N. Malleson puts it, 'In a rough and ready way one can say that anything which produces a major disturbance of consciousness without producing (or before producing) actual unconsciousness will precipitate a psychedelic state' [80].

Of all the substances mentioned, in this country and in other parts of the world, only two enjoy widespread and (on the whole, increasing) popularity, i.e. Cannabis and LSD 25. For example, mescaline produces a feeling of nausea, and is not widely used though one occasionally comes across addicts to other substances who have tried it. However, from the historical aspect, it may be of interest to note that a Mexican chronicler forty years after the conquest of Mexico by Fernando Cortez reported:

'The Teochichimekas ... know of peyotl. Those who eat peyotl take it instead of wine. They assemble somewhere in the prairie, dance and sing all day and all night. Then next day they meet again and weep to excess. With their tears they wash their eyes and clear their brains (i.e. return to reason . . .). The plant peyotl ... produces in those who eat or drink it terrible or ludicrous visions. The inebriety lasts two to three days and then disappears. (They) eat considerable amounts of the plant. It gives them strength, incites them to battle, alleviates fear, and they feel neither hunger nor thirst. It is even said that they are protected from every kind of danger.'

Some of this reads almost like a fairly contemporary description, and the last sentence reminds one of the danger inherent in the occasional omnipotent feeling of the LSD user who may step in front of a moving car feeling sure he would be able to stop it, or who may feel capable of flying out through a window. According to Lewin [20]:

'Until 1886 nothing was known as to the nature of this substance. At this time the plant came into my possession during my travels in America. (It was) recognised as a new species of anhalonium (and) received the name alhalonium lewinii. (It) contains four alkaloids, among them the vision-producing mescaline. ... Like the poppy, this alkaloid towers above the rest of the known plants on account of the special character of its effects on man. No other plant brings about such marvellous functional modifications of the brain. Whereas the poppy gradually detaches the soul and the body from all terrestrial sensations ... alhalonium procures . . ., by its peculiar excitation, pleasures of a special kind. Even if these sensations merely take the form of sensorial phantasms, or of an extreme concentration of the inner life, they are of such a special nature and so superior to reality, so unimaginable, that the victim believes himself transported to a new world of sensibility and intelligence ... Quite ordinary objects appear as marvels. In comparison with the material world which now manifests itself, the ordinary world of everyday life seems pale and dead. Colour-symphonies are perceived. The colours gleam with a delicacy and variety which no human being could possibly produce. The objects bathed in such brilliant colours move and change their tint so rapidly that the consciousness is hardly able to follow. Then after a short time coloured arabesques and figures appear in endless play, dimmed by black shadows or brilliant with radiant light. The shapes which are produced are charming in their variety; geometrical forms of all kinds, spheres and cubes, rapidly changing colour ... radiant tapestries, brilliant green, blue ... stripes, trees with light-yellow blossoms, and many things besides.

As well as these objects persons of grotesque form may frequently be seen, coloured dwarfs, fabulous creatures, plastic and moving or immobile, as in a picture. . . . These internal fantastic visions may be accompanied by hallucinations of hearings. These are far more rare than the former. Tinkling and other sounds ... are described as wonderfully sweet and harmonious. The general sensibility may be affected, and then the subject has the illusion of being without weight, of having grown larger, of depersonalisation, or of the doubling of his ego. The sense of time is diminished or completely lost.'

The modern apostles of the hallucinogens' cult are much less cautious than Lewin. For example, Huxley wrote on his experiences largely with mescaline and its derivatives and he called for experiments to decide whether all his visions might be no more than '. . . a hopeful utopian dream' [81, 82]. Timothy Leary, plays down the risks of the LSD 'trips' although many such 'trips' may end in terror and hell. But for a great many youngsters yearning for an 'opting out' on the one hand, and a state of greater awareness on the other, these timeless transformations and states of blissful experience prove an irresistible temptation. The contrast stated to exist between the harmful alcohol and opiates, on the one hand, and the harmless and helpful psychedelics on the other hand, to which Huxley alludes, has often been remarked upon. Thus William Burroughs [83] talks of cannabis as a drug that serves '. . . as a guide to psychic areas', whereas opiates by '. . . diminishing awareness of surroundings can only be a hindrance to the artist'. Similar points of view are often expressed by users of cannabis and LSD when they strongly condemn the stuporous state produced by alcohol. In a recent group session in which both alcoholics and hallucinogen-drug abusers participated, one alcoholic summed up the gist of the discussion in his concluding question: 'Is it that you drug takers want to be aware of life whereas we alcoholics want to forget it?' That this is not simply a question of black or white was illustrated at the same group session when the cannabis taker added that '. . . you may become aware of things too much ... doubt may become a fact and you become convinced that people are looking at you, talking about you'. The LSD user stated that '. . . sometimes, under LSD, things may become too much exaggerated for some people'. It is often said that the average LSD user may be quite a different person from the average heroin–cocaine addict, e.g. recently an American (heroin-addicted) patient talking about American conditions stated that, 'Most junkies do not like LSD which is the opposite to heroin.'

However, the modern young poly-drug abuser often takes any drug that he can get hold of, and youngsters in hospital because of the abuse of drugs, including cannabis and LSD, have not infrequently gone out into a pub and returned drunk. Thus one and the same person under different circumstances may make use of the effects of any or several of these drugs and there is not always a very clear-cut distinction between the different types of individuals attracted to the various drugs. In the USA '. . . not only marihuana but also psilocybin, LSD, peyote and morning glory seeds have been added to the drug repertoire of "beat" circles looking for "offbeat" experiences, often individuals who were formerly . . . involved with alcohol, marihuana, sleeping pills, wake-up pills, demerol and heroin' [84]. As regards the therapeutic value of cannabis and LSD, cannabis is no longer used medicinally in Western culture (although still administered by doctors in India) and the place of LSD in therapeutics has become increasingly problematic.

Cannabis

The Indian hemp plant (Cannabis sativa, Cann. indica) is known the world over under a great variety of names, the many aliases contributing to the confusion in the field. In this country the resin (hashish) is used more commonly than the leaves (marihuana – which is the form used in North America). Smokers of the 'reefer' cigarettes talk about it as 'pot', 'grass', 'weed', 'hash' or 'shit'. In India it is known as bhang or ganja, in North Africa as kif, in South Africa as dagga, as hashish or kief in the Middle East and as maconha in Brazil. The female hemp plant – the leaves and flowering top of this plant contain cannabis – is thus ubiquitous and can be easily cultivated practically anywhere in the world. Its widest growth is in India, Pakistan, Africa and south America. The law treats cannabis as a narcotic but it bears no chemical or functional relationship to the CNS-depressing opiates or the CNS stimulant, cocaine. Experiments in animals have usually found extracts of hashish to induce stimulation and excitement at first, followed later by general depression. At the request of the Commission on Narcotic Drugs of the United Nations it has been banned from pharmacapoieas the world over, though it is still used in some hospitals in India for purposes such as stimulating appetite in some patients. Like opium, cannabis has been employed in Indian systems of medicine for many centuries, and bhang, like opium, was used as a traditional folk medicine. The Chinese seem to have used it therapeutically years earlier than the Indians.

The use of cannabis as a euphoriant is said to have spread from India to the Middle East and North Africa [20], becoming known to the British and French in the nineteenth century. In Paris, hashish became fashionable in the middle of the nineteenth century among bohemian, artistic and literary circles following the publication in 1845, by the French neurologist, Jacques-Joseph Moreau, of his book, 'Du Hachich et de l'Alienation Mentale'. Two of the most famous 'Hashish Eaters' at the time were the poets Theophile Gautier (who founded the Club des Hashischins) and Charles Baudelaire.

The merits of hashish
An article published in 'Chambers's Journal' [85] towards the close of 1848 relates how a French doctor's glowing description of the merits of hashish brought about a kind of hashish epidemic among educated Frenchmen. The article includes rapturous descriptions of the delight of hashish intake and of the increase of musical perception, doubts and warnings about the ultimate danger, local endemic use following the enthusiastic reports of writers and doctors who tried out the drug on themselves and descriptions of the different effects of the drug on different individuals. Almost the whole article could be taken from a contemporary description dealing with cannabis use in Britain, but it is in fact dealing with the 1840s in Paris.

'Amongst several subjects of scientific inquiry in France, placed for the meantime in abeyance by the revolution of February, one of the most re-markable was the peculiar influence of certain drugs upon the human mind, and the alterations which they produce upon the perceptive powers, the imagination, and the reason. The attention of the French public was brought to this consideration by Dr Moreau, physician to the Hospital of the Bicetre in Paris, who, in the year 1846, published a short memoir upon the treatment of 'Hallucinations by the Thorn-apple, or *Datura stramonium*'. Whilst discussing the nature of eccentricities, of fantasias, and illusions, he was led to describe the singular power of a drug, the produce of the Indian hemp, called hashish, of awakening in the mind a train of phenomena of the most extraordinary character, entrancing the senses in delicious reveries, and modifying the organic sensibility. So invitingly did he paint the nature of the new impressions which arose from its use, that in a short time all the physicians and medical students were indulging in doses of this new addition to the charms of life. From them it rapidly spread to the poets, the idealists, and all the lovers of novelty. Each had a different tale to recount. Some saw phantasmagoric figures dancing more exquisitely than Taglioni; others heard sounds of music vibrating on their ears more impressive than Jenny Lind can produce; some of the simple vibrations of a few chords of the harp plunged into the sweetest melancholy; others felt a happiness such as language failed to describe – an exaltation of feeling, which raised them to joys far beyond what this sublunary world can offer. The opium-eater, and the devotee to the wine-bottle, declared that their favourite means of enjoyment possessed little power in comparison to the hashish.

In the year 1845, Dr Moreau gave to the world a work entitled 'Du Hashish et de l'Aliénation Mentale Études Psychologiques', in which we are furnished with the results of his experiences upon himself, upon his friends, and upon patients suffering under mental alienation. Since that period the drug has been subjected to various analyses, and the plant has been reared in France and in Algiers with a view of ascertaining its botanical character; but the ill effects that have followed upon its long-continued use, the uncertainty of the result that succeeds its employment, and the usual fate that attends upon the production of a novelty that everyone at first talks about, together with the late all-engrossing changes, have led to the abandonment of further trials. Still, the subject is worthy of attention, and we trust that its entire character will ultimately be ascertained.

The *Cannabis indica*, or hashish, has long been known in the Levant, as producing what is there called a fantasia. Our English travellers in Egypt, especially Lane, have devoted some attention to it, but rather as a matter of curiosity, than with a view either of trying it themselves, or learning what was the experience of others. The French Savants who accompanied Napoleon paid more attention to the matter. M. Virey, in a memoir published as far back as 1803, in one of the scientific periodicals, gave a medical view of it, and attempted to prove that it was the Nepenthes of Homer. Sylvestre de Lacy has taken a vast deal of pains to learn the ancient history that is to be gleaned relative to it, and has demonstrated that the word assassin is derived from the word Haschichin, which was given to the Ishmaelites who committed murder under its influence. He produces several Arabic texts, which bear out his interpretation, and then quotes the authority of Marco Polo, who tells us that the Old Man of the Mountains – so mysteriously known by our forefathers – educated young men, the most robust of his tribe, to execute his barbarous decrees. To those who delivered themselves up entirely to his will he promised future rewards of eternal happiness, of which he gave them a foretaste by placing them in delicious gardens, adorned with all that Asiatic luxury could imagine as rich and brilliant, and where every sensual gratification was at command. The young men, after having swallowed a certain beverage, were placed in temples within the gardens; and there, while under the influence of intoxication, indulged to the utmost in their degrading passions, till such was their rapture, that at a word they would throw themselves from the summit of a tower, rush through flames, or strike a poniard in the heart of their dearest friend.

Of those who have experienced the effects of the hashish in France, some have described their sensations in print. Amongst these is Theodore Gautier, one of the most distinguished writers of the day. He has, in the newspaper edited by Emile de Gerardin, *La Presse*, given the following testimony of its singular influence: 'The Orientalists,' says he, 'have, in consequence of the interdiction of wine, sought that species of excitement which the western nations derive from alcoholic drinks. The love of the ideal is so dear to man, that he attempts, as far as he can, to relax the ties which bind the body to the soul; and as the means of being in an ecstatic state are not in the power of all, one person drinks for gaiety, another smokes for forgetfulness, a third devours momentary madness – one under the form of wine, the others under that of tobacco and hashish.' He then proceeds to say that a few minutes after swallowing some of the preparation, a sudden overwhelming sensation took possession of him. It appeared to him that his body was dissolved, that he had become transparent. He clearly saw in his chest the hashish which he had swallowed, under the form of an emerald, from which a thousand little sparks issued. His eyelashes were lengthened out indefinitely, and rolled like threads of gold around ivory balls, which turned with an inconceivable rapidity. Around him were sparklings of precious stones of all colours, changes eternally produced, like the play of the kaleidoscope. He every now and then saw his friends who were around him disfigured – half-men, half-plants, some with the wings of the ostrich, which they were constantly shaking. So strange were these, that he burst into fits of laughter; and to join in the apparent ridiculousness of the affair, he began throwing the cushions in the air, catching and turning them with the rapidity of an Indian juggler. One gentleman spoke to him in Italian, which the hashish transposed into Spanish. After a few minutes he recovered his habitual calmness, without any bad effect, without headache, and only astonished at what had passed. Half an hour had scarcely elapsed before he fell again under the influence of the drug. On this occasion the vision was more complicated and more extraordinary. In the air there were millions of butterflies, confusedly luminous, shaking their wings like fans. Gigantic flowers with chalices of crystal, large peonies upon beds of gold and silver, rose and surrounded him with the crackling sound that accompanies the explosion in the air of fireworks. His hearing acquired new power; it was enormously developed. He heard the noise of colours. Green, red, blue, yellow sounds reached him in waves. A glass thrown down, the creaking of a sofa, a word pronounced low, vibrated and rolled within him like peals of thunder. His own voice sounded so loud that he feared to speak, lest he should knock down the walls, or explode like a rocket. More than 500 clocks struck the hour with fleeting, silvery voice; and every object touched gave a note like the harmonica or the Aeolian harp. He swam in an ocean of sound, where floated, like isles of light, some of the airs of 'Lucia di Lammermoor', and the 'Barber of Seville'. Never did similar bliss over- whelm him with its waves; he was lost in a wilderness of sweets; he was not himself; he was relieved from consciousness, that feeling which always pervades the mind; and for the first time he comprehended what might be the state of existence of elementary beings, of angels, of souls separated from the body; all his system seemed infected with the fantastic colouring in which he was plunged. Sounds, perfume, light, reached him only by minute rays, in the midst of which he heard magnetic currents whistling along. According to his calculations, this state lasted about 300 years; for the sensations were so numerous and so hurried, one upon the other, that a real appreciation of time was impossible. The paroxysm over, he was aware that it had only lasted a quarter of an hour.

A case, taken down in notes immediately after its occurrence, may be relied on as perfectly authentic, and as giving a notion of the varied nature of the influence of hashish. The individual, aware of its effects, not by experience, but by what he had heard, having swallowed some of the drug, sat down to the dinner-table; and, beginning the dinner in a true French style, ate some oysters, and then suddenly burst into a loud fit of laughter, which soon ceased. He was calm again until the dessert was placed on the table, when he suddenly seized a large spoon, to defend himself against a preserve of fruits, which he fancied was going to fight a duel with him, and then, with a shout of laughter, he rushed from the dining room. He seated himself in the saloon at the pianoforte, and com- menced an air, which was suddenly put a stop to by a horrible vision. The portrait of his brother, which hung over the instrument, became animated, and presented him a three-pronged staff, terminated by three lanterns – one red, one green, and one white. This apparition returned frequently in the course of the evening. Whilst seated on the sofa, he exclaimed suddenly, 'Why bind my limbs? I feel that I become lead! Oh, how heavy I am!' He was taken by the hands to lift him, when he fell upon the ground upon his knees, as if about to pray. Being lifted up, a sudden change came over him. He took the shovel from the fireplace to dance the Polka; he imitated the voice and gestures of the actors he had lately seen.

He fancied himself at the Opera; the people, the noise, and lights, elevated
his spirits to their highest pitch. He gesticulated, made a thousand in-
coherent speeches, and rushed into the next room, which was not lighted
up. Something frightful then came over him: he fell into an immense well;
it was unfathomable; he tried to lay hold of the stones that projected on
the sides of the well, but they fell with him into the abyss. The sensation
was painful, but of short duration, and again the scene of the Opera
appeared. He spoke of persons whom he had not seen for years; spoke of a
dinner at which he had been present five years before, although he was
conscious that he was at home, and that all he then saw had passed a long
time before, yet he saw before him two persons whom he had then met.
But a bliss that could not be described was the sight of an infant in a sky of
blue and silver, with white wings bordered by roses; he smiled, and
showed two beautiful teeth. He was surrounded by children with wings,
and flying in a blue sky, but they were not equally lovely. These all rapidly
vanished, after being a source of infinite delight; and suddenly the hashish
called up the land of lanterns. These were people, houses, trees, formed of
lanterns, in parallel rows; these lanterns marched, danced and jumped
about; in the midst of them appeared the three lanterns which belonged
to his brother's fork. One brilliant light seemed superior to all; this was
evidently produced by a piece of coal in the fireplace, for when it was
extinguished, the light disappeared with it. On drinking a glass of lemonade, the baths of the Seine rose up in view, where with difficulty he was
saved from drowning. A thousand fantastic visions floated across the mind
during the three hours of its influence, and there was a mixture of sensations such as only are felt in a dream.

Scarcely two people feel the same effects from hashish. Upon some it
scarcely acts at all; and there appears to be a power to resist within, which
can at pleasure be called into force. It generally has a striking action upon
females, sometimes producing a most extraordinary state of excitement;
but there seems to be no indication by which the intensity of its power can
be anticipated. There is something very analogous to the state of dreaming
through the whole progress of a paroxysm caused by it. A train of apparently
unconnected ideas rush across the imagination, and in their transition are so
rapid, that no chain that links them can be seized by investigation.

The ordinary physical effects of hashish are the feeling of a slight com-
pression of the temporal bones and the upper parts of the head. The respira-
tion is gentle; the pulse is slightly accelerated; a gentle heat, such as is felt
on going in winter into a warm bath of a temperature of about 98 degrees
is felt all over the surface of the body; there is some sense of weight, about
the fore part of the arms, and there is an occasional slight involuntary
motion, as if to seek relief from it. There are certain indefinable sensations
of discomfort about the lower extremities; they do not amount to much,

but are sufficient to render the body uneasy. If the dose, however, has been too large, it is not uncommon for several disagreeable symptoms to show themselves. Flashes of heat seem to ascend to the head, and even a boiling sensation in the brain has been felt; a sensation which not unusually creates considerable alarm. Singing in the ears is complained of; then comes on a state of anxiety almost of anguish, with a sense of constriction about the chest. Towards the epigastrium most of the untoward symptoms are referred. The individual fancies that he hears the beating of his heart with unaccustomed loudness, but on placing the hand on the region of the heart, it will be ascertained that its action is perfectly normal. Throughout the whole period it is the nervous system that is affected, no other part of the body being acted upon; hashish thus materially differing from opium, whose power is marked upon the muscular and digestive system, retarding the action of the organs, and leaving them in a complete state of inaction.

Under the influence of hashish, the ear lends itself more to the illusion than any other sense. It has been observed by those who devote their attention to the aberrations of intellect, that hallucinations of hearing are much more frequent than those of the eye or the other senses; for one diseased person who sees visions, there are three that are deceived by the ear; and the more intellectual are more generally prey to this affection. Luther held long conversations with a demon, and Tasso with an angel. The hashish gives to this sense an extreme delicacy and susceptibility; it is felt within the whole system; the sound seems to reach the heart; it vibrates in the chest, and gradually awakens remembrances and associations of ideas and imparts a feeling of increased sensibility. There is a species of ecstasy, a state of exaltation produced, that defies all explanation. The sight is seldom so much affected; there is rarely anything in the shape of a vision conjured up, but objects that are present are conveyed to the brain in a false view. Sometimes the face of a friend is multiplied, or an object of no striking character is converted into a beautiful figure – is metamorphosed in a thousand different forms; thus an old servant of 71 years of age, in spite of his wrinkles and grey hair, appeared before Dr Moreau in the form of a lovely girl adorned with a thousand graces; a glass of lemonade in the hands of a friend became a utensil full of burning charcoal; a hat and a coat placed upon a table were transformed into a rickety little dwarf, having the characteristic appearance of one of those hideous persons formerly employed to amuse the great, but not possessing the symmetry either of Sir Jeffrey Hudson or our inimitable Tom Thumb: the touch is occasionally modified, sometimes being endowed with a high degree of sensibility. The most singular hallucinations were those produced by the hashish in some cases of plague in which it was employed to allleviate suffering by Dr Auber: a young artist imagined his body endowed with such elasticity that he fancies that he could enter into a bottle and remain there at his ease;

one individual fancied that he had become the piston of a steam-engine; another felt himself growing into a balloon, ready to float upon the air. Some of the young Europeans at Cairo, on their way home after a feast of hashish, thought that the dark and dismal streets of the city had been suddenly illuminated; they persuaded each other that there was a magnificent fete going on, that the balconies of the houses were filled with crowds dressed in gala habits, and making loud noises, there being no real foundation for the supposition beyond the return home of some persons attended by Arabs carrying coloured lanterns.

Three persons had formed a party to try the hashish – an architect, who had travelled in Egypt and Nugia, Dr Aubert Roche, and Dr Moreau. At first the latter gentleman thought that his companions were less influenced by the drug than himself; then, as the effect increased upon him, he fancied that the person who had brought him the dose had given him some of more active quality. This he thought to himself was an impudence, and then he involuntarily reflected that he might be poisoned; the idea became fixed; he called out loudly to Dr Roche 'You are an assassin, you have poisoned me!' This was received with shouts of laughter, and his lamentations excited mirth. He struggled for some time against the thought; but the greater his efforts were, the more completely did it overcome him, till at last it took full possession of his mind; then a new illusion, the consequence of the first, drove all other thoughts from him. The extravagant conviction was uppermost that he was dead; that he was upon the point of being buried; his soul had left his body; in a few moments he had gone through all the stages of delirium. These fixed ideas and erroneous convictions are apt to be produced; but they are very evanescent, they last but a few seconds: it is only when there is any actual physical disorder that they remain for any length of time. The ordinary effect of this marvellous drug, however, is an ideal existence, so delicious that there is no wish to shake it off. The Orientalist, when he indulges in it, retires into the depths of the harem; no one is then admitted who cannot contribute to his enjoyment. He surrounds himself with the Almehs or dancing girls, who perform their graceful evolutions before him to the sound of music; gradually a new condition of the brain allows a series of illusions, arising from the external senses, to present themselves. Everything wears a fantastic garb. The mind is overpowered by the brilliancy of gorgeous visions; discrimination, comparison, reason, yield up their throne to dreams and phantoms which exhilarate and delight. The mind tries to understand what is the cause of the new delight, but it is in vain. It seems to know that there is no reality. The positive sensation of universal contentment is the marked feature of the state: it pervades every fibre, and leaves nothing to desire. The narrative of the monarch, so admirably told in the *Spectator*, who, though plunging his head for an instant only in water, lived during that short time several years in another existence, and went through numerous vicissitudes, seemed realised. On one occasion, when Dr Moreau, previous to his going into the opera house, had taken his accustomed dose, he fancied that he was nearly three hours passing through the lobby before reaching the boxes. This phenomenon attends equally upon opium-eating: centuries seem to elapse, during which long trains of visions stalk in endless line before the sight. Mr. De Quincey has furnished us, in his 'Confessions of an Opium Eater', with some most singular illustrations of this fact.

It is not with impunity that the brain becomes disordered with frequent indulgence in the delicious poison; at last it becomes weakened, and incapable of separating the true from the false; the intoxication too frequently repeated leads to an occasional state of delirium, but this is manifested in a manner almost as singular as the effects just narrated. It must be remarked that, during the dream of joy, there is a consciousness that all is illusion; there is at no period a belief that anything that dances before the senses, or plays upon the imagination, is real; and when the mind returns to its wonted state it acknowledges its illusions, and only wonders at the marvels that have been excited. But after these fantasies have too frequently presented themselves, there arises a permanent morbidity of mind, having for its manifestation a fixed idea – that of seeing beings belonging to an invisible world under various shapes. The Orientalists, and more especially the Arabians and the people of Egypt, believe, as is well known, in the existence of djinn or genii, a class of spirits forming an intermediate link between angels and man. There are in Egypt many persons who firmly believe that they have seen and held intercourse with these beings, nor can any attempt at reasoning persuade them that they have been deceived. The eaters of hashish are subject to such hallucinations. When Dr Moreau was in Egypt, the dragoman, who was a man of superior sense, having been selected by Champollion as his interpreter, the captain of the vessel in which he went up the Nile, and several of the sailors, had seen genii. The captain had seen one under the form of a sheep, that had lost itself, and bleating very loudly. He took him home with the intention of shearing him, and making the wool into a garment, and then eating him, when suddenly he rose up in the form of a man to the height of 20 feet, and with a voice of thunder spoke to him, telling him he was a djinn, and then disappeared. His dragoman had met an ass in the neighbourhood of Cairo that he wished to lay hold of; it ran with the speed of lightning, announcing itself a djinn with loud shouts of laughter. On another occasion he had been at the funeral of two holy men, Santons. He saw, and others saw very clearly with him, the coffins of the deceased lift themselves in the air, and place themselves on the height of Mokatam, a mountain near Cairo, in the mausoleum which had been destined for their reception. The individuals of whom Dr Moreau speaks passed three months in his service, during which they were in the complete possession of their senses; but such was the state to which they were reduced by this drug, that they would upon any trifling occurrence be affected with these illusions, and neither ridicule nor reasoning could shake their belief. The limited use of the hashish in France has as yet led to no derangement of this kind; but the knowledge that such consequences result from it is of the greatest importance, as it acts as a check to an indulgence in that which would soon become a vice. It may be emphatically said that none of nature's laws can be violated with impunity, nor can that reason which renders man pre-eminent be misapplied without a punishment.'

Alongside the many reports extolling the virtues of cannabis there have nevertheless always been voices crying out against its abuse. For example, 'In the year 1378 the Emir Soudoun Sheihouni tried to end the abuse of Indian hemp consumption among the poorer classes by having all plants of this description in Joneima destroyed, by imprisoning all the hemp-eaters and by ordering that all those who were convicted of eating the plant should have their teeth pulled out; many were subjected to this punishment. But by 1393 the use of this substance in Arabian territory had increased!' [20]. The views regarding the dangers of cannabis expressed by various authorities in the different parts of the world are still confused and contradictory even to this day. It has often been pointed out that even now there is not sufficient information available as regards the various forms of cannabis, that one does not know whether the plant cultivated in one part of the world is the same as in other parts, and that the proportion of constituents of the plant is dependent on its origin. Thus hashish and cannabis could really be essentially different products. They may denote in effect mixtures of different substances having completely different activities. The tetrahydrocannabinols are now held to be the active principle in cannabis, but the different methods of growing the plant and preparing hashish in the various countries produce differences in the proportion of active principles present which may to some extent explain the various effects observed. Thus it becomes essential to try to isolate the active pure substance and to carry out research with it. In the past the work done has been carried out on mixtures of unknown potency and constitution. 'The mode and site of actions (of cannabis), as well as its distribution, metabolism and excretion are still unknown. We are dealing with mixtures of active and less active chemical compounds, some of which may have their activity modified by their particle combustion when smoked. The yield of resin from the plant varies with the climate of its place of cultivation and with the method of harvesting. If tetrahydrocannabinol be the main active principle we still have the problems of mixtures of isomers, their stability, solubility, absorbability; no wonder, then, that few plant products are so variable and unpredictable in their effects as cannabis and its extracts. There remains plenty to do.' In this way Prof. A. D. Macdonald, then President of the Society for the Study of Addiction, summed up the proceedings of an International Hashish Symposium in 1965 [86]. Prof. Macdonald's statement that a lot remains to be done in this field is still true even today. However, the first isolation in 1964 in pure form of a natural tetrahydrocannabinol by Gaoni and Mechoulam [87] and the isolation of about 25 other natural cannabinoids have paved the way for systematic, scientific neurochemical, pharmacological and behavioural studies which are beginning to throw new light and to raise new questions. Δ'-THC is regarded as the major psychotomimetic principle in cannabis, with other constituents (cannabiboid or non-cannabiboid in nature) playing a minor part in determining the effects and side-effects. Authoritative reviews of present-day knowledge gained with the help of recent THC studies have recently been presented at the 1972 Second Symposium on Cannabis organised by the Institute for the Study of Drug Dependence [88]. An interesting early finding obtained with Δ^9-THC (equivalent to Δ^1-THC) was that of a highly significant, positive dose-effect relationship in man on pulse rate and subjective responses – and apparently also impairment of recent memory. Tests also showed that cannabis could have an adverse effect on cognitive functions. In mental tests those functions which were most dependent on recent memory were found to be most sensitive. In motor tests functions that required a high degree of concentration were not sensitive. Effects appeared with low amounts of THC, e.g. with the equivalent of one marihuana cigarette consisting of 500 mg of 0·7% THC-containing material. Cigarettes containing 2 mg THC were stated by Mechoulam to be effective, whilst those with a 5 mg THC content would give a 'pretty high' feeling. As at least 50% is destroyed on smoking, the effective doses might be as low as 0·5–1 mg. It is therefore of interest to note that a WHO Scientific Group Report [89] in 1971 estimated the daily THC consumption among North American marihuana users as 5–10 mg and the average daily dosage range in India and North Africa from 13–66 mg. Keeping in mind these marked regional differences in the amount of THC, and the findings about dose-effect relationship in mind, it would seem easier to understand the gross discrepancies in the effects of cannabis reported in the past from the various countries.

Cannabis 'habitues'

In many countries cannabis is the drug most widely used by young people. How widespread such cannabis smoking is, is impossible to say as its use is illegal, but the gradual rise in the number of prosecutions for smuggling the drug and for possession indicate a marked rise in its popularity in recent years. Originally in the 1950s, smoked in England by a section of the coloured population, jazz musicians and by unstable youngsters, its use has now been widely accepted by many stable young people, including students. In 1967 Abrams [90] reported that undergraduates had introduced the large-scale smoking of cannabis to Oxford in 1963, '. . . about the time that pop music, pop art and pop culture became a country-wide intellectual fad', and that, 'At least 500 junior members of the university . . . smoke cannabis when it is available'. According to information given at the time to the author, a similar proportion of 5% of Cambridge students smoked 'pot'. Nowadays the proportion of cannabis users throughout British universities is undoubtedly much higher. In England, marihuana is at present much less popular than hashish. Smokers who have tried both state invariably that hashish is the much more potent of the two. The personal experiences of many cannabis smokers have in fact been borne out by recent scientific studies, so much so that the United Nations' Laboratory has now prepared two different reference samples [88] of cannabis, i.e. the marihuana type, containing 2·6% THC, and the more potent hashish type, with 7·4% THC. The use of such reference samples by research workers the world over should greatly enhance the value of the comparison of the results obtained.

Smoking reefer cigarettes is the only popular way of using cannabis in this country; taking it by mouth and chewing or snuffing it seems uncommon. There seem to be certain differences between the effects of smoking and of eating cannabis. With smoking (the average cannabis smoker has been estimated to take about 4–8 mg THC) the effects come on and pass off more rapidly than with eating. The effects start within $2\frac{1}{2}$ hours and reach their peak in three hours. The intoxication period after smoking may last for about one hour as against 3–4 hours after eating [88]. Hashish smokers seem to be a fairly representative cross-section of the community, and whilst by and large unstable youngsters may be more attracted to the substance than the stable ones, clearly with more prevalent use there is now every likelihood of exposure and temptation coming across the path of the average youngsters. J. M. Watt [91] who worked with cannabis users in South Africa concluded on the basis of certain studies published in India by the Chopras, that personality traits were the primary cause of the cannabis habit and that cannabis habitues were unstable individuals, suffering from the same fundamental personality defects as other drug dependents. Impressions obtained in this country may possibly to some extent support this view as regards the habitual, very heavy smoker. One has to keep in mind that smokers who have progressed to taking of hard drugs, or who have acquired definite psychological dependence on it, or who have been found in possession (possibly because they have been smoking more regularly and exposing themselves more frequently to detection), do not constitute a representative sample of all smokers. A great many youngsters seem at present to smoke on certain occasions and at certain times only, apparently without coming to any harm and without escalating towards hard drugs. However, other factors being equal, it seems likely that the smoker with personality difficulties may be more tempted to become a habitual smoker than the otherwise normal youth who has no more than his fair share of personality problems and stresses. Availability and acceptance by the individual's own in-group or subculture must play an important part in introducing him to cannabis in the first place and attracting him towards regular use. Jellinek's hypothesis (see Section 2.3) as regards the acceptance of heavy drinking in a society and the prevalence of alcoholism [92] may also hold good for cannabis: in a society where cannabis use is widely accepted and regarded as normal or the done thing, even relatively stable members of this group may begin to take it more or less regularly. Where, on the other hand, the use of cannabis is frowned upon, mainly unstable individuals may expose themselves. Statements regarding the emotional instability or otherwise of the average cannabis user must therefore be read in association with the prevalence and acceptance of the habit in the country concerned and in particular the individual's own in-group.

The risk of escalation
Another aspect of the problem is the criticism often made that it is the illegality of cannabis that attracts certain youngsters to smoking, and that legislation would take away the glamour of the forbidden. Whilst

this may hold good for many individuals, there are certainly other youngsters who do not embark on smoking because they feel that there must be some good reason for the majority of medical opinion and for a law against cannabis smoking. Were such laws changed, this segment of the young population might then in all probability take up cannabis use. With advertising giving it glamour many more youngsters might become habitual smokers with the risk of the more unstable and vulnerable among them becoming psychologically dependent. Despite many popular pronouncements to the contrary it has certainly *not* been proven that hashish (and its various varieties) is free from any harmful effects. On the other hand, it is true that smoking as an illegal act may drive the smoker into the company of antisocial groups and into a delinquent subculture. Having started regular smoking such an individual may begin in time to look at himself as an asocial character – as society at large treats him in that way – and may respond by acting as such in an expectation-fulfilling manner. Having to acquire cannabis from pushers he may sooner or later also come into contact with people taking and selling the hard drugs. In this way cannabis users run a much greater risk than the average person of being introduced to heroin. Having already embarked on the illegal act of drug taking and having already discovered that one allegedly dangerous drug subjected to specific regulations – i.e. cannabis – had so far not produced any ill-effects, the step towards taking other drugs might not be too difficult. Thus it is not surprising that cannabis use may occasionally be the forerunner of heroin addiction. In fact in the initial period of the 'H–C' epidemic in this country in the early 1960s, practically all the young heroin-cocaine addicts we came across had previously taken marihuana. Almost all, incidentally, had also taken pep pills. (The average youth addicted to 'H–C' in the mid-1060s had started to smoke cannabis at the age of 16·5 years and to take pep pills at 16·9 years, before going on to 'H–C' at 18·5 years [93]. On the other hand we have come across a far greater number of regular cannabis smokers who had been at it for years without escalating to hard drugs. It would seem therefore that going on to heroin is certainly a greater hazard for the smoker than for non-smokers, but it is by no means inevitable and it happens only in a (probably relatively small) minority [94]. It would therefore seem wrong to base all education against the use of cannabis on the risk of escalation to heroin. It is also unwise as most young smokers know many veteran smokers who have used it for years without having gone on to heroin. Such youngsters could then write off any education coming from such quarters as incredible and biased.

Whilst much has been written on escalation from cannabis to heroin, little has been said on the much more likely escalation from cannabis to LSD. In its effects cannabis is, of course, much more like LSD than heroin which is basically quite a different type of drug. One hears some cannabis users say, 'A weak LSD trip is like smoking hashish to me – both exaggerate one's senses, one becomes more aware of what is happening to one'. In theory, escalation from cannabis to LSD – from a minor to a stronger hallucinogen – seems much more likely than from cannabis to the narcotic heroin. In practice, in the author's experience, when questioning addicts about the frequency of escalation from cannabis to heroin and to LSD respectively among their smoking friends, escalation to LSD was mentioned as a much more common occurrence [95]. The likelihood of a considerable proportion of cannabis users graduating to LSD should surely be kept in mind in any discussion on the question of legalising cannabis.

Drug dependence of the cannabis type

Reference was made above to the habit of cannabis smoking. The average smoker in this country when asked about the possibility of becoming dependent on cannabis immediately replies, 'No, it is not addictive', a statement which has almost become a slogan among the hashish users. They imply by such an answer that there is no risk whatsoever attached to cannabis, which they usually compare favourably with alcohol, the standby of their fathers and the middle-aged with whose values and attitudes they often disagree. Clearly a drug can have other dangers even if it is not addictive. Cannabis has occasionally been reported by some observers (mainly abroad) to lead to temporary psychoses, emotional maladjustment and crime (probably chiefly in the predisposed). At any rate, the statement that hashish is not addictive is true only if the term addiction is understood in the strictly pharmacological sense, i.e. as producing physical dependence. There are certainly no physical abstinence symptoms when the drug is suddenly discontinued. However, some smokers find the effects of the drug so attractive and the lure of returning to the state of relaxation and perhaps exhilaration so great that they seem to be unable to refrain from going on with their smoking whatever the risks involved. In many cases this behaviour seems to make nonsense of their claim that they could give up the drug whenever they wanted to. This reminds one of the alcoholics' perpetual claims that they could take or leave the alcohol at will. Thus whilst many smokers are able to give up the habit readily, some nevertheless find it very difficult and quite a few become psychologically dependent on it. Two examples that come to mind concern firstly a student who having been a gregarious, social marihuana smoker for a while, began to smoke it by himself whilst going through a period of stress and became strongly dependent on it [3]. Secondly, an 18 year old girl who apparently never before had ever dreamt of soliciting found herself on the verge of doing so when she no longer had any means of paying for her hashish supplies. It would seem therefore that the frequently made comparison between the regular cannabis smoker and the social drinker is not really correct. The average moderate social drinker – whatever his underlying unconscious motives – does not usually drink to get into a state of slight inebriation, though alcohol may act for him as a special lubricant. The average cannabis smoker, on the other hand usually aims definitely at feeling quite different and at getting 'high'. A more apt comparison would thus be between the hashish user and the regular relief drinker or the drinker in the prodromal phase who has started to use alcohol as a drug and no longer merely as a social drink. (See Figure 1 in Appendix.)

In the past it has often been said that unlike most other dependence-producing drugs cannabis does not lead to tolerance; i.e. that users do not need to increase the dose in order to obtain the effects they want to achieve. However, occasionally one comes across users who have been taking the drug for some time and complain that it no longer satisfies them, that they no longer get the kick and the thrill from it which they had before, and it is in this frame of mind that they may be tempted to try 'heavier artillery' in the shape of LSD or even heroin. Regarding the question of cannabis tolerance, as in other aspects, research now being carried out with the active constituents of cannabis rather than samples of unknown composition, seems gradually to be leading to some revision of formerly held views. As long as a century ago it was first noted that marihuana users may develop an increasing sensitivity on repeated exposure to the drug, thus experiencing a stronger effect (*reverse tolerance*). This is sometimes commented upon by cannabis smokers. On the other hand recent studies with laboratory animals have indicated that tolerance does in fact develop to certain effects of the drug though not to others [88].

The newer WHO substitution of the term dependence in place of the former addiction and habituation has much to recommend it, but bringing both cannabis and the opiates under one all embracing term, 'dependence', may have the disadvantageous consequence that youngsters having with relative impunity tried hemp may lose their fear of dangerous drugs in general. The harmful physical and mental complications of the opiates (and of the life style associated with their use) in the great majority of their users are clearly on a quite different scale from those produced by cannabis in a minority; and the goal sought by the cannabis and opiate users is often quite different. As the Chopras [96] expressed it, 'Unlike the opium, morphine or heroin addict who must have the drug to feel normal . . . . the hemp addict wants to recapture the pleasurable euphoric state into which the drug lifts him'. The pharmalogical nature of the drugs concerned is very different: in the case of the opiates the role of the drug is much more important (as a rule) than the users's make-up and the environment (except in the relatively infrequent 'stabilised addicts'—see Part 3), and the great majority of regular users taking an opiate regularly for a few weeks run a grave risk of becoming psychologically and physically dependent. In the case of cannabis the role of the individual's personality (and also of the environment) is of much greater importance than the nature of the drug, and, apart from the factors already mentioned – i.e. the regional variations in potency and composition of the extract, the strength of the preparation, the mode of application on the one hand, and the social setting on the other – the individual's personality make-up, his ego-strength, his expectations of the effect of the drug and his experience with it are all interacting factors which influence the outcome in the given individual. As far as cannabis as a dependence-producing drug is concerned our own experience by and large would tend to confirm the description given by Eddy and co-workers [8].

'Drug dependence of the cannabis type is a state arising from chronic or periodic administration of cannabis or cannabis substances (natural or synthetic). Its characteristics are:

(a) moderate to strong psychic dependence on account of the desired subjective effects,

(b) absence of physical dependence, so that there is no characteristic abstinence syndrome when the drug is discontinued, and

(c) little tendency to increase the dose and no evidence of tolerance.' (Though recent studies throw doubt on this question of lack of tolerance.)

The effects of cannabis
The effects of cannabis vary a great deal. The first Interdepartmental

Committee [39] described it as an intoxicant. In general, effects vary from earlier phases of excitement, loquacity, confusion and perhaps hallucinations, to later stages of irritability, drowsiness and sleep. Individual factors enter into the symptomatology and into the experiences a great deal. Trocchi states that, 'Perhaps the principal effect of marihuana is to take one more intensely into whatever experience' [97]. Patients have described its effects variously as:

'... smoking on one's own is not much good although you may be able to get high for a little while. Usually you can enjoy smoking only when you are in company.... Smoking is a state of mind. It is no good smoking when you are depressed although I can still enjoy it when I am in a state of apathy.... My smoking has gone down a lot since I started "fixing" heroin'.

(a girl, aged 19)

'I started to smoke marihuana when I was 16 from natural curiosity as I had heard such a lot about it.... It opened new fields for me... it made me feel "heady", it increased my awareness of everything and helped me to appreciate things better – paintings and music. ... It made me feel creative – ideas flow better to me.... I smoke alone sometimes but I prefer it in company.... Occasionally I have the "horrors" – great fears, but they do not deter me from smoking although I have no craving for marihuana. . .'.

(a girl, aged 23)

'I started marihuana when I was 15, gradually taking more and smoking up to four cigarettes per day. It was hard then to give it up when I was smoking regularly. But nine months ago I started "fixing" heroin and now I have no difficulty in leaving marihuana alone – I now smoke perhaps one a month. . .'.

(a youth, aged 20)

'I started marihuana when I was 19; now it is mainly hashish as there is not much "weed" about. I am always pleased to have a smoke but I do not find it a compelling habit, quite unlike the amphetamines for example; with them the more I take the more I want. . .'.

(a youth, aged 22)

'I tried kief when I was abroad; it made me buoyant and talkative at times; it brings the extreme of emotions; you are either very funny or very serious, depending on your mood and the company ... sometimes you laugh at the smallest things ..., but it may help you to concentrate on things. ...

In this country I have been smoking marihuana for the past two years. I find the effect pleasant and I enjoy it ... you can look at a puddle and when you concentrate it may assume the size of an ocean. I have never had hallucinations and I never become aggressive. ... But sometimes I feel that people are staring at me and policemen are taking a close look at me. ... I have come across smokers who become paranoid and who have had the "horrors" from marihuana. ... Time seems to take much longer, it feels as though a whole hour has passed and in reality it was only one minute...' When asked whether he considered this may constitute a danger when driving a car, this man stated that he 'believed there may be accidents from slower reaction: if something happens you may take much longer to react as you may be "paralysed"....

I think I could easily give up marihuana...'. This man had also tried nutmeg once when '... somebody gave it to me. I was told it would give me a "buzz", i.e. a "high".... I ate a little piece but it had no effect.'

(a youth, aged 21)

'I have been smoking continuously for three years, during the past year about half an ounce per day. I could give it up if I wanted to but I do not want to: it gives you a heightened perception of surroundings, music, colours, ... pleasant illusions ... quick thought and talk.... It gives you a nice feeling ... but I also had the "horrors" whilst taking hash: I thought people were talking about me ... that the room we were in was a prison cell ... a girl I was talking to was a policewoman ... I saw policemen coming up the stairs...'.

(a youth, aged 20)

'Shortly after having started on amphetamines in Paris I also began to have cannabis there – kief. The first time I had it it made me laugh, a good healthy laughter, and made me feel good. ... I did not smoke again till I returned to London where I usually smoked it with a group of people but occasionally also by myself. The group contained mostly 20 to 25 people, mainly artists and musicians but in my group there were no students or schoolboys. ... The main effects I got from hash were euphoria, a stimulation of perception of sound, sight, taste and of conceptual thought though the ideas may be quite superficial.... I was often depressed; cannabis sometimes helped to dispel the depression but sometimes it emphasised it. In company cannabis tended to make

me feel more depressed and paranoid, but when smoking by myself I did not usually get depressed, probably because I had more
control over my environment. Cannabis is definitely not dangerous but you can become psychologically reliant on it. . . . I need
something like this sort of drug or some sort of religious or
intellectual stimulus. . . . Normally it stimulated my perception
but not my action. . . . I was smoking large amounts of hash last
summer (1 ounce per week) and the stimulating effect became
deadened. I had reached a saturation point. This had happened
to me before but after leaving off cannabis for two weeks it
regained its former stimulating effect. This time however I went
over to heroin which is quite opposite to cannabis: "H" is more
of an escape, it produces its own feelings rather than cannabis
which exaggerates your own emotions.'

(student, aged 20)

Thus the smoker may often be euphoric and giggle without reason
and talk a lot. Memory may be impaired, reasoning confused and
perceptions distorted. Perception of music, painting and works of art
may be enhanced. Time seems to go very slowly and there may be
restlessness which later turns to drowsiness. Physically the eyes may be
reddened, the pupils dilated and there may be an obstinate cough.
Although smokers often claim to be stimulated by the drug they also
state that the stimulation is of thought only and not of action. Whilst
some continue working whilst regularly taking cannabis, in a great
many the drug by producing mental inertia, apathy and lethargy,
reduces the work drive (although some jazz musicians claim that they
are stimulated to better performances). In some individuals temporary
psychotic episodes may occur but this is often explained on the basis of
an unstable underlying mental make-up. As regards the use of the drug
by youngsters, their preoccupation with the drug and the type of life
that often goes with regular use – with the resulting neglect of interest
in furthering their education and vocational skill – their failure to
look at obstacles as challenges to be faced and overcome and thus as
opportunities for stimulating emotional growth and their concentration of attention on small subgroups to the exclusion of society at large
with the values and ideals completely at variance with each other, can
all in the long run prove to be a serious handicap.

The cannabis controversy

In various countries, such as the USA, Canada and the UK, many voices have been raised asking that the use of cannabis be legalised but the great body of international expert opinion is strongly against such a step. The Commission on Narcotic Drugs of the United Nations at its 20th session [98] in 1965 reiterated its view that, '. . . there could be no question but that cannabis presented a danger to society', e.g. by impairing the individual's social functions, by increasing tendencies to asocial and antisocial behaviour, and by disrupting interpersonal relationships. Special attention was directed to its possible effects on drivers, e.g. when smoked by taxi and lorry drivers, a habit reported to be not uncommon in Africa and Asia. A recent Danish study, using a car simulator and psychological tests, compared the effects of consuming cakes containing 8·16 mg THC to the effects of consuming fruit juice containing 70 g alcohol (producing a blood alcohol level of 100 mg/100 ml). It was concluded that the effects of cannabis on skills and judgements essential for driving were so pronounced as to make motoring during cannabis intoxication a risky procedure [88]. In some unstable people cannabis, by diminishing inhibitions, may allow underlying delinquent and aggressive tendencies to come to the foreground and thus lead to irresponsibility and criminal activities. Aggressive actions may also result from hallucinatory experiences (in smokers who are not experienced in the effects of the drug and who may panic), or from states of oversensitivity and extreme restlessness. However, in fairness it must be stated that Western observers by and large do not regard cannabis as an aggression-producing drug. There has certainly been no evidence of cannabis producing aggression among our patients, but rather of too much calming down with lack of initiative, too much relaxation and lethargy. An interesting hypothesis has recently been put forward in an attempt to explain the frequency of reports of cannabis panics and psychoses emanating from Asia and Africa as compared to Europe and the USA: environmental stress might increase the effect of cannabis, so that possibly poor living and other social conditions in North Africa and India, or also the combat situation of American soldiers in Vietnam, might more readily give rise to adverse reactions [88].

One interesting theory as regards the different cultural attitude of East and West to cannabis and alcohol has been put forward by G. Murphy [99]. In India, the Brahmin priesthood tolerates cannabis because social inaction is believed to have positive aspects, whereas alcohol is rejected as favouring the release of repressed impulses, thereby leading to disturbed behaviour. In Anglo-Saxon cultures on the other hand, Protestantism emphasises the work ethic and is hostile towards inactivity. Here overactivity carries social approval, even where, when as a consequence of drinking, it may be accompanied by disturbances. To some extent, this hypothesis is reminiscent of an older theory explaining the greater acceptance of opiates by the 'peaceful East' as against the popularity of alcohol in the 'competition-favouring West'. Protagonists of cannabis use often compare it favourably with alcohol, claiming that illegal hash is much less dangerous than legal alcohol. Whether this may turn out to be so or not in the long run, this comparison seems largely a 'red herring'. Cannabis should be judged on its own merits, and whether it should be legalised or not should depend on factors inherent in cannabis itself. There is no question that alcohol and nicotine are potentially dangerous substances, but this in itself is no argument for legalising yet another potentially dangerous drug.

In recent years, commissions in three countries have discussed and published reports on cannabis, the Wooton Committee in the UK, the LeDain Committee in Canada and the Shaffer Commission in the USA. Their reports showed quite a few similarities (all of them recommending some liberalisation of the cannabis laws) and had a similar fate. In the words of the leader writer in the magazine, 'Drugs and Society' [100], regarding the question of the harmfulness of the drug, they arrived at a verdict of '. . . not so much NOT guilty as NOT proven'. All these reports suffered from '. . . the same widespread publicity, liberal acclaim and governmental cold-shouldering . . .'. In all these countries, the governments failed to consider any far-reaching liberalising recommendations.

At the present time with increasing prevalence of cannabis use and clamour for its legalisation, the public debate is all too often dominated by emotionally coloured and biased statements, by '. . . little more than assertion and counter-assertion unsustained by accurate scientific knowledge' [88]. During public discussions, it is becoming more and more obvious that the cannabis controversy has come to centre less and less on the harmfulness or otherwise of cannabis but rather on its symbolic function, as a tool in the conflict between the young and the middle-aged, between non-establishment and establishment, between idealism and realism and between the value of the individual v. technology, etc. Yet in Western culture, cannabis is still a relative newcomer and in general people would be chary with the widespread use of a new drug until more accurate knowledge has come to hand regarding its

merits and dangers. To clamour for its legislation seems not only premature but irresponsible until further planned scientific research has
indicated which combination of active constituents may be relatively
harmless for what type of person under which social situation. Too
many overconfident assertions on the effects of cannabis have been
made on the basis of non-systematic observations with types of
cannabis of unknown composition, without any idea of their contents
of psychoactive constituents and without references to the amounts
taken.

Of the many uncertainties surrounding the problems of drug misuse
the subject of cannabis abuse is perhaps the most confused. For example,
controversy still surrounds such vital questions as to whether cannabis
can produce organic brain damage. Keeping in mind however the
differences between the more and the less potent derivatives of cannabis
and the likelihood of future research leading in time to different
assessments, possibly the fairest summing-up of a confusing situation
might be that there is no definite evidence of any harm coming from
occasional use of small amounts, apart from its leading to a 'braindrain
by preoccupation with the drug and the surrounding subculture and
the effects on the predisposed and unstable. However, chronic or
excessive use may lead to toxic changes, psychoses and antisocial
behaviour and emotional dependence – in particular when the more
potent derivatives are used, by the predisposed and perhaps especially
in situations of psychosocial stress.

All over the world it seems cannabis use is becoming more popular.
It has been estimated that in the USA this drug has been tried by 24
million people and used regularly by over 8 million. It may turn out
regrettably, in the present writer's view that as a consequence of
such widespread use and publicity, the drug may ultimately acquire
legal status. Most unbiased observers would probably agree that
cannabis should be legally clearly separated from the much more
dangerous narcotics, and that users – as different from pushers – should
not be treated as criminals. However, many facts about cannabis are
still obscure, and – as discussed above – it is only in the past few years
that research with the active ingredients have become feasible. With
alcohol and nicotine, it took a great many years before some of their
dangers became manifest; by then their popular use had become so
entrenched that it has proved virtually impossible to dislodge them
despite their undoubted dangers to health and life. One can only hope
that the same process may not be repeated in the case of cannabis.

Thus widespread use and clamour may have made the position of cannabis unassailable before research was given sufficient time to uncover its possible risks to the user's health. Obviously, wider social issues are involved but certainly the rapid spread has been greatly encouraged and fostered by what Dr Henry Brill [101] described as '... a highly articulate pro-drug movement with informal leadership and a highly developed pro-drug, anti-establishment dialectic'.

D-lysergic acid diethylamide (LSD 25)

Lysergic acid is the nucleus of the alkaloids of the parasitic fungus ergot, and the state of 'ergotism' – mental change resulting from ingestion of ergot – has been well-known for a long time. Lysergic acid itself does not produce illusions or hallucinations, and it acquires the mind-influencing properties which have made it famous only after a diethylamide group has been added. The psychedelic qualities of LSD were discovered by chance in 1943 by the Swiss chemist Hoffman who accidentally ingested a small amount. He felt dizzy and sank into a somewhat delirious state where he had, '. . . fantastic visions of extraordinary vividness accompanied by a kaleidoscopic play of intense coloration' – a state lasting two hours. Intent to find out what had caused this experience Hoffman proceeded to take a dose of 250 μg of crystalline lysergic acid diethylamide. Abnormal symptoms started after 40 min, becoming progressively worse. He felt dizzy, his field of vision was distorted, '. . . the faces of those present appeared like grotesque coloured masks', and at times he felt himself to be '. . . standing outside myself like a neutral observer and hearing myself muttering jargon or screaming half madly. . . . I heard someone screaming loudly in the room but after a while I recognised that I was the one who was doing the shouting'. After six hours his condition had improved greatly though the perceptual distortions were still present; the next morning he was quite well. In this way Hoffman had accidentally stumbled on this extraordinarily potent hallucinogenic drug, much more powerful than mescaline. To produce the same effects with mescaline much higher amounts would have to be taken. Both have been used by many investigators for purposes of research. The doses of mescaline employed have varied from 200 to 1200 mg, and from 25 to 1500 μg for LSD. The average LSD dose usually employed is about 100 μg (or gamma), about one tenth of a milligram. Most people embarking on a 'joy-trip' for the first time probably take 250 μg, but if they want to make sure that they will 'get there' they may take double this dose. Since the arrival of its synthetic and easily prepared rival – LSD, mescaline has lost much of its popularity, the more so as it is more likely to produce nausea and vomiting.

The effects of LSD
The effects of LSD may be extremely variable. To a large extent they depend on the make-up of the user, on the expectations and the degree of experience with the drug, the mood when embarking on the 'trip', the setting in which it takes place and the company. Effects may be quite different when taken in an impersonal, clinical setting, for purposes of treatment or research, from when the 'trip' takes place in the company of congenial fellow-travellers of 'trippers', all in search of new, visionary experiences. It is factors like these which may largely determine whether the trip will be a pleasant, joyful and happy one, or whether it may be unpleasant, anxiety or panic-producing, and accompanied by paranoid feelings. During the trip the mood may change rapidly as the LSD state produces heightened suggestibility. One patient described how he had felt very relaxed and happy until he realised that all the people previously in the room had left. Then he became panicky, started to scream and was greatly relieved when storm- ing out of the room he met outside people he knew well. Thus the LSD state may sometimes come to resemble an acute schizophrenic state, or to some extent the alcoholic DT, or it may be an extremely happy and joyful experience with the 'tripper' intensely fascinated by a highly delightful coloured picture, in which may be seen (or 'heard') beautiful, indescribable colours or music. Thus it is not only the effect of the drug itself which decides whether the trip leads to a mystic, vision- ary, ecstatic state, or whether it becomes a transport into a condition of temporary insanity. However, the 'joy-trippers' who are often highly immature and emotionally unstable personalities, attracted by the cult, report that as a rule the majority of their trips are very pleasant and most are only too keen to repeat the experience. Even the near- psychotic LSD-induced states, are different from a schizophrenic reaction, the 'tripper' usually retaining some measure of insight and knowing that the whole experience is not 'real' and will pass off sooner or later. The schizophrenic on the other hand, believes in the reality of the fantasy world. The LSD user's hallucinations are usually visual in nature, unlike the schizophrenic's predominant auditory hallucinations. In this way the LSD state resembles more the visual misinterpretations of organic mental states, i.e. conditions produced by

14

definite causative agents and not in an unknown functional manner as in schizophrenia. The best-known cause of visual hallucination is DT (in alcoholics) – and like the LSD 'tripper' the sufferer from DT too has occasionally some measure of insight. However, as a rule the LSD user enjoys his state; the alcoholic suffers from his DT. The LSD 'tripper' surrenders willingly and intensely to his experience; the alcoholic, terror-stricken, tries to escape from it and fights his tormentors and persecutors. The LSD user goes out of his way, searching for and looking forward to the experiences, whereas DT comes upon the alcoholic as a highly unpleasant, unwanted and feared side-effect. The LSD user is attracted by the glittering pictures, the beautiful scenery, which are for the LSD user the rich reward and the attractive goal, whereas DT for the alcoholic is the terrible price he has to pay if he wants to get the relief temporarily provided for him by alcohol.

Keeping in mind that LSD states may vary a great deal from each other the following is roughly what may occur to people taking LSD. Usually it is taken by mouth and things may then begin to happen on average within about 45 min. If the drug is mainlined straight into the vein the experience starts within a few minutes. After a few hours the intensity of the experience begins to fade and disappears altogether within 8–12 hours. Should there be very unpleasant experiences it is possible to cut them short by the administration of tranquillisers. On the other hand, the experience can be intensified by taking amphetamines. On the physical side, the pupil dilates, and the hands may tremble whilst temperature, pulse and blood pressure are usually only little affected. The individual may feel subjectively unable to walk, one patient saying that it came as a great discovery to him that he was in fact able to put one foot in front of the other [3]. The tripper then begins to have the distorted visions, the changes in perception of time and the alteration of emotions described above. He may also feel as if the environment and himself have become one and the same thing – i.e. 'loss of the ego through LSD' – so that memories usually kept repressed may be allowed in the LSD state to come to the surface. Apart from visual changes, hearing and touch may be heightened and appreciation of music increases. Occasionally the feeling of being unable to cope or of being overwhelmed by the experience can lead to states of anxiety, panic, terror or paranoidal states. Most users however experience many more good than bad 'trips'. The whole experience begins to fade after a few hours, for many trippers much too rapidly.

The following account, given by a 20 year old, illustrates some of the features described (as well as the way some 'trippers' talk about their experiences):

Case history

'... Ordinarily I feel like a drifter going around in circles ... there seems to be no point. ... Without drugs I feel like a machine but as I eat I must be living. ... I am on a circle from life to death: there is no point to this existence which is creating more and more neurotics and drug addicts. Being alive like this is hell. LSD puts you into infinity and eternity and when one has lost one's ego through LSD one feels much better. When on LSD you achieve peace of mind, By being in eternity, time ceases, you can comprehend infinity. You have lost your ego and there is no longer a duality between ego and the universe, and thus a guy on LSD has reached infinity and achieved peace of mind. ... Once you have reached Nirvana there is no point in living any more. Methedrine is the absolute opposite of LSD because it boosts the ego. ...

I had a number of LSD trips, 250 μg each, sometimes overlapping. ... It felt like stepping into the middle of the circle, but I felt apprehensive as I still like material life. ... I was no longer myself any more. I could hear the sound of every single leaf, I could see the oaktree beckoning me, I felt at one with the oaktree. I could see the grass growing and moving. I felt I could touch the clouds and the sky. ... I wanted to go further, to step into the void. I was not quite there – so I took more LSD. ... One cannot explain an LSD trip in words – you can see a chair as I do when we are both on LSD.

On another occasion I was developing a paranoia whilst on methedrine and LSD. I was with a girl friend and I wanted her but I did not want her to know. Meanwhile the LSD was building up and I felt like stepping out into the void again. My friend and I concluded that the only answer was death. I felt light and warmth ... but I became frightened. ... I began to feel that I had done wrong, and for the rest of my life I would be alone, in despair, in hell. ... That was the end and I collapsed into sleep.' Nevertheless, he added: 'With LSD I see beauty, and although I also sometimes experience "horrors", I would take it again ... to me, drugs give me something to live for.'

Whatever one may think of the risks or otherwise of the use of cannabis, there is no doubt that LSD is a highly dangerous drug – the more so as its effects are so unpredictable. Under heavy LSD dosage, the experienced 'tripper' may experience what he regards as exalting revelations, but the inexperienced may find themselves 'horribly alone in a dead, impersonal world . . .' and there are moments of terror. Quite stable people can develop an acute psychotic breakdown under LSD and paranoid episodes and panics are possible when the drug is taken by unprepared individuals in unsuitable surroundings. LSD users can experience terrors. They often feel that their heart is going to stop and have to wait for what seems like hours–because LSD increases the time dimension – for the second beat to appear; or they may feel that they are dead and not be sure whether they will come to life again.

The effects from LSD have been observed and described in this country from time to time and the present author has met patients suffering from short-term or longer-lasting psychoses, panics, 'flash-backs', depression, suicidal notions, and – in prison – one man who whilst on an LSD trip had killed a girl. This man – though perhaps somewhat immature – was an intelligent and pleasant person, the case illustrating that it is by no means only the very unstable individual who may come to grief through the use of hallucinogens (similar to our findings of psychological dependence on cannabis in intelligent, basic-ally fairly stable students). The occurrence of the phenomenon of the 'flash-back' can be very frightening. If the 'tripper' has unusual percep-tions and experiences shortly after taking the drug he is 'forewarned' and not unduly frightened; but if he has minor 'trips' weeks or months afterwards – long after he may have taken his last LSD dose – the effect of frightening visual hallucinations can be quite shattering. In the case of LSD-psychosis, one may sometimes find it difficult to decide whether the patient's state was primarily a consequence of his drug-taking, or whether LSD merely triggered off a previously latent state of schizophrenia.

In the USA, where there is much wider misuse of LSD, reports about the ill-effects of LSD are naturally much more common. For example, Louria and Sokolow [102] report that one New York hospital over a period of thirteen months admitted about 100 patients in a state of acute psychoses induced by LSD. They were suffering from symptoms such as terrifying visual hallucinations, feelings of overwhelming panics and fears, and marked agitation or bewilderment.

One subject debated a great deal in recent years is the possible risk of genetic and chromosomal damage arising from LSD use. Some years ago knowledge that such reports had appeared in the American press had got through to the British addicts' grapevine. Possibly due to this fear, LSD use in this country seemed to decrease for a year or two. However, at present the evidence incriminating LSD in this respect seems very slender.

LSD dependence

What about the possibility of developing dependence to LSD? A great many individuals find the experiences in the LSD state so attractive and so pleasant that they attempt to repeat them as soon and as frequently as possible. Five years ago the author came across an emotionally unstable and immature young American who travelled to and through various countries in Europe, in an attempt to find psychiatrists who were prepared to give him LSD. He usually obtained it from the illicit market, but he preferred to take it under psychiatric supervision. One General Practitioner who was frequently taking LSD denied that he was psychologically dependent on it. He regarded his tendency to take LSD as similar to the desire of a traveller to return again and again to the places which he found pleasant and beautiful on previous journeys. As regards tolerance this develops and passes off rapidly, the process in either direction taking about three days. There are no physical abstinence symptoms but some people feel disappointed and dejected when the LSD state has come to an end. Emotionally unstable individuals because of their underlying mental state are probably more likely to develop the LSD habit, but it can also develop in patients who have been given the drug in a treatment situation under skilled psychiatric supervision. As in other types of drug dependence it would seem that the underlying mental make-up and the goal which the LSD user seeks are important as regards the risk of becoming dependent on the drug. Thus no great risk of drug dependence seems involved when such hallucinogens are used in religious ceremonies and ritual fashion, as for example the use of peyote and morning glory seeds by American Indian tribes. However, the emotionally unstable and socially maladjusted may feel particularly attracted by these drugs, including, for example, 'arty' people such as struggling writers, painters and musicians, frustrated non-conformists and curious thrill-seeking adolescents and young adults [8].

Most LSD users seem to be able to go without LSD without great difficulties if it is no longer available. There is no physical dependence, but a minority of users may develop such strong psychic dependence that they wreck their careers by persisting in using the drugs despite strong social condemnations [8], despite occasional terrifying bad 'trips' and despite legal sanctions'

The use of LSD in psychiatric therapy
As regards the place of LSD in psychiatric treatment, reports are very contradictory and some therapists talk of excellent results whereas others declare it to have no value at all. Personality disorders, obsessional neurosis and alcoholism are among the conditions in which treatment by LSD has been investigated. As regards alcoholism, an excellent controlled study by research workers at the Ontario Research Foundation (1967) failed to provide any evidence '. . . that LSD is a useful adjunct to psychiatric treatment for alcoholism' [103]. Reviewing the earlier findings in the literature with different conclusions, the Canadian workers pointed out that '. . . the earlier studies failed to use any non-LSD control groups against which the effects of LSD could be compared'. Important changes had been claimed to follow LSD therapy in alcoholism, such as '. . . uncovering of the unconscious, integration of ego functions and . . . reordering of the emotional life'. In the Canadian investigation '. . . none of the expectations about psychological changes were clearly confirmed'. According to another view [80], 'LSD has a real, though a very limited, place (in therapy) . . . with substantially strong people whose neurosis is of a limited kind dimming their affective and colourful enjoyment of life . . .'. According to a recent psychiatric encyclopaedia [104], '. . . the therapeutic use of lysergide is now condemned by many psychiatrists. . . . The greatest danger of treatment lies in the production of a drug-dependent sociopathic individual . . .'.

Whatever its ultimate place in psychiatric therapy and as a research weapon, this odourless and colourless but extremely potent substance should only be available to qualified therapists and research scientists and is much too dangerous to be freely available to every oncomer. With this object in mind the importation, manufacture and distribution of LSD has rightly been severely curtailed. However, the fact that it can be easily synthesised by any competent chemist constitutes a great danger. One still meets many LSD users who feel that this drug has benefited them by giving them greater insight, self-awareness, etc. Nevertheless in view of the many risks attached to the abuse of LSD (and the same applies to other hallucinogens), the recommendations made in December 1966 by the Economic and Social Council of the United Nations' Commission on Narcotic Drugs make perfect sense.

The Council noted with deep concern, the increasing abuse of LSD. In view of '. . . the grave danger of this abuse to health and safety . . . to both the individual and society (it) requests governments to take immediate action to strictly control the import, export and production of LSD and substances producing similar ill-effects, either immediately or readily by conversion, and to place (their) distribution under the supervision of competent authorities'. It recommended that these substances should only be used for scientific research and medical purposes and only under 'very close and continuous medical supervision'; it condemned all other use and urged governments to take all steps to prevent it.

5.4 NARCOTIC DRUGS

'Among the remedies which it has pleased Almighty God to give to man to relieve his sufferings, none is so universal and so efficacious as opium.'

Thus wrote the famous English physician, Thomas Sydenham [105] almost 300 years ago. The opiates illustrate the principle that drugs which used in moderation and under skilful guidance can bring quick, complete relief from agonising physical pain and from terrible mental anguish, can when used unwisely and excessively in turn lead to the most severe mental suffering and physical decline.

Opiates are among the oldest drugs used by mankind and there is evidence that they were known in Asia minor six thousand years ago. In the times of Homer, 'nepenthes'—the drug of forgetfulness—was well-known and Louis Lewis had little doubt that it was in fact an opium preparation [20]. From the East and Asia minor where the opium poppy was first cultivated, knowledge about the plant spread to Europe, and, in the 8th century, to India and China. *Opium* was used as mankind's most important medicine for thousands of years and although in the East it had important social uses – comparable to those of alcohol in the West – its popularity was due to its unique powers of providing a feeling of extreme well-being. Thomas Sydenham was not the only doctor to be enthusiastic about opium. After all, at that time the actual cause of diseases was rarely known. Therefore doctors had to fall back on treating symptoms only and for this purpose there was no better drug, alcohol included, than opium. In fact, many doctors were such dedicated supporters of opium that they themselves fell victim to its dependent-producing properties in much higher numbers than members of any other occupational group. This illustrates the fact that intellectual awareness of the grave risks and consequences of one's actions does not necessarily protect one from foolhardy behaviour, such as drug misuse. At one time the proportion of doctors, the world over, among morphine addicts reached 40% and 10% of addicts were doctors' wives [20]. Today the proportion of professional addicts is not as high (see Table 4a in Appendix), but their contribution has at all times, and throughout the world, been disproportionately high. Clearly, the proportion of medical opiate addicts reflects the importance of ready availability of a drug as one of several important factors in the causation of drug dependence; and the relatively high percentage of doctors' wives who become morphine addicts reminds one of the disproportionately high standard mortality rate from liver cirrhosis in the case not only of publicans but also of their wives.

A now practically forgotten but once very popular opiate was *Laudanum* (a liquid extract of opium), a favourite and widely abused preparation. Among those who, to their cost, discovered not only the delights but also the tortures of laudanum were famous writers such as Coleridge and Francis Thomson. It had been popularised by De-Quincey's 'Confessions of an Opium Eater' (1821), to whom the '. . . divine poppy juice became as indispensable as breathing'. He had started taking the drug when, suffering from rheumatic pains, he obtained from a chemist in Oxford Street for the sum of 10½d, a sufficient helping of opium to 'hook' him for life [106]. Laudanum remained a favourite until the second half of the 19th century when its popularity was superseded by that of *chloral hydrate*. This drug, which is not an opiate, was then new, and its dangers were not initially recognised. Similarly, in 1898 heroin (diamorphine) was introduced as a 'safe' treatment for morphine addiction, apparently successfully until it turned out to be highly addictive itself. Again, many years later, in 1939, a newly-prepared synthetic substance with opiate-like qualities, pethidine, was hailed as a non-addictive drug, but soon proved very addictive (see Table 4a in Appendix), in spite of its relative lack of euphorinogenic effect. At one time the smoking of opium was popular among Chinese inhabitants of London's East End (among the Chinese in Hong Kong it is only in recent years that opium smoking has gradually been superseded by heroin). However, the favourite narcotics of English addicts (see Tables 4a and 5a–d in Appendix) were morphine and pethidine, but since the early 1960s their place has been taken by heroin, and, over the past few years by methadone (see

Tables 4a and 5a–d in Appendix).*

Opium is the dried juice obtained from the unripe seed capsules of the poppy – Papaver somniferum. The chief alkaloid of opium is morphine which is mainly responsible for its activity. *Morphine* was isolated at the beginning of the 19th century. Its positive effects are its pain-relieving property coupled with the feeling of calm and euphoria it produces, although these latter effects are largely responsible for leading to dependence. Its most dangerous action is the marked depressing of the respiratory centres. It may cause nausea and vomiting, sweating, and constipation. Another characteristic is the markedly contracted 'pin-point' pupil.

Codeine is another alkaloid present in opium, which, like morphine, is a phenanthrene derivative and is the methyl derivative of morphine. Unlike morphine, its narcotic euphoric and analgesic effects are very slight but it is effective against an irritating cough and diarrhoea. Like morphine it depresses the function of the cerebral cortex. Dependence on codeine is relatively rare but nevertheless from time to time one comes across people who habitually take codeine tablets (usually contained in analgesic compounds) to excess (see Section 5.2). As in the case of non-narcotic analgesics, the misuse of codeine preparations is partly due to their general availability without prescription. Free availability without prescription has also led some unstable individuals to occasional abuse of and sometimes dependence on certain cough mixtures such as 'paregoric' (the camphorated tincture of opium) [66] and Drimydril. Similarly, poppy heads (capsules of Papaver somniferum) – known to have been dependence-producing in certain parts of India for many years [107] – have in recent years also led to dependence among Indian immigrants to this country [108]. However, the most widely abused substance of this type which can be obtained in this country without prescription is *chlorodyne*, a tincture composed of chloroform and morphine. Its addictive properties were well-known many years ago and quite a few cases of dependence have occurred over the past few years. In common with many other easily obtained substances, women seem to be more often affected than men [109, 110]. The mixture is first taken for conditions such as diarrhoea or a cough. The user then finds that the drug gives both relaxation and some measure of euphoria, and thereafter begins to take it in ever increasing

* However, as Smart and Ogbourne have outlined in a very recent paper in the British Journal of Addiction (Brit. J. Addict, 1974, Vol. 2, 69) doctors differ in their method of notifying such addicts to the authorities. Under the circumstances it would therefore seem that the present notification system may tend to underestimate the number of misusers of narcotic drugs. Although the numbers involved are probably not very great.

doses, feeling unwell and developing withdrawal symptoms when attempting to leave off the drug.

Of narcotic drugs available on prescription only, those most frequently used in Great Britain in recent years are *heroin* (diacetyl morphine) and methadone (physeptone). The medical use of heroin has been suppressed in most countries as it is generally held to be even more addictive than morphine, but in the opinion of many British doctors heroin has unique properties that can be used for certain conditions. Compared to morphine, heroin holds a greater attraction for the addict. It produces a more intense euphoria and as a rule exhibits much less of the concomitants of constipation and vomiting which plagues the morphine addict. Because of its potency and as it is easily converted from morphine by a simple process, heroin has become a favourite of illicit manufacturers. Such illicit drug traffic still exists, e.g. in Marseilles where the 'stuff' smuggled in from the Far East and the Middle East is converted into heroin (see Figure 2 in Appendix). Heroin then finds its way mainly to the USA. All heroin in the USA is illicit, as American doctors do not prescribe it, and a huge black market has sprung up. The illicit black market in heroin in this country is much smaller but the fear of a large-scale imported black market was one of the reasons for the establishment of the Treatment Centres in Great Britain in 1968. The heroin peddled in the British illicit market is partly English heroin – i.e. an overflow from heroin tablets prescribed in the Treatment Centres – but at present is mainly the so-called Chinese heroin, coming from Hong Kong and sold in London's West End. Although the first large Court case involving Chinese heroin hit the headlines only a few weeks ago (May 1973), addicts have been talking about the availability in this country of 'Chinese heroin' for at least five years [3].

Synthetic narcotics

Other major narcotic drugs of addiction are the synthetic analgesics. For many years it has been the hope of manufacturing chemists to produce a drug which would be an analgesic, as effective a pain killer as morphine, but which would lack its addictive properties. In general these hopes were soon dashed, and the synthetic narcotics soon proved as addictive as morphine, the most obvious example being *pethidine* (introduced in 1939). A powerful analgesic and antispasmodic drug, its rapid withdrawal leads to symptoms such as anxiety, depression and cramps, and the higher doses then required bring about more severe withdrawal symptoms, such as confusional states, with hallucinations, misinterpretations and convulsion. Unlike morphine it does not lead to constipation or narrowing of the pupil. Pethidine dependence is frequently found amongst doctors and nurses who may have initially taken the drugs for its pain-killing effects, but it is hardly used at all by young, non-therapeutic addicts.

Pethidine addiction is much less common than dependence on another synthetic narcotic drug, i.e. *methadone*. This drug, synthesised in Germany during the last War also causes euphoria, tolerance and psychological and physical dependence. Withdrawal symptoms are less severe but more prolonged than in heroin dependence. Methadone is effective orally. For reasons such as these, methadone has been recommended as a substitution treatment of the withdrawal phase of heroin (and other narcotic) addiction (see Section 6.2). In recent years methadone has also been employed as long-term maintenance treatment for addicts because it produces cross-tolerance with heroin and diminishes the hunger and the hustling for heroin (see Section 6.2). However, methadone itself, in particular if mainlined, has also shown itself to be a highly addictive drug, which is at present very popular on the British illicit market.

The drawbacks of the opiates such as morphine and heroin, in particular their tendency to produce dependence, have for many years led to a search for substances which could have equally strong analgesic effects without their disadvantages. Pethidine and methadone have already been mentioned, belonging chemically to the phenylpiperidines and the diphenylpropylamines respectively. Other synthetic analgesics are chemically members of the morphinans (e.g. levorphanol) and benzomorphans (e.g. metazocine) [111]. However, as a rule all these narcotic analgesics have been found to be dependence-producing. The present author has, for example, come across, in this country, occasional (as a rule only one or two) cases of abuse of and dependence on dihydromorphine (Oilaudid), dextromethorphan (Romilar, which in form of a cough mixture has frequently been abused by unstable youngsters), dihydrocodeine (D.F.118), levorphanol (Dromoran) and dextromoramide (Palfium), a congener of methadone. This list is of course by no means complete.

Narcotic antagonists
However, the '. . . most promising lead to the long sought separation of desirable and undesirable morphine-like properties' [112] was the synthesis of analgesic drugs with antagonistic action to the narcotic

drugs. The first to be introduced was *nalorphine* (N-allylmorphine) which acts as a competitor to the narcotic drugs at the site of action. Given to morphine or heroin addicts, it rapidly leads to withdrawal symptoms, and, provided certain precautions are observed, can thus help in the diagnosis of opiate addiction – e.g. by dilating the pupils. (Diagnosis of opiate dependence – like that of amphetamine and barbiturate dependence – should as a rule also include laboratory testing of the urine by layer chromatography; on rare occasions gas liquid chromatography may be necessary). Nalorphine, however, is dysphoric, and is therefore not used as an analgesic; moreover it is short acting and has many opiate agonist effects. Other substances which have been studied belong to the benzomorphan group, ie. phenazocine (Narphen), cyclazocine, and pentazocine (Fortral). *Phenazocine* is a potent analgesic that can produce tolerance and a mild withdrawal syndrome and is thus itself dependence-producing. Pentazocine is less effective than morphine, it can be taken by mouth and was initially claimed to be non dependence-producing. However a few such cases have been described, and two cases – unstable personalities who had previously abused other drugs – were seen by the present author. The two antagonists which seem to hold out most promise are cyclazocine [113, 114] and naloxone [113]. *Cyclazocine* is an active analgesic, with occasional side-effects, such as dysphoria, vivid imagery and anxiety. *Naloxone* is an experimental opiate derivative, described as being '. . . 5–8 times more effective than nalorphine in antagonising opiate effects in animals'. Though cyclazocine has been described as having occasionally shown toxic effects, Fink *et al.* [113] have found the main drawbacks of cyclazocine and naloxone to consist in their short duration of action and not in their side-effects; and as – unlike in that case with cyclazocine – no secondary agonist effects have been so far observed with naloxone, these authors feel that naloxone '. . . uniquely satisfies the criteria-potent opiate antagonism without agonist or toxic effects'. Both cyclozocine and naloxone have been used clinically in the treatment of opiate addicts (see Part 6).

Narcotic effects
In spite of certain minor differences, the effects of the various narcotics are on the whole very similar to each other. Their main values lie in their powerful analgesic action, but they also have a marked sedative effect, leading to feelings of sleepiness ('nodding') and of detachment. It is the latter aspect which is often stressed by heroin addicts as the

effect of heroin which they value most. Naturally the effects vary with
the dose taken and with the way in which the drug is administered.
Today's young heroin and methadone addict usually prefers to inject
the drug intravenously (mainlining). Ten years ago, many young
heroin (and cocaine) addicts may have started with snorting (intranasal
administration) or skinpopping (hypodermic or intramuscular injection). With intravenous injection symptoms start after a few seconds;
if taken in other ways, a little later: the face begins to redden, the pupil
narrows, the skin begins to tingle, there is a feeling of relaxation,
freedom from anxiety, fears, inhibitions, followed by intermittent
drowsiness with drifting in and out of the dreamy state – the effects
usually passing off after a few hours. These narcotics are powerful
euphoriants, and by banning worry and anxiety, they transport people
readily into a pleasant dream world, so much so that the user likes to
re-experience these effects again and again. Relatively soon the users
of narcotics become psychologically and physically dependent on the
drug, and as tolerance develops even when relatively small doses (such
as those used medically in treatment of severe pain) are exhibited, the
user soon has to increase the amount taken to obtain the desired effect.
The development of dependence on relatively small therapeutic doses
after a relatively short period of administration of a few weeks is
characteristic of the narcotic drugs (see Section 2.4).

Drug dependence of the opiate type
Dependence on the opiates – now called by the WHO, 'Drug Dependence of the Opiate Type' – is both psychological (emotional) and
physical in nature. Emotional dependence is very pronounced so that
the user experiences an overwhelming desire or a compulsion to go on
taking the drug in order to obtain either positive or negative pleasure
from it – i.e. to heighten his pleasant feeling or to get away from feeling
miserable and anxious. Not only has the user to go on taking the dose
but he has to increase the dose more and more as tolerance develops
rapidly. In this way the addict to narcotic drugs can take enormous
doses which would kill the ordinary individual who is not used to these
drugs. For example, in the early 1960s it was not unusual to meet young
heroin addicts in London who were in the habit of taking five or ten
or even more grains daily (300–600 mg) – the ordinary dose used in
medical practice for the (non-addicted) individual being one-sixth of a
grain (10 mg).

Physical dependence likewise develops rapidly. As long as the addict is able to obtain supplies of his drug he may feel relatively contented and well. However, when his supplies decrease he begins to develop crippling and painful withdrawal symptoms. These start with mental symptoms and are followed later by physical symptoms, the latter denoting that a state of physical dependence has been reached by the individual. This abstinence syndrome starts within a few hours after the last dose has been taken. The addict becomes anxious, fearful and restless; irritable and unable to sleep. Aches and pains all over occur before the development of severe pains and muscular cramps; yawning, sneezing and eye-watering with rhinitis and excessive perspiration occurs. A few hours later the pupils dilate, muscles twitch, very painful cramps in the abdomen and in the calves result and vomiting and diarrhoea follow. (Diarrhoea and the dilated pupils are two examples illustrating that in many ways the withdrawal symptoms are the opposite from the features of chronic intoxication.) Blood pressure and temperature show a slight rise. The symptoms increase gradually in severity reaching their peak after about 24 hours in the heroin addict, and after about 48 hours in the morphine addict. Within about seven to ten days after the last 'fix' the addict has largely recovered from withdrawal illness. However, the process of recovery often takes many months, and many addicts complain of symptoms such as sleeplessness, depression and, in particular, inability to concentrate for periods of up to six months. Withdrawal symptoms are of course much more severe the more rapidly the addictive drug is withdrawn. Sudden, complete withdrawal of the drug without adequate substitution is inhuman and unnecessary (see Section 6.2).

As regards methadone, the development of euphoria and dependence (as with other addictive drugs) is a danger present much more in the case of intravenous injection than when given in oral form. Certain consequences of the prescribing of high methadone doses interfering with the effect of heroin, reduction of hunger for heroin and development of methadone dependence are well-illustrated in the following statement given by a young poly-drug abuser. In assessing the reliability of this statement, one has to keep in mind that it comes from a 20 year old addict who had only just stopped taking drugs after being caught by the police, that individual reactions vary a great deal, and that, of course, this statement only reflects his own experiences and may be challenged by others. On the other hand, it also illustrates certain historical and contemporary aspects of the British 'drug scene', and some problems arising out of the current practice.

Case history

'I have been receiving from a Group Practice doctor over the past five years, first 'H' (heroin), later methedrine, and then methadone as a linctus – initially 100 mg, then I was gradually cut down altogether for four months. I was also scoring when the linctus was being gradually cut down each day – 3–4 methadone ampoules (paying £1 each for them on the "market"), 20 Drinamyl (amphetamine and barbiturate combination, 10p–15p each) and was receiving from another doctor prescriptions of 30 mandrax (methaqualone combination) tablets, of which I was taking 3–4 per night. I also scored occasionally 30 mg "H" whilst I was taking 50 mg or less of methadone. With these smaller methadone doses, "H" had some effect, but when I had more than 50 mg methadone, "H" had no, or only a slight, effect. I then had no "buzz" or immediate "flash". I used to get the same effect, a "buzz" only, but no "flash" from methadone intravenous injections in higher doses. The "buzz" lasted for half to an hour; a serene, happy state and a beautiful taste, but there was no immediate "flash" or "bang", which I usually had after an intravenous "H" injection. Because I had no "buzz" after I had been reduced to 40 mg methadone, I went back to scoring "H". Higher methadone doses (e.g. 80 mg) took away the "H" feeling. On high doses of linctus methadone I had no desire for "H". I was then satisfied with, and addicted to methadone. Methadone withdrawal is worse than "H" withdrawal; with "H" you crave for the needle, with methadone, you crave for the "buzz". At first, three and a half years ago, the Group Practice put me on 150–200 mg linctus methadone, perhaps more. I felt a beautiful "buzz", equal to "H"; then didn't crave for the needle or for "H". Later, when down to 30 mg methadone, I still did not desire "H", but as methadone did not do much for me, I was tempted to score. To get the same "buzz" as 100 mg linctus, you need 7–8 ampoules (i.e. 70–80 mg). Yet linctus methadone has little market value and nobody sells it. Ampoules are easy to buy any time. When the Group Practice started to cut me down to 5 mg and below, I failed to get the lovely beautiful feeling in my stomach, mouth, head, everywhere, which I had got from doses above 60 mg. Most of my acquaintances were registered, receiving methadone ampoules, but sometimes they scored "H" on top of it (which is now selling at about 125p per 10 mg tablet). I never touched Chinese H – there are too many

Police Inspectors watching, and it is too easy to take an overdose. Linctus methadone (70–100 mg) gave me a "buzz", coming on gradually after 30–40 minutes, a strong feeling of well-being and I was satisfied with it. But not with doses of 40 mg or so of methadone. When I was given 40 mg it didn't do anything, apart from stop me from being sick. I then took double the dose, in order to get the strong "buzz", although I did not get the sudden, momentary "flash" that hits you and lasts about 30 seconds. Even intravenous methadone gives me a slight "flash" only after I have taken at least 6–7 ampoules (60–70 mg), but the "after-buzz" was better with linctus than with the ampoules. That is why I stayed so long – 3 years – on linctus. It is easy to get addicted to the linctus in high doses. The sickness when coming off linctus methadone is worse than coming off "H", and worse than coming off intravenous methadone: you feel very sick, with phlegm in your mouth, like a double dose of "flu", you are very drowsy and sleepy. I was very addicted to linctus methadone, and when the doctor tried to get me down, I started to score about 4 ampoules of methadone, and later on I went back to "H".'

Incidentally, this method of carrying out heroin withdrawal with the help of methadone must not be confused with methadone maintenance, the technique of using the drug for a much longer period. The latter method aims at helping the heroin addict to keep off heroin by giving him regular doses of methadone which are less disabling than 'H' and allow the addict to continue with his work (see Section 6.2).

What effect has the continued self-administration of narcotic drugs on the addict? He may often present a picture of physical and mental deterioration. Emaciation, a sallow complexion and skin showing scars, discolouration, or even abscesses as a result of frequent injections taken without observing sterile precautions are almost constant findings. Trophic disturbances include brittle nails and loss of hair. Loss of appetite and obstinate constipation also occur. Mentally, the addict may become lazy, unreliable, insincere and dishonest. Any effort he makes becomes more and more restricted to the over-riding object of securing drug supplies. In this way the addict neglects personal hygiene and food intake, and begs, 'cons', steals, forges prescriptions or cheques or becomes a prostitute in order to get the money to obtain drugs. Through his habit of neglecting sterile precautions he may suffer not only from local but also from general infection (septicaemia, endocarditis). The usual custom of sharing needles etc. among many addicts may cause viral hepatitis. His average life span is much shorter than that of his contemporaries, as he is prone to take (often accidentally) overdoses, to get involved in accidents, and to suffer from under-nutrition with accompanying lack of resistance to intercurrent infections etc.

Naturally the addict's family and society also suffer. The youngster becomes a cause of extreme anxiety and worry to parents. (Societies have been established in which parents of young addicts have banded themselves together in an attempt to support and to help each other, similar to the Alanon movement in the case of alcoholism.) Society suffers from the loss of potentially productive members by having to look after dependents, or by having to maintain the addict in hospital or prison. On the other hand, the notions that the heroin addict is an aggressive dope-fiend and a sex-maniac belong to the realm of legend. He may be driven to crime because of the overwhelming need to obtain the drug at any cost and at any price, but the addict's crimes are directed against property rather than against persons. As regards sex, the addict soon loses all sexual desire and interest. It has even been said that one of the reasons for individuals developing a liking for heroin may be connected with their desire to get away from the anxiety caused to them by their lack of aggressive and sexual instincts. Certainly aggressive acting-out is much more common under the influence of alcohol than under the influence of the opiates. The question of how best to prevent narcotic addiction remains unanswered. Neither the punitive American approach nor the overpermissive, old British system have succeeded in preventing the emergence of epidemics with harmful and often disastrous effects on individual and society alike.

Some American statistics
Reference has already been made to current poly-drug abuse by youngsters in the UK. This involves in the main soft, non-narcotic drugs. A few statistics relating to the non-medical use of non-narcotic and narcotic drugs by youngsters and adults in the USA are contained in Tables 6 and 7 in the Appendix.

The statistics contained in Table 6 in the Appendix are based on a nationwide survey of 2411 adults (aged 18 years and over) and 880 youngsters in the age-groups 12 to 17 years. The survey was carried out by the American Commission on Marijuana and Drug Abuse, whose chairman, Raymond P. Shafer [115] discussed the findings at length at a recent Conference on Alcoholism and Drug Addiction in Eagleville (one of the few places in the USA treating both these conditions in the same set-up). The survey showed that 3·5 million youngsters had smoked marihuana (i.e. 14% of youth) at one time or another. Thirteen million individuals described themselves as current users. However, within the week prior to the survey, many more people had taken alcoholic drink, i.e. approximately one-fourth of all youth (6 million) and over a half of all adults (74 million). During the same period 4 million youngsters and 53 million adults had smoked tobacco. But in spite of the vast use and abuse of alcohol, '. . . the vast majority of Americans don't recognise alcohol as being a drug'.

One and a half million youngsters and 3 million adults had at some time experimented with inhaling volatile solvents (such as glue). Five and a half million adults and 3/4 million youngsters had taken sedatives for non-medical reasons. Similarly the proportion of adults (i.e. 8·5 million) who had taken tranquillisers non-medically was much higher than the 3% of youth. Almost equal proportions of youngsters (6%) and adults (7%) had taken over-the-counter sedatives, tranquillisers and stimulants for non-medical purposes; and the same (just under 5% of youth and adults) applies to the use of hallucinogens.

Shafer felt that the 'H' and 'C' figures arrived at by the Survey underestimated the real amount of abuse. Most 'H'-dependent and 'C'-using street drug-takers were unlikely to be counted in a household survey. Nevertheless it is interesting to learn that as many as 3·2% of adults and 1·5% of youth were found to have tried cocaine. Not so long ago – i.e. 1960–1968 – abuse of 'C' was very popular among youngsters in London. At the time it seemed that North American heroin addicts coming to this country had only rarely taken cocaine at home, and were introduced to this drug not infrequently by the prescribing London doctors. In London the abuse of 'C' has practically vanished since the advent of the Treatment Centres (although the author has been told that over the past few weeks it has again become readily available on the illicit market). In the USA, on the other hand, the abuse of cocaine over the past few years seems to have become an increasing problem.

Table 7 in the Appendix summarises the findings of a number of American studies as regards drug use amongst students in the late 1960s [116]. Comparison with the proportion amongst youngsters smoking cannabis in the 1972 survey shows a high percentage of smoking students. One might perhaps have also expected a clearly higher proportion of LSD 'tripping' students compared to other youngsters. The percentages of students smoking cannabis and having occasional LSD 'trips' might not be very different in England from those shown among American students. However, one only rarely comes across students in this country taking amphetamines (apart from possibly a few tablets before examinations) [117]. This makes the very high proportion of amphetamine users among Californian students seem rather surprising.

REFERENCES

1. Dally, P. J. (1967). *Chemotherapy of Psychiatric Disorders* (London: Logos Press).
2. Connell, P. H. (1958). *Amphetamine Psychosis* (London: Chapman and Hall).
3. Glatt, M. M., Pittman, D. J., Gillespie, D. G. and Hills, D. R. (1969). *The Drug Scene in Great Britain* (London: Edward Arnold) (Revised Reprints).
4. Scott, P. D. and Willcox, D. R. C. (1965). *Brit. J. Addict.*, **61**, 9.
5. Kalant, O. J. (1966). *The Amphetamines* (Univ. Toronto Press).
6. James, I. P. (1968). *Lancet*, **i**, 916.
7. Glatt, M. M. (1968). *ibid.*, **ii**, 215.
8. Eddy, N. B., Halbach, H., Isbell, H. and Seevers, H. M. (1965). *Bull. WHO*, **32**, 721.
9. Wilson, C. W. M. and Beacon, S. (1964). *Brit. J. Addict.*, **60**, 81.
10. Angrist, B. M. *et al.* (1967). *N.Y. St. J. Med.*, **67**, 2983.
11. Annot (1968). *Practit.*, **200**, 202.
12. Oswald, I. and Thacore, V. R. (1963). *Brit. Med. J.*, **2**, 427.
13. Eysenck, H. J. (ed.). (1963). *Experiments with Drugs* (Oxford: Pergamon Press).
14. Glatt, M. M. (1957). *Brit. Med. J.*, **1**, 460.
15. Glatt, M. M. (1959). *Lancet*, **i**, 887.
16. Bejerot, N. (1970). *Addiction and Society* (Illinois: Charles C. Thomas).
17. Clein, L. J. and Benady, D. R. (1962). *Brit. Med. J.*, **2**, 456.
18. Oswald, I. *et al.* (1971). *Brit. Med. J.*, **2**, 70.
19. Laurent, J. M. (1962). *Ann. Medico-Psychol.*, **120**, 649.
20. Lewin, L. (1964). *Phantastica*, 247, 260, 268 (London: Routledge and Kegan Paul).

21. Emboden, W. (1972). *Narcotic Plants*, 84 (London: Studio Vista).
22. Malcolm, A. I. (1971). *The Pursuit of Intoxication*, 251 (Ontario, Toronto: Addict. Research Found.).
23. Laurence, D. R. (1966). *Clinical Pharmacology*, 336 (3rd ed.) (London: J. and A. Churchill).
24. *Lancet*, (1972). ii, 1278.
25. Nichols, A. B. (1973). *ibid.*, i, 480.
26. Fischer, E. and von Mering, J. (1903). *Ther. Mh.*, 17, 208.
27. Willcox, W. (1913). *Lancet*, ii, 1178.
28. Willcox, W. (1934). *Brit. J. Inebr.*, 31, 131.
29. Locket, S. (1973). *Practit.*, 211, 103.
30. Bartholomew, A. A. (1961). *Med. J. Australia*, ii, 51.
31. Isbell, H. *et al.* (1950). *Arch. Neurol. Psychiat.*, 64, 1.
32. Glatt, M. M. (1956). *Lancet*, i, 313.
33. Glatt, M. M. (1955). *Brit. Med. J.*, ii, 738.
34. *Lancet*, (1954). Editorial, ii, 75.
35. *Brit. Med. J.*, (1954). Editorial, 2, 1534.
36. Glatt, M. M. (1962). *Bull. Narcot.*, 14 (2), 19.
37. Brooke, E. M. and Glatt, M. M. (1964). *Medicine, Science and the Law*, 4, 277.
38. Zacune, J. and Hensman, C. (1971). *Drugs, Alcohol and Tobacco in Britain*, 55 (London: Heinemann).
39. Interdepartmental Committee Report on Drug Addiction (1969). (London: H.M.S.O.).
40. Glatt, M. M. (1969). *Lancet*, ii, 429.
41. Fox, R. (1971). Paper at *6th Int. Congr. Suicide Prevention*, Mexico.
42. Locket, S. (1957). *Brit. J. Addict.*, 53, 105.
43. Barraclough, B. M., Nelson, B., Bunch, J. and Sainsbury, P. (1971). *J. Roy. Coll. Gen. Practit.*, 21, 645.
44. Lader, M. (1972). *Drugs and Society*, 17 (March).
45. Stengel, E., Cook, G. and Kreeger, I. S. (1958). *Attempted Suicide* (London: Inst. Psychiat.).
46. Matthew, H., Roscoe, P. and Wright, N. (1972). *Practit.*, 208, 254.
47. Fraser, H. F. *et al.* (1958). *J. Amer. Med. Ass.*, 166, 136.
48. Hunter, R. A. and Greenberg, H. P. (1954). *Lancet*, ii, 58.
49. Glatt, M. M. (1954). *Lancet*, ii, 143.
50. Willcox, W. (1934). *Lancet*, i, 370.
51. Desmond, M. M. *et al.* (1972). *J. Pediat.*, 80, 190.
52. *Brit. Med. J.*, (1972). Editorial, 2, 63.

53. Isbell, H. and Chrusciel, T. L. (1970). *Dependence Liability of Non-Narcotic Drugs* (Suppl. to *Bull. WHO*, **43**) (Geneva: WHO).
54. Glatt, M. M. (1955). *Lancet*, **i**, 308.
55. James, I. P. (1962). *ibid.*, **2**, 277.
56. Nyswander, M. (1965). *Drug Addiction in Youth*, 126 (E. Harms, editor) (Oxford, N.Y.: Pergamon Press).
57. Glatt, M. M., George, H. R. and Frisch, E. P. (1965). *Brit. Med. J.*, **2**, 401.
58. WHO Expert Committee Addiction-Producing Drugs (1964). *WHO Techn. Rep. Ser.*, 273
59. Glatt, M. M. (1958). *Brit. Med. J.*, **2**, 1100.
60. Glatt, M. M. (1959). *ibid.*, **1**, 587.
61. Glatt, M. M. (1967). *ibid.*, **i**, 444.
62. Parish, P. (1972). Drugs and Society, 11 (April).
63. (1973). *Lancet*, **i**, 1101.
64. Kryspin-Exner, K. (1966). *Brit. J. Addict.*, **61, 283.**
65. Peters, U. H. and Seidel, M. (1970). *Arzneimittel-Forsch.*, **20**, 876.
66. Kielholz, P. (1957). *Schweiz. Med. Wschr.*, **87**, 1131.
67. Battegay, R. (1958). *Nervenarzt*, **29**, 467.
68. Abrahams, M. J., Armstrong, J. and Whitlock, F. A. (1970). *Med. J. Australia*, **57** (11), 397.
69. Kato, M. (1969). *Int. J. Addict.*, **4** (4), 591.
70. Battegay, R. (1963). Vom Hintergrund der Süchte, 2nd ed., 9 (Blaukreuz Verlag, Bern; Blaukreuz Verlag, Wuppertal-Barmen).
71. Bell, D. *et al.* (1969). *Brit. Med. J.*, **2**, 378.
72. Kerr, D. N. S. (1973). *Med. News*, Feb. 19, 9.
73. Murray, R. M. (1971). *Lancet*, **ii**, 1260.
74. *Med. News*, (1973). April 23, 1.
75. Holmstedt, B. (1964). Foreword to Lewin, L. *Phantastica* (London).
76. Cohen, S. (1964). *Drugs of Hallucination* (London: Secker and Warburg).
77. Blatherwick, C. E. (1972). *Canad. J. Publ. Hlth*, **63**, 272.
78. Krug, D. C., Sokol, J. and Nylancer, I. (1965). *Drug Addiction in Youth*, 36 (E. Harms, editor) (Oxford: Pergamon Press).
79. Louria, D. B. (1968). *The Drug Scene*, 48 (N.Y.: McGraw-Hill Book Co.).

80. Malleson, N. (1972). *Drugs and Society* (Feb.). 1 (5) p. 17 for GPs, Appendix on Drugs (1972). 32 (D. Leigh, C.M.B.)
81. Huxley, A. (1967). Culture and the Individual, Quoted from *The Book of Grass*, 192 (G. Andrews and S. Vinkenoog, editors) (London: Peter Owen).
82. Huxley, A. (1954). *The Doors of Perception and Heaven and Hell* (N.Y.: Harper and Row).
83. Burroughs, W. (1967) Quoted from *The Book of Grass*, 207.
84. Cohen, S. (1969). *The Drug Dilemma* (N.Y.: McGraw-Hill Book Co.).
85. *Chambers' Edinburgh Journal* (1848). The Hashish (W. and R. Chambers Ltd).
86. Macdonald, A. D. (1965). *Hashish: its Chemistry and Pharmacology.*
87. Gaoni, Y. and Mechoulan, R. (1964). *J. Amer. Chem. Soc.*, 86, 1646.
88. Paton, W. D. M. and Crown, J. (1972). *Cannabis and its Derivatives* (London: Univ. Press).
89. WHO Working Party on Cannabis (1971). *WHO Tech. Rep. Ser.*, **478.**
90. Abrams, S. (1967). Quoted from *The Book of Grass*, 235.
91. Watt, J. M. (1965) in *Hashish* (Ref. 86), 54.
92. Jellinek, E. M. (1960). *The Disease Concept of Alcoholism* (New Haven, Connect.: Hillhouse Press).
93. Glatt, M. M. and George, H. R. (1967). *Brit. J. Addict.*, 62, 147.
94. Glatt, M. M. (1969). *ibid.*, 64, 109.
95. Glatt, M. M. (1967). *Lancet*, ii, 1203.
96. Chopra, R. N. and Chopra, I. C. (1965). *Drug Addiction* (New Delhi: Council of Scientific and Industrial Research).
97. Trocchi, A. (1967). Quoted from *The Book of Grass*, 108.
98. Economic and Social Council (U.N.) (1965). *Commission on Narcotic Drugs*, 20th Session (N.Y.: U.N.).
99. Murphy, H. B. M. (1965). *Bull. Narcot.*, 15 (1), 15.
100. (1972). *Drugs and Society* (April), 1 (7), 1.
101. Brill, H. (1970). *Communication and Drug Abuse*, 111 (J. R. Wittenhorn et al., editors) (Springfield, Ill.: Charles C. Thomas).
102. Louria, D. B. and Sokolow, M. (1966). *Nightmare Drugs* (N.Y.: Pocket Books Inc.).
103. Smart, R. G., Storm, T., Baker, E. F. and Solursh, L. (1967). *LSD in the Treatment of Alcoholism* (Univ. Toronto Press).

104. *Encyclopedia of Psychiatry for GPs, Appendix of Drugs* (1972). (C. H. Leigh, B. Pare, and J. Marks, editors) (Roche Products Ltd).

105. Sydenham, T. (1680). Quoted from Laurence, D. R. *Clinical Pharmacology*, 3rd ed. 224 (London J. and A. Churchill).

106. Pearsall, R. (1965). *Addictions*, **12**, 20.

107. Chopra, R. N. and Ghose, N. N. (1931). *Indian J. Med. Res.*, **19**, 415.

108. Glatt, M. M. and Hoxssain, M. M. (1963). *Brit. Med. J.*, **2**, 102.

109. Sister Patricia (1964). Quoted from Glatt, M. M. *Brit. Med. J.*, **2**, 308.

110. Glatt, M. M. (1964). *ibid.*, *Brit. Med. J.*, **2**, 308.

111. May, E. L. (1972). *Agonist and Antagonist Actions of Narcotic Analgesic Drugs*, 17 (H. W. Kosterlitz, H. O. J. Collier, and J. A. Villarreal, editors) (London: Macmillan).

112. Eddy, N. B. (1972). *ibid.*, 3.

113. Fink, M., Freedman, A. M., Resnick, R. and Zaks, A. (1972). *ibid.*, 266.

114. Brill, L. and Jaffe, J. H. (1967). *Brit. J. Addict.*, **62**, 375.

115. July 1 (1973). *The Journal*, Toronto, p. 13.

116. Young, J. and Crutchley, S. B. (1972). *Drugs and Society* (Oct.).

117. Glatt, M. M. (1967). *Pax Romana Journal*, **6**, 18.

PART 6

PART 6

TREATMENT AND REHABILITATION*

6.1 GENERAL PRINCIPLES IN THE TREATMENT OF ALCOHOL AND DRUG DEPENDENCE

Before describing the therapy in some detail, a few general principles should be briefly discussed. This it is hoped, will, despite certain overlapping, greatly simplify later discussion and general understanding.

Treatment of physical and psychological dependence

The division of dependence-producing drugs into those producing psychological dependence only and those also capable of producing physical dependence is of considerable therapeutic significance. Drugs which stimulate the CNS, such as cocaine, the amphetamines and khat, as a rule produce psychological dependence only and clinically there is no evidence of physical dependence (see Part 2). Likewise LSD and cannabis apparently produce psychological dependence only. In view of the lack of risk of a physical abstinence syndrome, cessation of drug intake in people dependent on such drugs can be sudden and complete, although an eye should be kept on such mental withdrawal symptoms as depression etc.

Drugs which depress the CNS often produce a state of physical dependence as well as a state of psychological dependence. In these cases because of the danger of a physical abstinence syndrome on sudden withdrawal, the drug should either be tapered off gradually (e.g. in the case of barbiturate dependence) or temporarily replaced by an adequate

---

* This chapter is largely based on a contribution to the *International Handbook of Medical Science*, 2nd ed. (D. Horrobin and A. Gunn, editors) (Lancaster, England: Med. and Tech. Publ. Co.)

substitute (e.g. by methadone in the case of heroin addicts). Physical (as well as psychological) dependence-producing drugs include opiates, the hypnotic–sedatives (in particular barbiturates, but also most non-barbiturate hypnotics), the tranquilliser meprobamate, the benzo-diazepines, chlorodiazepoxide and diazepam only in very high doses and when administered for a long period [1, 2], alcohol and possibly also nicotine. In alcoholics and addicts to hypnotic drugs, the physical abstinence syndrome includes withdrawal convulsions and delirium tremens, and therefore requires the prophylactic administration of anticonvulsants and powerful tranquillisers. Provided this precaution is taken, alcoholics as a rule can be – at least in hospital – suddenly and completely taken off alcohol.

It is popularly assumed that physical dependence is more dangerous than psychological dependence. However, whilst it is true that as regards risk to life the physical abstinence syndrome is more important than the psychological withdrawal symptoms, from the aspects of relapse and rehabilitation following completion of withdrawal, psychic dependence is more important. Thus alcoholics, barbiturate and opiate addicts relapse as a rule not because of physical but mainly because of psychological dependence. Alternatively they may relapse as a consequence of factors such as the original psychological conflicts or a simple social situation which invokes drinking. Social dependence is often a cause of relapse e.g. the addicts' involvement with their sub-culture, which exerts a strong attraction on them, may induce them to return to their former drug-taking habits [3].

Therefore sobering-up the drunk and detoxifying the drinker and the drug taker are by themselves no more than first-aid measures or curtain raisers which have always to be followed up by long-term and rehabilitation measures. Otherwise all that will have been achieved is to render the alcoholic and the drug addict fit to resume drinking and drug taking in a better physical state, with renewed vigour and fervour. To put it another way, initial therapy of the state of physical depen-dence and intoxication by means such as tranquillisers, vitamins, fluids etc. is vital, but must always be followed up by the therapy aimed at neutralising and removing the effects of psychological and social dependence [4]. For example, if drug takers after treatment in hospital are sent out without provision being made for their living in a drug-free environment, without having been put in touch with new friends, without attempts at vocational guidance and assistance, they will drift back to their old haunts, their former drug-taking friends and subculture and to certain return to their drug-taking habits [3]. No treatment programme for alcoholics and drug addicts can be regarded as complete and to have any reasonable chance of long-term success unless adequate provision is made for planned comprehensive after-care. This is most urgent and absolutely imperative in the case of the young non-therapeutic drug abusers.

The combined approach

While there are many dissimilarities between alcohol and other drugs, there are also many similarities. In view of the similarities, e.g. in causation and treatment [5, 6], the WHO Committee on Services for the Prevention and Treatment of Dependence on Alcohol and Other Drugs (1967) [7] recommended a *combined approach* to problems of alcoholism and drug dependence. Such a combined approach, in the Committee's view, would apply most usefully to research, least usefully to control measures, with treatment and education taking an intermediate position. One important reason for recommending a combined approach was the feeling that in recent years the approach to alcoholism as an illness and to the alcoholic as a sick man had become increasingly accepted – e.g. in England and North America – whereas in many parts of the world (including North America) drug addicts were still mainly regarded as criminals. It was hoped that such a combined approach would in time also make drug dependence more widely acceptable as an illness. In the UK drug addicts have in principle for many years been considered to be sick people in need of help, whereas in the USA 'dope fiends' have been widely approached as criminals, with medical men until recently taking very little active part in their management. In very recent years, however, whilst in the UK, addicts to the opiates are still treated as sick men, their treatment has become somewhat less permissive in the sense that only specially licensed doctors can prescribe such drugs [3], whereas in the USA quite a few centres have recently begun to treat heroin addicts by such means as methadone maintenance [8, 9] or blockade with opium antagonists, such as cyclazocine [10]. Again, differences in national and local situations, in public image and in legal provisions offer an opportunity for research, comparing and contrasting the methods and results obtained under varying conditions in these two countries.

A comprehensive approach

In the aetiology of alcohol and drug dependence (as discussed in Part 2) many factors are usually involved. Therefore, in the prophylaxis and the management of the health problems involved, it is obviously not enough to limit oneself to measures directed at the legal control of the drug (agent) but attention has also to be directed to the personalities involved (host) and environmental conditions (11, 12).

In view of the multifactorial causation, clearly one and the same treatment cannot be the best for every individual involved. Different types of personalities take drugs of widely varying composition and effect, for varying reasons, under widely different conditions, for varying lengths of time, in greatly varying amounts. Therefore, treatment, too, should be as far as possible individualised and tailored to the requirements of the individual patient. Treatment should always be preceded by an investigation and an assessment of the causative factors involved in the individual patient. The question is therefore not as sometimes debated, whether in general to adopt the Pavlov approach, or that of Freud. Whether to employ methods based predominantly on Freud or on Pavlov, should be decided only after an assessment of the individual patient's needs, and very often there may be a need for combining various techniques based on different therapeutic philosophies [13].

Though often expected by patients or their relatives, there is in fact no hope for a miraculous cure by chemotherapy at the present state of knowledge. In general, most observers would regard treatment by drugs as adjuncts to the more fundamental task of an emotional re-orientation of the patient's attitudes and life-style. This involves relatively brief psychotherapy – individual or in groups – and social therapy, giving assistance to the patient's social problems such as domestic, housing and occupational difficulties. In most cases a comprehensive approach, combining psychological, social and pharmacological techniques, is nowadays regarded as the best form of treatment in alcoholism and dependence on other drugs.

Clearly such multidimensional comprehensive therapy cannot be carried out by members of one therapeutic discipline, but is the responsibility of a well-integrated multidisciplinary team, whose members have to work in close cooperation with each other. Medical men, social workers, sociologists, nurses, priests, probation officers, the alcoholic's family, recovered alcoholics (AA) and addicts, personal managers, employees of local authorities and voluntary welfare agencies, at times also magistrates, lawyers, police etc. are all members of the therapeutic team [11]. Sometimes the team member first approached by the patient or his family may not be the best one to help in this individual case. He must then be prepared to refer him to a member of the team who may be better qualified or in a better position to assist him, such referral serving the purpose not of shifting responsibility but of sharing it. There is no place here for interdisciplinary rivalry, jealousy or warfare, but a need for the closest interdisciplinary collaboration and pooling of experiences and forces. In fact, representatives of one discipline should have a fair notion of the functions of the other team members, e.g. the psychiatrist must have some idea of the work and the role of the sociologist and *vice versa*. He must not only consider the psychological aspects of the problem, but must also be aware of the social causative factors involved.

Alcoholism and drug dependence are both illnesses of the whole family. Treatment cannot be regarded as complete without also including other members of the family in the treatment situation [11]. Often the family constellation may have greatly contributed to initially setting the patient on the road to excessive drinking or drug taking. In the case of the alcoholic, sometimes the wife (who may frequently be older or the more dominating partner compared to the emotionally often much more immature alcoholic husband) may have married him primarily because of unconscious personality needs of her own. In the case of the young drug addict he often, rightly or wrongly, blames the lack of understanding shown by his parents for his opting out of the family circle, his tuning in to the gang subculture and turning to drugs. Whatever the cause the alcoholic's or drug addict's behaviour must exercise considerable influence and have wide repercussions on the attitudes, feelings and behaviour of the whole family. Thus, the family often needs help as much as the patient himself. Moreover, among environmental factors – which are so important in the patient's success or failure in the tasks of resocialisation and rehabilitation – none is more important than his family's attitude. His relatives – like the patient himself – have to become acquainted with and learn to accept emotionally the illness concept of these conditions, so that they are in a better frame of mind to understand his otherwise unpredictable and incomprehensible behaviour, and to help him ease his way back to family and the community as a whole. Faulty attitudes of both patient and family can otherwise lead to a persistence of mutual misunderstanding and recriminations.

Is dependence on alcohol or other drugs a *symptom* of underlying psychological or social problems or a *disease* in its own right? In the past, psychiatrists usually regarded alcoholism solely as a symptom of the underlying psychopathology. They therefore tended to neglect the symptom – excessive drinking – as being of relatively minor interest, hoping that by diagnosing and remedying the underlying psychological cause the need for excessive drinking would disappear. However, it is only fair to say that approaches based on such reasoning as a rule failed to get anywhere, and there is little evidence that orthodox psychoanalysis had any success with alcoholism [14]. In practice, AA, who look at alcoholism as a disease without (in theory) caring much about the underlying psychopathology, had much more success in the treatment and rehabilitation of alcoholics.

There seems, at any rate, no reason why these two approaches could not be successfully combined. Alcoholism and drug dependence can therefore both be looked at as conditions which, in many (certainly not all) cases, may have started as symptomatic of underlying psychological problems (Jellinek's alpha alcoholism) [15], but which in the course of time may have outrun their original purely symptomatic function, and have assumed the extent and the importance of a disease in their own right, therefore in group sessions with alcoholics and function, and have assumed the extent and the importance of a disease in their own right, e.g. causing in turn physical and mental complications. Therefore in group sessions with alcoholics and drug-dependent individuals at the Alcoholism and Drug Dependence Unit at St Bernard's Hospital, discussions deal with psychological (and social) problems which may originally have caused excessive drinking or drug taking, as well as with difficulties in interpersonal relationships which quickly become manifest when patients live in close proximity in a therapeutic community and with events arising during, and as a consequence of, their drinking or drug-taking career [4]. Thus psychiatrists, GPs etc. can work together with AA, their work often being a good and frequently necessary complement to each other.

The role of the medical profession
Whether one regards alcoholism and drug dependence as essentially a symptom or as an illness or disease, there is no doubt that they are (though not exclusively) the responsibility and province of the healing professions, and that doctors are – or should be – vitally interested. (see Section 7.1). Naturally these conditions also constitute a social problem (economic, financial, theological and criminalogical), but they are also an important medical problem. This, of course, does

not mean that doctors should make a take-over bid – a fear that was expressed at a recent conference by the well-known Finnish sociologist Kettell Bruun regarding conditions pertaining to alcoholism in his country. However, this fear of a take-over bid by doctors in problems of alcoholism and drug dependence can certainly be discounted as far as the UK and probably also as far as the USA is concerned. Unfortunately the danger here is that doctors have all too often opted out from taking an active and leading interest in these conditions (though fortunately to a gradually decreasing extent). This may have been to a large extent the consequence of inadequate teaching of these subjects in the medical curriculum [11]. For instance, alcoholism, if mentioned at all to undergraduates, was often only referred to in terms of its rare complications, such as liver cirrhosis. This results in doctors, who later on in their professional life, only think of a possible diagnosis of alcoholism when a patient exhibits these late (and fortunately relatively rare) complications. Thus the great majority of cases of alcoholism (in England perhaps 13–14 out of 15 alcoholics on the average GP's list) are never known to their GPs. Regarding other types of drug dependence, until recently the term 'opium addiction' probably often conjured up notions of some exotic, oriental affliction, hardly ever seen in Western countries. Thus in the 1960s, the UK doctors and the general public had a rude awakening for which they were totally unprepared. Then again, the fact that respectable drugs, such as barbiturates and amphetamines, could produce dangerous states of drug dependence was until recently hardly known to the great majority of doctors. A consequence of this was that quite a few GPs by their liberal and generous prescribing habits contributed greatly to the spread of epidemics [3].

There is therefore a great need for adequate teaching at undergraduate level in the subjects of alcoholism and drug dependence (and equally, of course, of students of other professions concerned with alcohol and drug-dependent individuals). This would not only lead to earlier diagnosis and detection of cases of alcohol and drug misuse, thus allowing earlier treatment with prevention of further complications – (*secondary prevention*) – but would also gradually alter the attitude of doctors. They would no longer look at these people as time wasters who could do better if they only tried, but rather as sick human beings in need of help. This would also have the effect that alcoholics and addicts (and their families) would no longer keep away from the GP as long as they could (or present themselves under the guise of sufferers from headache, backache, stomach-ache, injuries etc.) because they fear

1 6

moralising lectures, but would come forward at an earlier phase. At this stage the chance of successful help and rehabilitation would be much greater than later on when easily irreversible complications might have set in. Such a positive attitude by the medical profession towards these sufferers, would in time, alter the attitude of the community at large, so that the stigma attached to these conditions would gradually fall by the wayside. Again this would lead to patients seeking help much earlier [11].

The patient's attitude to himself – e.g. his guilt feelings and the need to project them on to his family and the community at large – is to a large extent a reaction to family and community attitudes. Therefore a change in medical attitudes, by changing family and public attitudes, would also constructively influence the alcoholic's and addict's attitude to himself. He might then no longer regard himself as a hopeless misfit, unable to live up to society's prophecy about himself. Instead he will come to look at himself in a more hopeful light and be encouraged to co-operate actively in his own rehabilitation.

From the point of view not only of treatment but also of prevention (education of the general public, changing public attitudes, research) it is vital that the medical profession takes a leading, active part in the management of problems of alcoholism and drug dependence [11].

The inadequacy of the education of medical practitioners in regard to these conditions, can be seen from the relatively high proportion of doctors who themselves become alcoholics and drug addicts. As regards other drugs, doctors are easily exposed to constant temptation and opportunity (as are nurses, pharmacists, etc,), though in theory their knowledge should prevent them from taking unnecessary risks. Exposure does not explain the relatively high incidence of alcoholism in doctors in spite of their knowledge. This is not really reflected in the standard mortality rate – in England, two and a half times that of the average population, and probably kept low artificially by the unwillingness of doctors to certify liver cirrhosis as the cause of death in a colleague.

Treatment facilities
Neither alcoholism nor dependence on other drugs is a respecter of social class, occupation, race or religion. A comprehensive programme must therefore cater for everybody, in particular for all social classes. For some reason or other in England it is in the main alcoholics from Social Classes I and II who turn up at the treatment agencies. This does

not necessarily mean that there are proportionately more alcoholics among these classes but that the illness concept of alcoholism and the knowledge that alcoholics can be greatly helped has as yet not become widely known among other social classes. Conversely, in the USA it used to be mainly the slum area youngsters who became drug abusers and dependents. In recent years this situation has begun to alter. In England, youngsters from all social classes were always represented among those becoming dependent on drugs in the 1960s. At any rate, any (comprehensive) treatment programme for alcoholics and addicts has therefore to make provision for the care and management of alcoholics and drug dependents of all classes and all types, by in-patient facilities, out-patient facilities, halfway houses, community treatment, connections with other treatment and after-care agencies etc.

In 1962 the Ministry of Health recommended the establishment of regional alcoholic units for the hospital treatment of alcoholics [11]. There are now in the UK eighteen such regional units, one in Scotland, and one in Wales, apart from a number of smaller units. The Ministry memorandum rightly stressed the need for such in-patient units to work closely together with GPs, social services, local authorities and voluntary organisations such as AA. In our own view, the whole complex of in- and out-patient facilities, halfway houses, domiciliary visits etc. should be regarded as the 'unit' and not merely its in-patient facility [11, 16]. In such a way, the unit should be able to cater for all types of alcoholics in all phases of the condition, even if such patients may not fit into a therapeutic community geared to group discussions. It is obvious that it must not limit itself to the treatment of patients who seem to have a fair prognosis.

The question is often raised as to whether in-patient or out-patient therapy is preferable for alcoholics and drug addicts. This seems however, to be no more than an academic problem [11, 16], as there will always be patients who, at least to start with, will require hospitalisation. The lesser the stigma, the more likely will be the number of those who will present themselves at such an early stage of development that the whole treatment can be carried out without hospital admission – e.g. by the GP, possibly with the help of health visitors, AA etc. The questions should rather be, 'Which type of person requires in-patient treatment?' and 'Which type requires out-patient treatment?' To this purpose much further research will be necessary. The answer to these questions may be determined not wholly by the type of patient and the stage of the development of the condition, but also by the number and type of specially-trained staff or suitable facilities available. Where, for example, special hostels are available, many patients who otherwise would have had to stay in hospital for longer periods could leave hospital earlier; and quite a few homeless and friendless patients might avoid hospitalisation altogether. Such hostels should probably cater exclusively for alcoholics and drug addicts respectively as it has often been found that they do not fit in well into therapeutic communities consisting in the main of other types of patients. The same principle also holds good, very probably, for the treatment of alcoholics in hospital. However the question of forming communities consisting exclusively of drug addicts probably requires much further research.

The length of hospitalisation may also depend largely on the type of after-care available, including assistance from voluntary organisations and local authorities. For example, in areas where there is a strong and good AA group, patients can often be discharged earlier from hospital, and where out-patients clinics or treatment centres have at their disposal a sufficient number of well-trained and experienced social workers and other helpers, hospitalisation can sometimes be avoided altogether.

Not all alcoholics, and perhaps not all addicts, require medical care and attention, though probably in all such cases the GP could be of the greatest help. The GP is in a key position, in as far as he knows the family background and often the history of such a patient from childhood onwards. He is in a position to explain the illness concept of dependence to the patient and to his family, and thereby remove certain psychological obstacles which stand in the path of their applying for help. He could carry out a certain part of the treatment himself, or refer the patient to the facility best suited to his condition and he could collaborate with out-patient and in-patient facilities, local authorities and with bodies such as AA. He could also supervise the after-care (e.g. disulfiram administration in the case of alcoholics) after discharge from hospital. He has the chance, based on his intimate knowledge of the home situation and the family background, to spot early behavioural changes and thus to make an early diagnosis, to win the patient's confidence and co-operation and to impress on him and his family the need for treatment and the likelihood – provided there is co-operation – of recovery or at least marked improvement. In helping the families of alcoholics and drug addicts to regard the conditions as illnesses rather than as a vice, crime, character weakness etc., the GP can do a great deal to alter a negative home atmosphere into one that is constructive and helpful [11].

Treatment goals

The treatment goals should be realistic and aim at the optimum attainable in each given patient. The ideal goal is, of course, total abstinence from alcohol or addictive drugs, combined with effective and satisfying social-occupational functioning. The goal of total abstinence from alcohol in the case of alcoholics should in general be strictly adhered to, notwithstanding occasional reports of ertswhile alcoholics having become moderate drinkers. Helping alcoholics to achieve total abstinence is usually the first step in therapy, because as a rule only after he has stayed sober for some time, is the alcoholic in a fit state to understand, and to grapple with, his underlying psychological and social problems. On the other hand, in drug addicts as in alcoholics, personality defects may prevent such people from being helped beyond a certain potential, and in such people one has often to be satisfied with a more modest goal, falling short of life-long abstinence and full, independent socio-occupational functioning. Chronic drunkenness offenders, for example, who never in their life had been socialised, may sometimes require life-longe motional and social support. They certainly are always in need of a much more comprehensive and wider rehabilitation programme (including, e.g. vocational guidance and training, help with finding suitable lodgings or hostels, etc.) than the average alcoholic (17).

The task of establishing a realistic attainable goal becomes even more complex in the case of drug-dependent individuals. Ideally addicts should be weaned off their drugs and be helped to learn to live fully and happily without them. But so many young drug addicts are emotionally so unstable, immature and dependent that sometimes one wonders whether they will ever be in a position to function without drugs. Similarly, in the case of certain amphetamine or barbiturate users, who function fairly well for years as long as they are given a moderate maintenance dose of their drugs, but who go to pieces if their drugs are discontinued, it is difficult to decide whether insistence on total abstinence from their drug in such exceptional cases is essential [18]. In the case of narcotic addicts the question of stabilised addicts is sometimes brought up. They must be few and far between, as tolerance usually forces the addict to push his dose upwards, and so many narcotic addicts do not function well anyway whilst taking these drugs. Rarely one comes across addicts who seem to function reasonably well on small doses of heroin (and even cocaine) or – in the USA – frequently on high doses of methadone. On the other hand, it is clear that before agreeing to such maintenance therapy in the case of young newcomers who claim that they could not live without their drugs, stringent precautionary clinical and laboratory investigations should be carried out. In the UK, for example, the present drug epidemic amongst youngsters was directly helped on its way by the ease with which a few London GPs agreed to prescribe large amounts of amphetamines, heroin, cocaine and more recently barbiturates to youngsters appearing on their doorsteps and clamouring for such drugs [3, 19].

Thus whilst as a rule ideal goals should be aimed at, one has sometimes to be satisfied with less complete, intermediate goals, e.g. with the patient's improvement rather than full recovery, with reduction of drug amount as far as possible, and with his functioning at a level of socio-occupational and emotional stability, that is not too unsatisfactory for him and that frees him from the need to indulge in subsocial activities.

The treatment procedure and the phases of treatment in cases of alcoholism and other forms of drug dependence follow in general a similar order. Treatment starts in general with the gradual or abrupt withdrawal of the drug and detoxification. This is followed by long-term treatment and finally the rehabilitation phase, though clearly no strict demarcation line exists between them. In fact, the rehabilitation task begins in most cases the first time such a patient is seen. After-care is the most important phase. In many patients it will be necessary also to treat complications, such as malnutrition, overdoses, injuries etc., so that any treatment facility specifically dealing with these conditions should have immediate and rapid access to medical and surgical establishments. Very often – i.e. as a rule in drug addicts and commonly in alcoholics – the withdrawal and detoxification treatment will require hospitalisation, whereas the long-term and rehabilitation treatment will take place in the community. Whether the immediate post-withdrawal and the initial steps of the long-term therapy will be carried out on a residential or non-residential basis, will depend on a number of factors, such as type of drug dependence, severity of individual case, treatment philosophy (e.g. therapeutic community facilities aim at much more than mere drug withdrawal, such as emotional re-orientation etc.), availability in the community of adequate after-care facilities or self-help organisations etc.

Compulsory treatment

The question of compulsory treatment in patients suffering from alcoholism or drug dependence is complex and controversial. It is often said that it is of no use to treat such patients unless they are 'ready', yet, on the other hand, the former view that alcoholics cannot recover until they have reached 'rock bottom' has now been abandoned. 'Rock bottom' is not a static point and does not mean that a sufferer must have lost family, home and health, but is an individual experience at a juncture at which the sufferer realises that he cannot any longer continue with his drinking or drug taking in his old way. Everyone agrees, of course, that it would be preferable that such patients come voluntarily for treatment, but what is one to do if one sees such people going downhill rapidly, adamantly refusing treatment despite their obvious urgent need for it. In fact, probably the great majority of so-called voluntary (in the UK, informal) alcoholic and drug-dependent patients are voluntary in name only; very often they come pushed along by the threat of divorce, loss of job or court proceedings. In such cases the 'rock bottom' experience has been hastened by external agents, and one wonders whether this principle could not with advantage – and sometimes possibly with health and life-saving effect – be employed more often. Use is made of a similar principle for example, in the case of many American firms whose constructive policy in regard to their alcoholic employees consists in helping them to have treatment whilst keeping their jobs open, but in threatening dismissal if they fail to undergo and to co-operate with treatment [20].

It is often maintained that treatment is useless unless patients are motivated, but many experiences have shown that even patients who at the beginning were totally unmotivated, sooner or later acquired insight into their illness and their need for treatment [11]. Likewise the argument that treatment results with compulsorily treated patients were poor, does not dispense with the occasional need to consider the possibility of compulsory therapy in individuals who refuse treatment where it is obviously imperative. Many alcoholic patients have in fact recovered although their treatment was initiated without their consent [11]. As regards people dependent on other drugs, at the present juncture results unfortunately are often equally unsatisfactory whether they are treated voluntarily or compulsorily [18, 21].

Finally, there is the often used argument of the 'liberty of the subject'. Yet it is difficult to see how one could speak of the freedom of an habitually intoxicated alcoholic or a continually 'stoned' drug addict to make a rational choice. Such people are more or less continually prevented by their intoxicated state from making any free decisions. Only if treatment has helped them, for several weeks at least, to abstain from alcohol or drugs would they be rendered rational enough to take such a decision.

It is sometimes argued by sociologists [22] that psychiatrists calling for compulsory treatment measures hide their essentially punitive attitudes and authoritarian techniques of social control behind a mantle of humanitarianism. However, those professional workers not directly involved in active therapeutic measures might easily overlook the need for active steps which are necessary both in the interests of the individual's own health as well as (often) that of his family. After all, the alcoholic and drug-dependent individual destroy not only their own health but also that of those nearest and closest to them, and desperate appeals for help coming from the family are only too well-known to those charged with looking after such patients.

Clearly, care will have to be taken that compulsory treatment does not degenerate into mere custodial care, that as far as possible the therapy within the hospital or unit is carried out exactly as for voluntary patients (e.g. within the framework of a therapeutic community), and that the compulsory label is discontinued as soon as possible. Such compulsory treatment should be followed by an adequate period of after-care and supervision after discharge, and hospital treatment could possibly often be cut short by a system of parole, e.g. to a hostel. As in all such schemes, built-in research evaluation should be part and parcel of such programmes.

However, in general, arguments and discussions about the need or otherwise for compulsory treatment measures are usually shelved on the grounds that there is no adequate proof that it would work, and that voluntary measures would be better. While everyone would agree that voluntary treatment would be preferable – if patients would agree to have it – the present laissez-faire policy, in this writer's view, means that quite a few sufferers from alcoholism and drug dependence, whose health could at least be temporarily restored or at least greatly improved, may die prematurely or unnecessarily.

One difficult point in this connection must still be remembered. Like voluntary treatment, compulsory therapy could be expected to work best in the case of those people for whom one would be most reluctant to employ it, e.g. the middle-aged, fairly stable alcoholic who in the past has achieved a fair degree of socio-economic stability and has since fallen on bad times. On the other hand, little success could be expected in the case of the young antisocial alcohol or drug user suffering from an underlying character disorder, who usually can expect little help from voluntary treatment either.

In the UK under the Mental Health Act 1959, Sections 25, 26, 29 and 60 provide in certain cases grounds for the hospital admission of alcoholic or drug-dependent patients – though not primarily because of alcoholism or drug dependence but because of their disturbed mental state in general [17]. Similarly Section 4 of the Criminal Justice Act makes it possible, with the consent of the sufferer, to impose a Condition of Residence in hospital of up to one year.

Although alcoholics and drug addicts are sick people, requiring rehabilitation and not punishment, for some reason or other there will always be those among them who, because of offences related to their compulsive drinking or drug taking, will find themselves in prison. A recent Home Office Working Party Report on Habitual Drunken Offenders [17] recommended a whole series of changes, including sobering-up stations and varying types of hostels for such people, which should replace the present useless cycle of repeated fines or short-term imprisonment. However, it is clear that some time will elapse until these suggested changes can be implemented. Until then such people – of whom a considerable proportion are genuine alcohol addicts with evidence of chemical dependence [23] – will often be sent to prison, as may be other alcoholics and drug-dependent individuals who run foul of the law. It should be possible to establish in a few selected prisons, proper units for their treatment, to be run on the lines of therapeutic communities, with a well-trained and sympathetic, understanding staff, possibly with the provision that a certain period, in the case of co-operative offenders, could be spent in hostels whilst working outside prison; any misdemeanours would automatically lead to loss of privileges. In this way a more constructive regime could be established which might help in the rehabilitation of a certain proportion of these people [11, 21].*

* Such a unit – comprising alcoholics, drug addicts, compulsive gamblers etc. and working on the principle of a therapeutic community with extensive group therapy – has recently been established in a London prison. As the experiment is still in its initial phases, it is of course much too early to draw too many inferences at this stage. However, thanks very largely to the enthusiasm and the great interest of the (mostly) self-selected staff, so far one witnesses a surprising amount of co-operation and initiative from the inmates who participate very actively in the regular and frequent group discussions and other activities. Once more it has to be stressed that whatever the effect on these addicts whilst they are in prison, such experiments cannot succeed unless they are followed up by a comprehensive after-care programme

Drug therapy

In the host, predisposition or vulnerability often plays an important role in the causation of alcohol and drug dependence, therefore care has to be taken whilst treating such patients not to substitute one type of drug misuse and dependence for another. For example, the psychogenic alcoholic – in contrast to the sociogenic alcoholic – may often act as if he feels two tablets might do him twice as much good as one. Thus a practitioner who prescribes barbiturates in an attempt to wean him from his alcoholism, might possibly succeed, but only at the high price of substituting a state of barbiturate dependence in place of alcoholism. However, alcoholics have also been found to readily abuse non-barbiturate hypnotics, such as glutethimide, methylprylone paralde-hyde, methaqualone (in the form of the proprietary preparation mandrax) etc., the tranquilliser meprobamate, and the stimulating amphetamines. Thus great care must be taken in the treatment of alcoholics to minimise or to avoid the prescribing of these dependence-producing agents, and as far as possible non-dependence-producing drugs should be prescribed instead. Naturally the same principle holds good for addicts to other drugs. It is interesting to note that many of the drugs more recently favoured by young drug addicts are the same ones which years ago were (and still are today) abused by alcoholics. Thus in recent years on the English drug scene many youngsters have abused amphetamines (including Drinamyl, methylamphetamine), bar-biturates and mandrax – often refusing the alternatives offered to them by the doctor, such as the benzodiazepines (chlordiazepoxide, diazepam or the hypnotic nitrazepam). Likewise in our experience among alcoholics such abuse of amphetamines, barbiturates, mandrax, and glutethimide (Doriden) was common in the past, but abuse of the benzodiazepines was very rare [11]. Changing over from alcohol to the opiates among recovered alcoholics and *vice versa* seems much less common in England than in the USA. But quite clearly the possibility that emotionally unstable and vulnerable personalities, with a psycho-logical readiness [15] to escape into drug abuse, may easily switch from one addictive agent to another must always be kept in mind in the treatment of these people.

Naturally the therapeutic use of tranquillisers, hypnotics and anti-depressants cannot always be avoided (and may often be of great value) in these patients who so often suffer from anxiety, tension, depression, insomnia etc., especially in the early post-withdrawal as well as during the withdrawal period. Probably no CNS-affecting drug is quite free from the risk of producing dependence, especially in unstable personalities, and in particular in those individuals who have already proven themselves prone or predisposed towards the development of dependence in the past. But care should be taken to choose those drugs which seem, so far, to have shown relatively less abuse liability; for example among the tranquillisers the phenothiazines and the benzodiazepines; among hypnotics the non-barbiturates, in particular (at the present state of knowledge) nitrazepam; and the modern non-stimulating antidepressant drugs (see Part 5) in place of the CNS-stimulating amphetamines. Care should also be taken to discontinue all such drugs used as soon as possible.

Another question to be considered is the use of these drugs in later phases, during the after-care and rehabilitation period (as different from the withdrawal and immediate post-withdrawal period). For example, they may be used in the alcoholic who from time to time may be assailed by what AA members call *dry-drunk* episodes of tension or depression. These episodes also occur in drug addicts who try to keep away from their drugs of dependence. In principle, it would of course be better to keep away from CNS-affecting agents altogether in the long-term therapy of such people. However, although 'hope is better than dope' [24], sometimes judicious, temporary, moderate employment of mild tranquillisers and antidepressants may help these patients to get over periods of tension and depression which might otherwise carry a great risk of provoking a relapse into drinking. From his knowledge of the patient's personality and vulnerability, the doctor has to assess (a very difficult task) whether the patient is capable of tolerating this particular episode of tension and of overcoming the hurdle without the help of drugs, or whether the tension would prove too much and the patient would be more likely to fall by the wayside, so that for a period tranquillisers or antidepressants may be indicated [25]. However, in the long run, clearly the alcoholic's and the drug addict's hope of a happy future rests on the foundations of re-education and emotional reorientation, rather than on chemical tranquillisation, sedation or stimulation [25].

Psychological and social therapy
In the hands of various observers, quite different therapeutic techniques have achieved success in the case of some alcoholics and drug addicts, only to fail abysmally in the hands of others. It has therefore been

argued that possibly all these different techniques may work on the basis of a common denominator, i.e. the breakdown of old-established, long-cherished attitudes to such an extent that the way is free for the development of diametrically opposed attitudes, and a totally changed outlook [26, 27]. Such personality disruption might, for example, possibly result from the chemical aversion therapies for alcoholism by apomorphine or emetine, which have also been used occasionally for other forms of drug dependence), the fear-of-death provoking experience of the disulfiram–alcohol reaction, Wesley's technique of frightening his listeners with 'hell and brimstone' before offering them a way out, the conversion experience of some AA members, and also the 'rock bottom' concept of AA. Similarly, there is the uncovering process of analytic psychotherapy, and the frequently very aggressive, possibly often traumatic techniques employed by the self-help organisation of drug addicts such as Synanon and the encounter groups of Phoenix. Possibly all these techniques may be so traumatic to the patient's ego that his old attitudes become shattered and he becomes ready and motivated to search for alternative, more constructive ways of trying to cope with his inner (emotional) and external problems and obstacles.

However, a common denominator might also lie, perhaps, not so much in the type of therapeutic techniques used but in the attitude of the therapist, i.e. his ability to get through to the patient and to build up a helping relationship [11]. After all, the same techniques which proved so valuable in the hands of some therapists, failed with others. Many wonder-drugs and techniques which were found extremely helpful by their initiators, who had extreme faith in them, have come and gone, because others lacking belief in their value failed to reproduce the successful results of the originator of the new technique. Nobody adopting a censoring, moralistic, or even ridiculing attitude, in a 'holier-than-thou' spirit is likely to have much success in treating alcoholics. On the other hand, an approach based on understanding and genuine emotional acceptance (which implies much more than just paying lip-service to the disease concept of alcoholism or drug dependence) will often get a long way. Understanding and accepting such patients does, of course, not mean that all their activities are approved. On the contrary, the therapist who has been able to build up such a genuine, helping relationship with the patient, will often be in a good position to convey to him that certain behaviours are in fact not in his best interest – and the patient will be willing to accept such strictures from this therapist whilst rejecting them scornfully when coming from another therapist.

Whether social or psychological therapy [28] is relatively more important, may to some extent depend on the circumstances in which a person becomes dependent. In countries [15] or occupational groups [11] in which drinking or drug taking is widespread and socially accepted, even emotionally relatively stable personalities may become heavy drinkers (and some among them alcoholics) or become dependent on drugs, without necessarily feeling very guilty or secretive about it (see Part 2). Such personalities may require less psychotherapy, though supportive advice or counselling may be necessary, and attention will have to be directed to their social or occupational environment, as, for example, removal from the influence of their subculture. On the other hand, in countries, or socio-occupational groups where heavy drinking is taboo (and similar considerations may apply to heavy drinking in women), in the main psychologically vulnerable personalities will expose themselves to the risk of social censorship and become excessive drinkers or drug takers. In such cases, psychotherapy will play a more important role – e.g. such people may also be beset by guilt feelings, depression, and their prognosis as a group will be less favourable than that of the first group.

Pharmacological therapy

In general it may perhaps be said that in the withdrawal and post-withdrawal phases, drug therapies are relatively more important (although the rehabilitation process and the attempt to establish a helping relationship with the patient should already have started by then), and that psychological and social methods of therapy become relatively more important in subsequent phases. However, certain specific pharmacological therapies are employed in the long-term treatment, i.e. the alcohol-sensitising treatment in the case of alcoholism using disulfiram or CCC (citrated calcium carbimide) and the use of narcotic-blocking agents (methadone) and narcotic antagonists (e.g. cyclazocine) in narcotic dependence. The modes of action in these therapeutic approaches to alcoholism and drug dependence are quite different from each other. However they are similar in that in both cases the specific drug therapy aims at dissuading the alcoholic or the narcotic addict from continuing with his drug of dependence, by pharmacological interference with the effect of his addictive drug on him. In the case of the alcoholic this occurs by (the fear of) producing a very unpleasant and dangerous reaction through stopping the further metabolic breakdown of alcohol (at the acetaldehyde stage). In the case of the narcotic addict it occurs by (a) producing cross-tolerance between methadone and the opiate (such as heroin) on which the addict had become dependent, and by reducing the craving for the opiate, or (b) by preventing through the use of narcotic antagonists, the opiate addict from finding relief when taking his narcotic, through the precipitation of abstinence symptoms, and by helping to forestall the development of dependence in those dabbling and experimenting with opiates.

Treatment with alcohol-sensitising agents, such as disulfiram, is not based on conditioning as repeated disulfiram–alcohol tests would be too dangerous (e.g. ECG changes have been noted after such tests). However, another pharmacological therapy for alcoholism depends largely on the establishment of conditioning, i.e. the aversion treatments by the use of emetine, and probably also apomorphine, or by electric shock. The treatment of narcotic dependence by antagonists is based on conditioning theory [29]. Narcotic antagonists by interfering with the relief, or the 'reward' – otherwise obtained by the addict's recourse to his narcotic during his enforced abstinence period – might lead to extinction of physical dependence and of drug-seeking behaviour [30, 31].

Self-help organisations

It is not too much to say that the approach to alcoholism has been revolutionised since the advent in 1935 of the fellowship of Alcoholics Anonymous [11] which to a large extent has also been a forerunner of and (with several modifications) the model for several self-help organisations for addicts formed over the past few years. Whatever other methods may be used in the treatment of alcoholics, the therapist will find an invaluable ally in AA, the fellowship of recovered, and recovering alcoholics. Here the alcoholic – feeling misunderstood, rejected and ostracised by society – finds a body of people who have undergone similar experiences to his own. He feels understood, accepted, and experiences a feeling of belonging and by helping other alcoholics he gains self-confidence, self-respect and satisfaction. Meeting in AA other alcoholics who have in the past used over time the same defence mechanisms as he has done, he soon finds he can no longer get away with these rationalisations, projections, repressions and denials. He is thus encouraged to allow his façade to disappear and learn to face up to reality.

In principle the same basic approach is employed not only by Gamblers Anonymous and the Weight Watchers but also by the drug addicts' newer self-help organisations [32] – Synanon, Daytop, Phoenix and Odyssey – indeed, the first, Synanon, was started by a recovered alcoholic. Compared with AA, they are more aggressive in the sense that the attitude change – which takes place more gradually in those alcoholics who stick to the AA programme of recovery, involving the '12 steps' – is helped along more actively by such means as the encounter groups of Phoenix and Marathon. During these group sessions accusations pour forth, there is a controlled release of anger and verbal aggression, with the purpose of encouraging members to become honest and to express emotions, and so to acquire new modes of behaviour, attitudes and values. Another difference between AA and these addicts' self-help groups is the fact that AA is non-residential (although there are now all over the world also many AA groups in hospitals and prisons). AA meetings are attended, as a rule, by alcoholics who live in their own homes, who often follow their occupations etc., and who usually meet at closed meetings (for alcoholics only) or at open and public meetings, which are open to family, friends and the general public. Compared to alcoholics, in narcotic addicts there is usually a greater disturbance of personality and of the mode of living. This may be due to the narcotic addicts' dependence on a potent narcotic drug, their greater degree of immaturity and their greater social disruption (estrangement from parental home, lack of residence etc.). As such, the addict's self-help communities are usually residential, being run (like units and hostels for alcoholics and addicts) on the lines of a therapeutic community. Apart from Synanon, the aim of these self-help organisations (and the most difficult task) is usually – after dependency on the drug has been altered temporarily to a dependence on the therapeutic community – to assist their members towards a re-entry into the community at large.

Both AA and the addicts' self-help groups are also of great value as means of education and enlightenment of the general public. AA, for example, has shown to the professional and lay public (as of course also to alcoholic newcomers) that alcoholics in their thousands can recover, and has thus helped to change the former picture of doom and gloom into one of hopefulness. In time, one may hope, these addicts'

self-help organisations may assist, too, in the gradual change of the
public image of the drug addict.

The therapeutic community

The principle of the therapeutic community – employed by the
addicts' self-help organisations – is also the basis of the approach in
alcoholism and addiction units and hostels [11, 21]. For example, in the
UK two Government Memoranda have recommended – for those
alcoholics who require hospitalisation – treatment in regional alcoholism units which are to work in association with GPs, local authorities, voluntary organisations, AA etc. The therapeutic community
approach – introduced into psychiatry by Maxwell Jones [33] – in such
units is combined with another basic principle, discovered by AA, i.e.
the ability of alcoholics easily to identify with each other and thereby
to learn from and to help each other by mutual understanding. In a
therapeutic community the old hospital hierarchical system has been
abandoned, and all grades of staff and patients work together towards
a common goal. This involves as much active patients' participation,
initiative, responsibility and self-government as possible. Everything
occurring during the 24 hour day in close living, working and playing
together can be observed and discussed, and thus used to therapeutic
purpose. The aim of treatment in such a therapeutic community goes
thus far beyond mere dry withdrawal and detoxification, which is
largely a chemical process. It also deals with post-withdrawal and the
early rehabilitation phases, though it is impressed on the patient that it
still constitutes only the first step in a much longer drawn-out, long-
term rehabilitation process [6].

Obviously, such units – which should have out-patient and hostel
facilities etc. – should also provide help with social and occupational
problems. Thus they should have access to facilities for vocational
guidance and possibly occupational training, facilities for education,
etc. They also provide excellent opportunities for professional and lay
education and for research [11, 16].

Similarly, alcoholic hostels, such as those for discharged hospital
patients, for ex-prisoners or for habitual drunkenness offenders (for
example Rathcoole House in London [23]) are largely based on similar
considerations. As already discussed the therapeutic and management
regime needs to be tailored to the different types of alcoholics with
their varying socio-occupational and educational backgrounds and
potentialities etc.

Post-alcoholism and drug-dependence units and group-therapy sessions nowadays probably mix male and female patients, but should treatment facilities, for example residential units, cater both for alcoholics as well as for addicts to other drugs, or should they be treated, separately? Should those dependent on soft drugs (amphetamines, barbiturates, hallucinogens) be treated alongside opiate addicts, or not? Should those injecting the drugs – skinpoppers (i.mu.) and mainliners (i.v.) – be mixed with those taking them orally?

Clearly these are all questions which require much more planned research. At present opinions vary greatly. Most therapists separate alcoholics and drug addicts but in our units where they have been mixed [34], despite initial difficulties – arising for example from the great differences in age and general outlook between the middle-aged alcoholics and the younger addicts – in the course of time certain advantages were observed. For example, quite a few of the more mature alcoholics were able to relate well to, and to help the much more immature addicts. Tensions which may often arise between the more conforming alcoholics and the non-conforming addicts, created by different age groups, values and life styles, abound with therapeutic opportunities which can be utilised [35] – including the possibility of bridging the generation gap. Obviously the risk of bringing drugs into open establishments (and nowadays the units for alcoholics are usually open) create additional surveillance problems, which in at least one instance led to the abandoning of one such experimental programme in the USA [36]. However, in our experience the mixing in the same unit at Warlingham Park Hospital and at St Bernard's, of middle-aged, therapeutic (i.e. with the drug originally prescribed by a doctor), amphetamine and barbiturate addicts with middle-aged alcoholics – with often similar psychopathology – never produced any real difficulties. We now have in our set-up alcoholics and all types of addicts living in the same wards, i.e. in the same therapeutic community, but we include the middle-aged amphetamine and barbiturate addicts in the group-therapy sessions of the alcoholics, and have separate group sessions for the younger addicts.

Likewise different views are held about the advisability or otherwise of mixing soft and hard drug users [37]. Some observers feel that amphetamine users of the adaptive type (i.e. essentially middle-aged abusers bolstering up their otherwise conventional social functioning) should not be treated in proximity with 'escapists' (i.e. usually younger amphetamine abusers escaping from conventional social functioning),

1 7

or with most narcotic addicts, but in proximity with other 'medicine abusers' (of tranquillisers and antidepressants) and some analgesic addicts who had medical or accidental onsets. It has been claimed that because of the risk of 'seduction', amphetamine abusers should not be treated alongside narcotic addicts, and 'fixers', who inject their drugs (for example methylamphetamine) should not be treated alongside oral amphetamine abusers. In our experience – administrative reasons forced us in the early 1960s to mix soft and hard drug addicts – cases of such seduction were extremely rare, and did not really produce any great problems, but certainly, as already said, much further research is necessary in this field.

Care must be taken in each case not to overlook complications which may have arisen as direct or indirect consequences of drug abuse. Physical complications may include, for example, overdosage (common in the case of hypnotics and narcotics), possibly leading to respiratory depressions (necessitating resuscitation, narcotic antagonists etc.); neglect of personal hygiene and food intake; the mimicking of many neurological diseases by habitual barbiturate overdosage; infections (often – in the case of injections – a consequence of unsterile 'gear') with local and general sepsis or viral hepatitis; or injuries. Mental complications may include paranoid psychosis (amphetamines), anxiety, tension, aggressive behaviour (stimulating drugs) or depression (LSD and 'come down' from stimulating drugs) with risk of suicide attempts or gestures; or states of confusion, disorientation (e.g. hypnotics, LSD) and anxiety, paranoid states, panics (cannabis, LSD) and 'flash-backs' into a hallucinatory state days or weeks after LSD has been taken etc.

Long-term therapy and rehabilitation

In all types of drug dependence withdrawal treatment must be followed by measures aimed at long-term therapy and rehabilitation. Here measures will often have to be quite different. Thus, the modern type of unstable, immature, young multi-drug abuser, the more stable, middle-aged therapeutic or professional addict and those individuals whose drug abuse was precipitated by episodes of extreme stress, or by social pressure, such as subcultures encouraging drug use cannot be treated in the same way. Factors depending on host, environment and agent have all to be taken into consideration when mapping out rehabilitation programmes in individual causes. The task is often much less difficult in the middle-aged, educated, skilled individual who has the support of family and the sheet anchor of a steady interesting job. This addict often may require no more than help from an understanding family doctor and possibly temporarily a regime of tranquillisers and antidepressants, perhaps combined with counselling of the family; and similar conditions may prove helpful in the case of the middle-aged, barbiturate- (or amphetamine-) dependent housewife. Much wider rehabilitative efforts – occupational training, finding of congenial homes and friends – may be needed in the case of the younger, non-therapeutic drug abuser, in particular the young non-therapeutic narcotic addict, who has in recent years become so much more common at the cost of the therapeutic, middle-aged drug abuser [3].

6.2 TREATMENT OF ALCOHOL AND DRUG DEPENDENCE

ALCOHOLISM

Acute stage

Although sudden withdrawal of alcohol – a CNS-depressing drug – occasionally leads to a severe physical abstinence syndrome, including epileptiform convulsions in the first 12–36 hours, and subsequent delirium tremens, abrupt, sudden cessation of alcohol, rather than gradual tapering off is now the method favoured by most therapists for hospitalised alcoholics. In heavy drinkers, where the possibility of such complications is feared, it is wise to give prophylactically such medication as phenytoin (epanutin) 100 mg t.d.s., and tranquillisers (phenothiazines, benzodiazepines or possibly chlormethiazole [11]) (see below).

Dehydration, salt depletion, malnutrition and restlessness require methods such as liberal administration of fluids and salt orally or parenterally, vitamins (especially the B complex) at first parenterally (parentovite is a favourite preparation) i.v. or i.mu., and later orally, and tranquillisers to calm the tense, anxious, agitated and restless patient. Among tranquillising drugs all major and minor tranquillisers have been used, such as chlormethiazole and the phenothiazines: chlorpromazine (Largactil, Thorazine) 50–100 mg t.d.s. (despite the theoretical risk of liver toxicity which in practice does not seem to have provided a great problem), promazine (Sparine) 50–100 mg t.d.s., trifluoperazine (Stelazine) 5–10 mg t.d.s. and thioridazine (Melleril) 50–100 mg t.d.s. (in higher doses an anti-Parkinsonian drug should be given with the phenothiazines, e.g. benzhexol (Atrane). Of the minor tranquillisers the benzodiazepines, chlordiazepoxide (Librium) 10–30 mg t.d.s. or diazepam (Valium) 5–10 mg t.d.s. have been widely used, apparently in the USA all of them in somewhat higher dosage than in the UK. A recently recommended drug is Doxepin (25 mg t.d.s.) [38]. All these tranquilliers can in an average case be gradually withdrawn within about one week.

Insomnia may require the administration of hypnotics at least for the first few nights, and as barbiturates and other non-barbiturates (the latter to a somewhat lesser extent) have proved addictive, nitrazepam (Mogadon, 0·5–1·5 g nocte) seems at present the safest drug for that purpose.

DT

In prevention and treatment of DT the same drugs can be used, though in somewhat higher dosage or parenterally. On the European continent, especially Sweden and Germany, and also in our own experience, both for prevention and treatment of DT, chlormethiazole (Heminevrin) has proved an excellent sedative–hypnotic (39, 40). It is derived from the thiazole part of the vitamin B_1 molecule, and is available as 0·8% solution for i.v. injection or infusion, and as 500 mg tablets. In severe cases of DT, treatment starts by i.v. injection of 40–60 ml of the 0·8% solution over a period of 3–5 minutes, and continues with an oral regime of 2–4 tablets (in less severe cases treatment starts here), to be repeated within 1–2 hours, the aim being to produce profound sedation or sleep; ordinarily a maximum dosage of 9–10 g a day should not be exceeded. We have used this drug also as our routine in ordinary cases of alcohol withdrawal in alcoholics [40]. The drug should be discontinued after 6 days, as, like other CNS-depressing drugs, it carries a risk of psychological and also, more rarely, physical dependence. For this reason it should not be employed as a routine hypnotic or daytime sedative in alcoholics or drug addicts. Because of some evidence that alcoholics prone to develop DT are less likely to develop dependence on other drugs [41], chlormethiazole could be employed for somewhat longer periods in DT patients if required.

A point probably not sufficiently stressed and as yet not widely appreciated even in medical circles, concerns the risk of dangerous physical withdrawal symptoms supervening in heavy drinkers. Such alcohol abstinence syndrome, like the barbiturate abstinence syndrome, is possibly more dangerous than the much more widely known opiate abstinence syndrome. One often hears of alcoholics who have suddenly made up their minds to give up drinking and to 'sweat it out' at home.

Unless skilled medical help and nursing supervision is available at home, in the case of heavy drinkers it seems much safer under such circumstances to 'taper off', by gradually reducing the amount of drink over the next few days, than to cut alcohol out suddenly. Much more preferable, of course, would be the admission of such a patient to detoxification centres [17] (pioneered in Czechoslovakia and Poland and proved of value in the USA – e.g. in St. Louis – and which, one hopes, will be established in the UK in the near future) or to a general hospital for a few days.

Another point concerns the frequent tendency of many (particularly the mainly psychogenic) alcoholics to also take other drugs habitually to excess, especially barbiturates. All alcoholics should therefore be questioned about their drug-taking habits. Should they also habitually have taken barbiturates to excess, these should be tapered off gradually. Where they deny taking barbiturates but where there is some suspicion or doubt, phenobarbitone 100 mg t.d.s. (rather than phenytoin) should be given for the first 3–4 days and then gradually reduced and stopped. The fact that, like alcohol, barbiturate withdrawal can lead to DT must be kept in mind.

Long-term treatment and rehabilitation [11]

Following withdrawal and detoxification, the earlier phase of the long-term treatment and rehabilitation programme could be carried out with the alcoholic remaining as an in-patient, for example in a therapeutic community set-up. On the other hand, after initial withdrawal and detoxification the alcoholic could leave hospital and continue treatment as an out-patient whilst living in the community. The principles were all discussed in Section 6.1. Treatment involves a combination of psychological and social approaches with physical therapies as adjuncts.

Psychotherapy and supportive counselling

There is in general no need for a deep form of psychotherapy and psychoanalysis has not proved successful in the treatment of alcoholism [14]. Brief eclectic psychotherapeutic techniques (often based on psychoanalytic principles) have found widespread employment. The large number of alcoholics in need of treatment practically precludes individual psychotherapy for the great majority anyway, but anyhow, partly because of the urgent need of alcoholics for resocialisation, group psychotherapy is being increasingly employed as a valuable, acceptable (to patients) and effective method. The aim is for the alcoholic to gain some insight into his problems and personality difficulties – which he has tried to solve by taking recourse to drink (or drugs) – and to learn to cope with tensions, anxieties etc. in a more mature and less self-destructive manner than searching oblivion in drink or drugs. That social class is often a factor in alcoholism treatment has recently been stressed by Canadian research workers [42] who found that current clinical treatment of alcoholics favours patients from higher social classes, perhaps partly because of verbal skills involved in psychotherapy and the middle-class background of most therapists. Clearly care should be taken to make allowances for this, possibly by forming a greater variety of socially more homogenous groups presenting fewer social barriers to interaction. On the other hand, we never experienced any difficulties arising from mixing all social groups of alcoholics in our units at Warlingham Park and St. Bernard's.

Social methods [11]
Social support is necessary in a great many alcoholics, its extent depending on the lack of social adjustment, home and occupational circumstances etc. The need to include the patient's family in the treatment situation, to assist the patient in finding suitable accommodation (including hostels), a congenial job, etc. has already been stressed.

In some alcoholics support within the community may have to be very prolonged. At any rate family attitudes are of the greatest importance, as may be the attitudes of an understanding factory Medical Officer and personnel officer. Altering the alcoholic's environment where possible (e.g. finding a circle of friends who are not heavy drinkers etc.) would often help but is frequently not feasible so that alcoholics will have to be assisted towards learning to live with reality and the world as it is, and accepting their own personality limitations.

Physical treatments
Two different types of approaches have found more or less widespread use:

(a) Drugs which sensitise the body to alcohol, such as disulfiram (antabuse) and citrated calcium carbimide (abstem, temposil).

They act as conscious deterrents against drinking, provided the alcoholic has become fully convinced that if he were foolish enough to risk drinking within 3–4 days or 36 hours of taking disulfiram or CCC respectively, he would be likely to suffer extremely distressing (and dangerous) symptoms; e.g. flushing, feeling faint and sick, breath-lessness, feeling like dying etc. Most observers no longer regard a preliminary alcohol–disulfiram test as necessary. The procedure is for alcoholics to regularly take a maintenance dose – for example 1 tablet of antabuse (i.e. 200 mg) in the evening, or a tablet of abstem (1 g) in the morning. CCC is slightly less effective than disulfiram; its protective effect starts more rapidly and also wanes earlier than that of disulfiram. Given such minimum maintenance dosage, serious side-effects from taking these drugs, for example peripheral neuropathy, are rare. Obviously it is easy for the alcoholic to stop taking these tablets and, as in the case of any other method, its success depends on the therapist's ability to arouse a motivation in the alcoholic to try to abstain from drinking. Thus these drugs, like other physical treatments, are no more than adjuncts to the more fundamental socio-psychological techniques. Yet in the hands of the GP who is able to establish a positive relation-ship with his alcoholic patient, his use of such drugs, perhaps combined with referral to AA, may in many early-stage alcoholics provide a very efficient and successful approach.

A more recently introduced drug – metronidazole (Flagyl) – claimed to have some disulfiram-like properties and to diminish alcohol withdrawal symptoms and craving [43], has not yet been sufficiently evaluated to allow more definite conclusions.

(b) Aversion techniques.

Pharmacological methods – apomorphine [44] or emetine [26] and, more recently re-introduced, electric shock techniques – have been employed to induce in the alcoholic a conditioned aversion towards the sight, smell and taste of alcohol. The principle consists in associating the taking of alcohol with an unpleasant experience. These methods have, of course, to be carried out in hospital. Although at one time very popular, especially in private practice, nowadays consensus of opinion is probably that at best such conditioning techniques are no more than adjuvants to psychosocial methods.

Clearly, before carrying out any of these physical techniques, a thorough physical and laboratory investigation is required, including urinalysis, liver function tests, ECG and probably blood analysis; and in the case of the aversion techniques, nursing staff well-versed in these particular methods must be available.

(c) Other drugs are sometimes employed.

LSD for some time enjoyed a certain vogue in the treatment of alcoholics, but again it is probably fair to say that few therapists would

now feel that there is a real indication for it in the treatment of alcoholics – although further research is indicated [45].

The occasional use of tranquillisers and antidepressives [46] (but not
barbiturates or amphetamines and related drugs) to tide alcoholics over
occasional emotional crises and periods of difficulties has already been
referred to [25].

Alcoholics Anonymous

AA and its sister organisation, Al Anon (and also Alateen, for the
adolescent relatives of alcoholics), are the most valuable allies of the
doctor in the rehabilitation of alcoholics. On its own AA – without
any professional help – has assisted more alcoholics to a contented
state of sobriety than all professional disciplines taken together. AA
regards alcoholism as a sickness of body, mind and spirit, social (group),
psychological and spiritual factors all entering into the AA programme
of recovery. Some of its principles have been discussed above. AA is
only too happy to co-operate with doctors and other professionals.
There are now groups all over the British Isles (and even more in the
USA, where it was founded nearly 40 years ago). Two additional points
must be made. As the image of 'the' alcoholic is based on the loss-of-
control alcoholic – the person who, having had one drink, cannot be
certain of being able to call a halt on that occasion – the GP when
recommending other types of alcoholics to join AA, should explain
the difference to his patient so as to forestall misunderstandings. Also
the GP who has recommended disulfiram or CCC to his patient, should
warn him against being put off these tablets by the occasional ill-
informed adverse comment from a few overenthusiastic AA members
who feel that because they have done well with AA alone, any drug
treatment is superfluous. Just as doctors have no monopoly in treating
alcoholics and should co-operate with AA as far as possible, it is likewise clear that by itself no single agency – not even AA – can successfully treat all alcoholics. By itself, AA is probably the most successful
single agency, but as there are so many different types of alcoholics,
there is an absolute need for close, integrated collaboration of all
interested agencies.

The GP will also find the greatest help from close co-operation with
Al Anon, the organisation for families of alcoholics. By referring the
desperate wife of an alcoholic to that organisation, she will find kindred
souls with similar experiences, frustrations etc. and will find great help
in meeting others in a similar position. She may thus develop a dif-

ferent attitude, find new hope, and in this altered frame of mind may be able to approach her alcoholic husband in quite a different way from before – which in turn may have positive consequences on his behaviour in the future.

Complications
Prior to establishing a treatment programme, a full physical examination and certain laboratory tests should be carried out. Alcoholism, like all other forms of dependence, can lead to physical complications. Some of these complications are reversible, e.g. polyneuropathy (treated by vitamin B complex in high doses to start with parenterally, later orally and then with physiotherapy etc.). Polyneuropathy is sometimes associated with memory defects and confabulations (KorsaKoff's syndrome – which may improve to a major or lesser extent), Wernicke's syndrome (high vitamin B complex parenterally), reversible fatty infiltration of the liver, or irreversible liver cirrhosis – which, however, under a regime of total abstinence and balanced diet, may be stationary for many years. These physical as well as the mental complications (alcoholic paranoia, dementia etc.) require separate treatment – quite apart from the over-riding need for lifelong abstinence.

Can alcoholics learn to drink in moderation?
In spite of the publication of occasional case reports of a few 'cured' alcoholics apparently having managed for years to drink in moderation, at the present state of knowledge the rule must still remain that alcoholics have to learn to accept, without resentment or bitterness, the fact that drink is definitely out for them. Quite a few alcoholics manage in fact to drink moderately for short periods, by clinging to certain rules: such as beer or wine only, drinking with meals and in company only, drinking very small amounts only, or only when in a cheerful, relaxed frame of mind etc. [11]. But sooner or later in almost all cases these attempts are doomed to failure. It is true that for an alcoholic who for so long had considered alcohol as practically his only ally and standby, the future may sound bleak and miserable indeed without alcohol, but the GP can make use of a technique used by AA, i.e. for the alcoholic to live a day at a time. He may find the task of living without alcohol for one day easily manageable; tomorrow is another day which will be tackled when it comes along. In this way the sober days will mount to weeks, then to months. The doctor will be able to assure the alcoholic that once he has managed six and more

months without a drink, the going will become easier [47], though every alcoholic must for ever beware of neglectful overconfidence. The doctor can also reassure his alcoholic patient that many thousands of male and female alcoholics have found life without alcohol not only tolerable but also happy and full. Naturally when joining AA he will meet numerous examples of recovered alcoholics, a visual demonstration which will give him hope. By helping other alcoholics, once he himself has been off alcohol for a certain period, he will also do a great deal to help himself (AA's '12 step' Work, Sponsorship).

In the overall approach to alcoholism the family doctor has a key role to play, not only as a very important member of the therapeutic team but also by setting an example to the general public in accepting the alcoholic as a sick man who can be helped and who is well-worth helping.

DEPENDENCE OF THE BARBITURATE TYPE

Whilst the protagonists of this type are the barbiturates, very similar features occur also in the case of dependence on non-barbiturate hypnotics and sedatives, and the minor tranquillisers [2]. Though not yet included in the WHO descriptions, chlormethiazole dependence seems to belong to the same type (as does paraldehyde). There is development of psychological dependence and also physical dependence, with the supervening of a dangerous physical abstinence syndrome when dosage is suddenly reduced below a critical level. Because tolerance is irregular and incomplete, there is disturbance of behaviour and a state of chronic intoxication which often resembles that seen in long-standing alcoholism. Treatment in all these forms of dependence resemble that described for alcohol dependence.

Acute stage

These drugs must never be suddenly withdrawn but tapered off gradually, for example, in the case of barbiturates by about $0 \cdot 1$ g every second day. Reduction should be stopped temporarily for a few days when signs such as tremor, anxiety, insomnia etc. appear. In cases of persistent anxiety and depression following withdrawal, smallish doses of benzodiazepines and antidepressants (not amphetamines) could be given. Vitamin medication is indicated where there is evidence of undernutrition, as for example in the modern type of young main-liners of barbiturates. In cases of insomnia, nitrazepam seems the most suitable drug at the moment. During barbiturate withdrawal watch should be kept for evidence of serious depression and possible suicide attempts.

In the modern cases of multiple drug dependence, withdrawal of the various drugs can be carried out simultaneously. In the case of dependence on the popular barbiturate–amphetamine preparations (e.g. Drinamyl) the drug should be tapered off as described above.

Withdrawal DT
The best method is probably to reintroduce smaller doses of the drug concerned, and withdraw it slowly after a few days. Alternatively, high doses of a phenothiazine (e.g. chlorpromazine 100–150 mg t.d.s.) or paraldehyde 10 ml i.m.u., or, perhaps best, chlormethiazole (as described in the alcoholism section) can be given.

Post-withdrawal phase, long-term treatment and rehabilitation
The principles have been outlined in previous sections. There is, of course, a great difference here between the rehabilitation needs of the modern young addict and of the middle-aged addicts, who usually have been introduced to the drug by their GP (therapeutic addict). The latter may often still have the stabilising influence of home, husband and family, and although in their case, too, the condition may tend to relapse, their chances are not too bad.

The state of chronic intoxication – with features such as ataxia, confusion, disorientation, slurred speech etc. – usually responds fairly rapidly to the regimen of rest, gradual reduction of barbiturates (or the drugs involved), vitamin medication (if there is evidence of neglect of nutrition), non-barbiturate hypnotics when an hypnotic is needed, possibly followed later on in states of continuing tension or depression by minor tranquillisers and/or antidepressants. In as far as, to a certain extent, the psychopathology of middle-aged barbiturate abusers resembles that of alcoholics, we have for many years included such patients in groups formed predominantly by alcoholics. There seemed little difficulty in mutual identification, in particular as the alcoholics' groups always included a certain proportion of drinkers who also had habitually misused barbiturates.

Individual psychological support, counselling, or brief psychotherapy may occasionally be required to help these patients to cope with inner stresses and outer problems (domestic, marital, business etc.) from which they had initially sought refuge in excessive drug taking.

In general, as with alcoholics, the outlook for middle-aged barbiturate addicts is not too bad, though probably less good than in the case of alcoholics. This depends mainly on the ego strength and stability of the underlying personality, his or her history of residential, domestic and – in male addicts – occupational stability, and the support available from family, friends and occupation. No drug therapy comparable to disulfiram is available in the case of dependence on barbiturates (or on other soft drugs).

Complications
The complications arising from intravenous self-injections are worse in the case of barbiturates than with methylamphetamine, opiate and cocaine injections. However, in the UK, practically all youngsters taking barbiturates to excess are multi-drug abusers, as a rule also taking cannabis and amphetamines, and often heroin, methadone and LSD. After the gradual withdrawal of the barbiturates and attention to the physical state and complications, the treatment and rehabilitation problems are therefore the same as discussed in the case of other young drug abusers in the following chapters. As a rule, young British barbiturate abusers claim they have been driven to the use of 'sleepers' as a consequence of the policy of the specialised Treatment Centres which did not provide them with as much 'stuff' (heroin, or more recently, methadone) as they need. The problem of barbiturate abuse by British youngsters is therefore intimately bound up with the approach to the problem of the young heroin addict.

DEPENDENCE OF THE MORPHINE TYPE

This type, with strong psychological dependence and rapid development of physical dependence and tolerance, is seen in habitual misusers of opium, morphine, heroin etc., as well as of synthetic products, such as methadone, pethidine, dextromoramide etc. As in the case of the barbiturates, there is in many ways a fundamental difference between young non-therapeutic addicts on the one hand and the relatively more stable middle-aged addicts on the other. The latter may have started their drug-abusing career as a consequence of being prescribed opiates during the course of a painful illness (therapeutic addicts). A few of these may have managed to keep on a relatively stable dosage and to function fairly well (stabilised addicts), although such occurrence by and large seems to be relatively rare. The group of (usually middle-aged) professional addicts (doctors, nurses etc.) also differ from the young non-therapeutic group. Similarly the largely middle-aged opium smokers in the Far East seem a very different group from the young, modern type of narcotic addicts in the UK and in the USA. In this middle-aged group, opium smoking in the 'dens' is to a large extent related to long-standing customs and poor material living conditions (in this respect resembling the heroin misuse among New York's slum dwellers) rather than to marked personality problems. Given the possibility of some change of environmental conditions, in cases where such dependence is mainly a consequence of environmental, social and cultural factors (e.g. acceptance of drug taking among a certain group), many such addicts could be regarded as being 'easily amenable to treatment' [48].

The problem is much greater in the group of young heroin addicts in whom personality instability may have been a marked contributory factor in the escalation from soft drugs (cannabis, amphetamines) – used widely among their peers – to the hard drugs (from which the great majority of their drug-taking peers had shied away). Subcultural factors often also play a role in these young drug abusers. In treatment both sets of factors – personality and environment – require urgent and often long-continuing attention by such means as psychotherapeutic support, counselling, help with social problems etc. It must be remembered that addicts, in particular narcotic addicts, do not revert to ordinary normal functioning for some time after withdrawal. Effects of prolonged opiate abuse may last six months (prolonged abstinence) [49] and psychological after-effects may linger on for a very long period.

Withdrawal phase
After full assessment of the personality and environmental factors in the given individual and after physical examination (complications) and laboratory investigations, it may occasionally be decided to delay withdrawal. This decision could be the result of certain physical complications (infections, severe malnutrition etc.) or because for some reason or other a maintenance or a very gradual method of withdrawal is adopted. Where it is decided to proceed with withdrawal immediately, the addict's fear of the 'cold turkey' – i.e. withdrawal without any adequate substitution drugs – should be allayed. Narcotic withdrawal symptoms (diarrhoea, severe abdominal cramps, aches all over etc.) can often be very severe, and it would seem inhumane to subject

addicts to such a regime when today adequate, humane and effective methods of withdrawal are available. It is necessary to state this clearly, as very often addicts use their fear of the 'cold turkey' as an alibi not to come for withdrawal treatment at all, and to continue their drug taking. It is remarkable, however, that the narcotic drug self-help organisations manage to tide their newcomer addicts over these very distressing withdrawal phases without the help of drugs. This is mainly a result of support from the groups, which of course reflects the very high motivation of addicts who have decided to join these organisations. However, in hospital or in prison there is no place for such severe regimes.

Methods of withdrawal
Of the regimes formerly described in textbooks and, for example, in a report of a Study Group of the WHO in 1957 [48] most have been abandoned. These include such regimes as the withdrawal of narcotics under cover of such substances as barbiturates or meprobamate (a treatment regime which itself carried the hazard of additional forms of dependence), scopolamine, or with the help of ECT or insulin. In certain circumstances gradual withdrawal under cover of pheno-thiazines – as mentioned in that report – may possibly still be tried. Certain supportive therapy, such as intravenous fluids, cardiovascular stimulants etc., will be required occasionally and should be readily available. However, the method usually employed nowadays for rapid withdrawal, which is very effective and carries little risk, is the substitution method with methadone.

Methadone (known in the UK under its proprietary name Physep-tone) is a synthetic opiate analgesic with similar actions to morphine, but longer lasting. It produces psychic and physical dependence and withdrawal symptoms are probably by and large less severe (though more prolonged) than those of morphine or heroin dependence. In the withdrawal treatment of heroin and morphine addicts, methadone is temporarily substituted for 'H' or morphine and then is itself gradually withdrawn over a period of roughly 7–10 days. The amount and the duration of the medication depends on objective abstinence signs and not on the history obtained from the patient. Methadone is usually given orally (parenteral medication only rarely being necessary) – for ex-ample as syrup of methadone in a dose of 10 or 20 mg, to be repeated when abstinence signs persist. According to Blachly [50] American addicts only rarely require more than 40 mg during a 24 hour period;

English addicts who at least in the past may have taken a higher heroin dosage may sometimes need a greater amount of methadone. When withdrawal symptoms subside methadone is gradually withdrawn, the dose being reduced by 5 mg every 12 or 24 hours. 1 mg methadone is said to equal 1 mg heroin or 3 mg morphine (and 30 mg codeine) [50].

Methadone, of course, is itself an addictive drug. At present the number of known and unknown English addicts using methadone is probably higher than that of heroin addicts. A drug found to carry only a slight addictive risk and, because of its unsuitability for parenteral injection, having a much smaller hazard of misuse, is the antidiarrhoea agent, diphenoxylate, a congener of pethidine [51]. Trials of diphenoxylate (in form of Lomotil), combined with the hypnotic-sedative drug chlormethiazole, have shown it to be a possible alternative to methadone in the withdrawal treatment of opiate addicts. The dosage employed was 1 to 2 Lomotil tablets (diphenoxylate hydrachloride 2·5 mg plus atropine sulphate 0·025 mg), and 2–4 chlormethiazole tablets (0·5 mg) (not exceeding 16 chlormeth tablets per day) every 4 hours, for a period of 4–7 days [52]. In our experience this combination of Lomotil with a tranquilliser has proved effective in the treatment of the heroin abstinence phase over the past eight years, but requires – and deserves – further trials [52, 53], (as does perhaps the possibility of using Lomotil in long-term ambulant therapy of addicts).

Long-term treatment
The withdrawal treatment will always have to be followed up by the much more important long-term and rehabilitation treatment. This should enable the addict, as far as possible, to cope with life without recourse to dependence-producing drugs. He will as a rule require long-continued support from professional workers, local authorities, voluntary agencies, family, friends, and the Church etc. Often a gradual process of weaning from reliance on the security and shelter of the hospital, such as transfer from closed wards (in cases where they have been found necessary) to open wards, then to halfway houses and later to a controlled and supported home environment before complete independence at home, may be advisable and necessary. The final phase of adjustment will have to take place in the community, and long-term support and assistance from many community agencies (which, for example, could help in vocational rehabilitation and finding suitable employment) may often be required. Individual and group

counselling of addicts and their families may often be very helpful, apart from educational and vocational training. Long-continued out-patient supervision by parole officers has proved helpful in civil commitment programmes for narcotic addicts. A *rational authority approach* (as contrasted with the *punitive approach*) has been described by L. Brill and Jaffe [30, 54]. Here a court agency and a Rehabilitation Centre work in close co-operation, sharing information, casework planning and decision making. Coercive measures and controls are also employed (or kept in the background as possible deterrents) in order to anchor the addict firmly in the treatment situation. Some units in England have used Section 4 of the Criminal Justice Act – Probation Order with a condition of Residence and/or Attendance at an out-patient clinic – with a similar purpose in mind [21].

Comprehensive programmes aiming at rehabilitation of narcotic addicts all include a variety of psychological, pharmacological and social approaches. The two most widely employed approaches nowadays are the chemical methods (maintenance or, more rarely, antagonists) on the one hand, and the self-help organisations on the other.

Chemotherapy

(a) *Methadone maintenance* [8, 9] – This method was introduced in 1964 by Dole and Nyswander [9]. High maintenance doses of, for example, 80–120 mg of methadone prevent the addict from getting any kick from heroin, cross tolerance leading to a *blockade* of the heroin effects; somewhat smaller doses, moreover, eliminate narcotic drug hunger. Thus the way is paved for effective rehabilitation. In a methadone maintenance programme addicts report once daily to receive their dosage of 100–180 mg in orange juice. This large dosage is effective for about 24 hours. The heroin addict is thereby helped to keep off heroin, to take up employment and to readjust his life. Many former heroin addicts have thus been helped to function within the community and to adjust socially and occupationally without further criminal involvement. Not much research seems to have been done as yet to decide whether after a period of methadone maintenance it might be possible to take the addict off the methadone as well so that he may live free from addictive drugs – and to what extent it may be advisable or otherwise to try to achieve this goal.

Not all American clinics employ high methadone doses in their maintenance programmes. Professor A. Goldstein, chairman of the fourth National Conference on Methadone Treatment (1972) preferring 'as low a dose as will do the job', employs doses of 40–50 mg/day, which his blind dose comparisons have shown to be as effective as much higher amounts [55]. (Incidentally, Goldstein deplores the term blockade to describe cross tolerance produced by methadone – as cross tolerance '. . . has nothing at all to do with the true blockade produced by antagonists, which prevent opiate actions without raising the tolerance threshold or producing physical dependence, and which produce no "high" themselves' [55].

It has been stressed that methadone maintenance should be employed only under the auspices of clinics or hospitals which have the required wide range of services needed at their disposal. It is therefore unsuitable for use by the individual medical practitioner. Much further research is required in regard to methadone maintenance. For example, under present circumstances this approach is probably more suitable under American than under British conditions, as in Britain it might often be difficult to establish that the newcomer – when first appearing at the out-patient Treatment Centre – has in fact been dependent on a narcotic for any length of time [21].

(b) The so-called British Approach – Until 1968 any British medical practitioner was allowed to prescribe heroin to addicts. To a large extent, because of the overprescribing of heroin (and cocaine) by a small number of London GPs under this now abandoned overpermissive 'British System', a heroin–cocaine epidemic arose in England in the early 1960s [3, 56]. Since 1968, only doctors at the newly established Treatment Centres (of which there are about fifteen in the London area and a few in the provinces) are permitted to prescribe heroin and cocaine to addicts. In general the policy adopted by the Treatment Centre doctors is (apart from virtually eliminating the prescribing of cocaine) as far as possible to cut out the prescribing of narcotics altogether, or at least to substitute methadone in place of heroin. As a consequence of such a policy, the number of methadone addicts notified to the authorities was for a short period (1969) greater than that of heroin addicts. Methadone is used in these British clinics by and large in much smaller doses than in the American maintenance programmes [57] and probably not so much with the aim of a prolonged maintenance programme, but rather in the hope that at some time in the future at least some addicts may become motivated to stop all addictive drugs. Moreover, probably more addicts receive methadone in the form of ampoules than in the form of the oral tincture – largely perhaps, because addicts resist giving up 'fixing' and the therapist may fear that if he insisted on oral

1 8

medication, the addict may stop coming to the Centre, with the loss of any hope of establishing a therapeutic relationship.

As it is, although the number of known narcotic addicts in the UK (which kept on rising until 1968 and then began to drop) has since been largely contained (see Table 4 in Appendix), addicts are buying and selling drugs on the black market – among them methadone. The risk of addiction is of course much greater when methadone is injected (as is often the case in England) than when taken in oral form (as in the American maintenance programme) [9]. It seems that in the UK very few addicts are by a deliberate prescribing policy stabilised on heroin, so that it is quite wrong to compare and contrast American methadone maintenance programmes with a policy of 'heroin maintenance' in the UK. At any rate, because of differences between conditions in America and the UK (for example, sociocultural and legal differences, differences in personalities of drug abusers and in doctors' prescribing habits), methods proving successful in one country may not necessarily be so in another. Careful assessment, close supervision (including urinary monitoring) and controls are necessary in the British Treatment Centres as in the American Maintenance programmes to minimise the danger of abuse, for example in avoiding the 'spilling over' of prescribed drugs to the black market.

According to Home Office figures by the end of 1969 of the total number of 1466 known addicts to hard drugs, 499 were taking heroin and more than double that number, i.e. 1011, were taking methadone (either alone or in combination with other drugs) – so that '. . . methadone had supplanted heroin as the drug most commonly used by addicts' [57]. However, at the time (as nowadays) the number of those buying Chinese 'H' or methdaone on the Black Market was not known, and in the 1970s first notification of heroin users shows that they have again outstripped the methadone users, as confirmed by the official Home Office figures. Thus the ratio between heroin and methadone notifications, which was about 10:1 in 1968, had been reversed into 1:2 by the end of 1969 (see Table 5a in Appendix). As this Table shows, over the whole three year period 1969/1971 (despite the predominance of known methadone users in 1969) the 'H:M' ratio as regards first notification, again indicated a clear preponderance of 'H' users (over 2:1) which became more marked in 1972 (over 4:1) and even more so in the first quarter of 1973 (5:1). The increase of first heroin notifications can hardly be ascribed to an altered policy of the Treatment Centre doctors who probably would not prescribe heroin to newcomers not already taking this drug. Thus these rising 'H' notifications probably reflect the increased use of Chinese heroin, a drug first reported to be misused by youngsters in about 1967 [3]. Since then poly-drug abusers have continually talked about the availability of this drug in London's West End, but it is only over the past few months that one has begun to read about a number of Court cases involving the peddling of Chinese heroin. It is difficult to know whether the rising first notifications of 'H' addicts since 1972 indicate an increase of absolute numbers of abusers of Chinese 'H', or whether they merely reflect a greater police activity in the part of London's West End where this drug has been peddled for at least six years or so. In spite of this recent rise in the abuse of Chinese 'H' its import seems sporadic. There seems to be no organised illicit drug trade in the UK and no great increase in crime as a result of reduction of heroin prescribing in 1968. Clearly as in the USA the situation is very fluid and requires constant vigilance as the drug scene is changing continually.

Narcotic antagonists

Cyclazocine is an orally effective narcotic antagonist, whose regular administration (on an out-patient basis) to volunteer heroin addicts of good motivation has been found helpful (in the USA) in preventing return to narcotic drug use, as it reduces the mental and physical effects of heroin and other opiates [10, 30, 31]. A single oral dose of 4 mg cyclazocine was found in the USA to prevent the effects of heroin administration for a period of 20–28 hours, with its peak effects after 6–8 hours. As long as the addict continues to take cyclazocine, heroin – unless taken in large amounts – will have little effect on him. Thus, it is hoped in time to bring about the extinction of conditioned physical dependence and of drug-seeking behaviour (see Section 5.4). Before starting the antagonist, the narcotic must first be withdrawn.

Cyclazocine has a number of unpleasant side-effects. These are not present with another opiate antagonist, naloxone, which, however, is too expensive, and is even shorter acting than cyclazocine, its antagonism to opiates lasting 3–4 hours [10]. Research is being carried out to develop new drugs which lack cyclozocine's side-effects and are longer acting and to develop a long-acting naloxone depot injection [57]. The final place of the antagonists in the treatment of narcotic drug dependence cannot yet be assessed.

When considering the value of all these chemotherapeutic approaches, it should be kept in mind that nowadays many addicts are multi-drug abusers, and that cured heroin addicts may continue to abuse or start abusing soft drugs, such as amphetamines or barbiturates or also alcohol. All such forms of chemotherapy should be regarded as part and parcel of an overall comprehensive rehabilitation programme (for which indeed, they may sometimes pave the way) and which – as already said – should include vocational guidance, educational training or retraining, resocialisation and assistance by welfare, social workers or probation officers etc. As drug dependence is commonly symptomatic of underlying psychological or social problems, psychosocial therapies will have to accompany or follow methadone or cyclazocine treatment.

Self-help organisations

In contrast to the chemotherapeutic approaches, the therapeutic community approach treats alcoholics and drug addicts essentially as people suffering from underlying psychological problems, such as emotional instability or immaturity. However, drug abuse, having started as a symptom, has in time led to secondary changes, so that later on addicts have many common features – even if originally their personalities varied a great deal. Because of such changes brought about in the course of their drug-taking career, drug addicts find that they have a lot in common which enables rapid and easy identification with each other. This principle, as already discussed, is made use of in special units, halfway houses etc. by professional workers, but also in self-help organisations, run by addicts themselves, often with the help of recovered addicts.

The principles have already been discussed above: as a rule they form residential groups, members helping each other; no drugs are given, even during drug withdrawal and the addicts participate in often very outspoken group discussions in which members severely criticise each other. However, it is hoped that group support will enable the criticised member to survive such critical remarks and in time benefit from them, leading to a change in his immature outlook and behaviour and to emotional growth. New members start at the bottom, being called upon to perform the most onerous and menial duties, but are gradually able to work their way up towards positions of trust and responsibility. There are now quite a number of such organisations, varying slightly in their approaches and in their co-operation with professional bodies. Visitors are certainly impressed by the way in which formerly antisocial and irresponsible individuals co-operate with the groups code.

However it is probably much too early to try to assess the long-term fate of those who have left the residential communities and returned to ordinary living, where they are no longer able to depend on the support of the group.

DEPENDENCE ON STIMULANTS, HALLUCINOGENS AND CANNABIS

As these drugs produce no physical abstinence syndrome there is no need for any special withdrawal regime. As regards long-term therapy of the state of psychological dependence, no specific chemo-therapy is available that could be compared with the methadone maintenance programme or the antagonists in the case of the opiates, or with the sensitising drugs in the case of alcohol. The general principles applicable to the withdrawal phase and the long-term approach have been outlined above. As in other forms of drug dependence, after the withdrawal and detoxification phase is over, attempts must be made to establish a long-term after-care and rehabilitation regime by a combination of physical, psychological and social approaches.

Certain features sometimes observed among these types of drug abusers deserve brief mention. The amphetamine 'high' is often fol-lowed by a psychologically painful 'come-down' experience, so that a watch should be kept for depressive symptoms possibly accompanied by suicide attempts in this phase. Antidepressant (but not the CNS-stimulating) drugs may have to be used at the time in spite of the delay of action, although in general they are not greatly appreciated by such patients. Impulsive, irresponsible, aggressive and violent behaviour sometimes noticed in habitual amphetamine abusers may require the administration of tranquillisers. Paranoid psychosis – a not uncommon complication of habitual amphetamine abuse – necessitates treatment by major tranquillisers such as phenothiazines. Fortunately the prog-nosis is good, the psychosis as a rule clearing up rapidly when the consumption of amphetamines comes to an end.

Whilst, as already discussed, there are very few indications for start-ing amphetamine medication in new patients, the question may some-times arise as to whether middle-aged people who have for years functioned satisfactorily on slightly excessive doses of a drug such as Drinamyl (dextroamphetamine combined with amylobarbitone) should be given further maintenance doses or not. One might feel that in such cases – with the number of tablets perhaps no greater than 4–5 per day, with no evidence of a desire for increase of dosage etc. and where attempts at reducing and withdrawing these tablets lead to persistent complaints of lethargy, depression, inability to work etc. – it might perhaps be better to leave things well alone.

The acute and prolonged reactions which may occur in LSD users [32, 58] may necessitate – apart from such general measures as attempts at reassurance ('talk down') and psychological support – medicinal treatment in the form of tranquillisers, for example phenothiazines (chlorpromazine i.mu.) during the acute panic reactions, during the 'flash-back' phenomenon following some time after the drug has been taken and during an acute or prolonged LSD psychosis etc. Prolonged psychological support will be necessary in such patients for some time after the acute manifestations have passed off. Phenothiazines are said to be contra-indicated in cases where STP (and not LSD) has been consumed because of the danger of potentiation [58]. Untoward reactions following cannabis use (as a rule much milder and much less common than in the case of LSD) require similar symptomatic treatment as the LSD reactions.

Where individuals in states of psychological dependence on amphetamines, LSD and cannabis ask for help, they are initially probably best treated in hospital, to be followed by prolonged medical and social supervision after discharge. In as far as habitual cannabis users as a rule see nothing wrong with this drug and (rightly or wrongly) claim that they could give it up at any time [3], they usually lack any motivation to co-operate with any treatment suggested to them.

CONCLUSION

Much progress has been made during the past decades in the understanding and the treatment of alcoholism and drug dependence, but a great deal more remains badly understood and requires much further research. Much remains to be done, for example, in the fields of treatment, education and prophylaxis. Alcoholism and drug dependence are problems of multifactorial causation requiring an integrated multi- and interdisciplinary approach; for example, as regards treatment, by the employment of psychological, social and pharmacological techniques.

6.3 PROGNOSIS

The prognosis is in general better for alcoholics than for people dependent on other drugs – perhaps partly for the reasons discussed in the preceding section.

In Western culture alcohol has become a 'domesticated drug' [15] its consumption sanctioned by tradition and culture, and encouraged by society. Thus even relatively stable people can become excessive drinkers and thereby run the risk of alcoholism. Because of this, their personality and social stability will on average be better than that of the hypothetical average drug addict who, in Western culture, had to break social taboos and the law (e.g. forge prescriptions) in order to acquire drugs (e.g. opiate, cocaine) or to manipulate doctors into prescribing excessive amounts for him etc. Thus often the future addict's personality may have been from the beginning more unstable than that of the future alcoholic. For similar reasons, women alcoholics may be on the average more unstable personalities than male alcoholics, and in general young alcoholics and drug addicts more unstable than the middle-aged. After all, it often took the middle-aged alcoholic many years before his personality resistance was so broken down that he became an overt alcoholic, whereas the resilience of the younger alcoholics was probably slight from the beginning.

Again, on the whole, prognosis will be better in such persons who have become alcoholics or drug addicts mainly (or at least partly) because of occupational temptation and exposure, or because of social pressure exerted by a subculture. But clearly this may again depend largely on the possibility to change the noxious environment, as otherwise the temptation and exposure will continue. As a rule, such a change is not possible in the case of people whose livelihood is involved. Therefore treatment in these cases may mainly consist of helping them to adjust, and learn to adopt better coping mechanisms than in the past.

In general, prognosis for alcoholics is much better than generally believed by the lay and professional public alike; roughly two alcoholics in three – in an unselected sample – can be expected to improve greatly under an adequate therapeutic regime [11]. This knowledge, if imparted by doctors to alcoholics and their families, should give them hope and encouragement. Many female alcoholics too – though their outlook may be less good on the whole – can also recover or improve greatly. Unemployed, single, homeless alcoholics etc. naturally require a more comprehensive regime of support and after-care than employed, skilled alcoholics with family support. The length and strength of support and after-care required in alcoholics and addicts is inversely proportional to the stability of personality, and to the presence of stabilising factors in terms of family, employment, residence etc.*

The prognosis of addicts to other drugs, as a whole, is by no means as hopeless as often assumed. Some years ago a WHO Study Group [48] pointed out that the majority of addicts the world over belong to the category of 'easy amenability to treatment', i.e. those whose drug dependence was 'not due to a primary personality disorder'. In these addicts, drug dependence originated from incidental stress, especially in countries where the drugs used were freely available and inexpensive, or from social, environmental or cultural factors, or where drug taking started during the course of serious illness. Fortunately the second category of drug-dependent individuals, i.e. those who were 'less amenable to treatment' and whose drug dependence was superimposed on 'a basically pathological character structure' was held to be numerically smaller. This category consists of immature, narcissistic personalities with low frustration tolerance and 'poorly developed ego and superego'.

However, even in the young, immature narcotic addict – with possibly the worst prognosis of all forms of drug dependence – one has to remember that only recently have definite attempts been made to learn more about them and to carry out proper research into adequate methods of treatment and rehabilitation. Various, newer techniques have helped in the recovery of a minority among them. Possibly, as suggested by Winnick [59], some narcotic addicts may in their thirties mature out of their addiction. Therefore, even methods which provided temporary help and a 'breathing space' only may help them to stay alive up to this age and may therefore assist greatly in their ultimate recovery. Here again, better training and greater interest of doctors should in the future play an important role.

---

* The personality of the hypothetical average alcoholic is much more mature than that of the usually much younger and inexperienced 'average' drug taker. The 'average' alcoholic is often in a better emotional state and social position—in spite of his precarious physical state, malnutrition, physical complications, advanced age etc.—than the young drug abuser who has 'dropped out' from family and ordinary society. Inexperienced, educationally and vocationally unskilled, devoid of home, friends and means, he is all too often left to fend for himself. To keep up a bridge of continuing communication and dialogue with the 'dropped out' addict is as vital for the young as for the older drug abuser

Problem of relapse

Doctors, like all other healing professions, should keep in mind that all forms of drug dependence are essentially *relapsing disorders* and that many patients only recover after a number of unsuccessful attempts. Early failures should therefore not be regarded by the doctor as a failure of all therapeutic attempts but as a challenge to try again and again. Such failures should not be taken by the doctor as a personal affront. Again, as already stressed before, in many patients with a very limited personality potential, even partial successes and realistic goals are important.

Certain factors important for success or failure in the treatment of alcohol- and drug-dependent patients have already been discussed, such as, for example, the ability of the therapeutic team to establish a therapeutic relationship with such patients by adopting an understanding, accepting attitude, and the adequacy of a planned after-care programme and community support. A very important factor is naturally the emotional stability of the underlying personality of the addict, and – to a certain extent correlated with it – the history of his past social (domestic, occupational, residential) stability. Obviously the greater such stability, the better is the prognosis, provided other factors are equal. For reasons such as these it is impossible to compare the treatment results obtained by different authors, in particular if no details of the composition of the case material is available. For example, most therapists will have a high proportion of therapeutic successes if the great majority of their patients are basically well-adjusted, relatively stable personalities whose alcohol or drug misuse had started at a time of abnormal severe internal or external stress. Such people may often give a history of having coped well and having done fairly well at home and at business before starting their drug abuse. Their alcohol or drug abuse may have followed severe emotional stress (e.g. death of a close relative) or may have arisen as a consequence of severe social pressure (e.g. the need to conform to local, subcultural customs). Other responsible factors in basically stable individuals may have been continual occupational exposure and temptation. Yet even in such occupational groups, or among those under severe stress, clearly only a certain proportion exposed to the same experiences and influences become dependent, so that the personality or host factor must play a role even under such circumstances.

Whereas in general with this type of alcohol- or drug- dependent type of patient the outlook is not bad, all therapists will have a high proportion of failures if among their patients there happens to be a majority of psychopathic patients with serious character disorders. These individuals may have shown evidence of marked adjustment problems even before they embarked on their drug abuse. In such patients, alcoholism or drug dependence is no more than one – and possibly not the most important – facet of their emotional disturbance.

Thus psychological, social and pharmacological factors may be important in prognosis, just as they are in the aetiology of alcoholism and drug dependence. Personality stability, and the stability and support that can be provided in the addict's environment have been discussed in the foregoing. But prognosis is also dependent on the type of agent. Once having become 'hooked', individuals dependent on drugs such as heroin or cocaine may find giving up such drugs more difficult than persons dependent on many other types of drugs – given other factors being equal. On the other hand, factors pertaining to host, environment and agent, as we have seen, work in close dynamic interaction with each other. For example, a middle-aged therapeutic morphine addict, whose addiction is to a strong addictive agent but whose pre-addictive personality may have been relatively stable, may have a much better prognosis than a very unstable non-therapeutic youngster dependent on amphetamines (although pharmacologically they are weaker agents than morphine) and having no stabilising domestic or occupational support. In prognosis, as in aetiology, the relative importance of factors pertaining to host, environment and agent cannot be evaluated in isolation from each other.

REFERENCES

1. Chambers, C. D. and Brill, L. (1971). *Narcot. Control Commiss. N.Y. State*, NACC Reprints. **4,** No. 1.
2. Essig, C. F. (1968). *The Addictive States*, 188 (A. Wikler, editor) (Baltimore: William and Wilkins Co.).
3. Glatt, M. M., Pittman, D. J., Gillespie, D. G. and Hills, D. R. (1969). *The Drug Scene in Great Britain*, 19, 43, 80, 101, 106, 115 (Revised reprint) (Edward Arnold).
4. Eddy, N. B., Halbach, H., Isbell, H. and Seevers, M. A. (1965). *Bull. WHO*, **32,** 721.
5. Glatt, M. M. (1967). *WHO Chron.*, **21,** 293.

6. Glatt, M. M. (1970). *World Dialogue on Alcohol and Drug Dependence*, 311 (E. D. Whitney, editor) (Boston: Beacon Press).

7. WHO Expert Committee (1967). *WHO Tech. Rep. Ser.*, **363**, 8.

8. 2nd Nat. Meth. Maint. Conf. (1970). *Int. J. Addict.*, **5**, 341.

9. Dole, V. P. (1970). *ibid.*, **5**, 359.

10. Brill, L. and Laskowitz, D. (1970). *Cyclazocine, Eastern Psychiat. Res. Assoc. 15th Ann. Meet., New York City*

11. Glatt, M. M. (1972). *The Alcoholic and the Help He Needs*, 2nd ed., (London: Priory Press).

12. Halbach, H. (1959). *Brit. J. Addict.*, **56**, 27.

13. Glatt, M. M. (1961). *Lancet*, **i**, 1112.

14. Alexander, F. (1949). *Fundamentals of Psychoanalysis*, 24 (London).

15. Jellinek, E. M. (1960). *The Disease Concept of Alcoholism* (New Haven, Conn.: Hillhouse Press).

16. Glatt, M. M. (1967). *New Aspects of the Mental Health Service*, 115 (H. Freeman and J. Farndale, editors) (Oxford, N.Y.: Pergamon Press)

17. Home Office Report of Working Party (1971). *Habitual Drunken Offenders* (London: H.M.S.O.)

18. Glatt, M. M. (1969). *Brit. J. Addict.*, **64**, 165

19. Glatt, M. M. (1969). *Lancet*, **ii**, 429.

20. C. D. Smithers Foundation (1968). *Understanding Alcoholism*, 138 (New York: Scribner and Sons).

21. Glatt, M. M. (1969). *Brit. J. Addict.*, **64**, 165.

22. Cohen, S. (1971). *Images of Deviance*, 11 (Penguin Books).

23. Cook, T., Gath, D. and Hensman, C. (1969). *The Drunkenness Offence*, 9, 51, 99, 109 (Oxford, N.Y.: Pergamon Press).

24. Asher, R. (1958). *Lancet*, **i**, 954.

25. Glatt, M. M. (1959). *Brit. J. Addict.*, **55**, 111.

26. Williams, L. (1956). *Alcoholism*, 39 (Edinburgh, London: Livingstone).

27. Sargant, W. (1949). *Proc. Roy. Soc. Med.*, **42**, 3.

28. Glatt, M. M. (1970). *Brit. J. Addict.*, **65**, 51.

29. Wikler, A. (1972). *2nd Int. Symp. Drug Abuse, Jerusalem* (Abstracts), 85.

30. Brill, L. and Jaffe, J. H. (1967). *Brit. J. Addict.*, **62**, 375.

31. Fink, M., Freedman, A. M., Resnick, R. and Zaks, A. (1973). *Agonist and Antagonist Actions of Narcotic Analgesic Drugs*, 266 (H. W. Kosterlitz, H. O. J. Collier and J. E. Villarreal, editors) (London: Macmillan).

32. Louria, D. B. (1968). *The Drug Scene*, 182 (N.Y., Toronto: McGraw Hill Book Co.).
33. Jones, Maxwell (1968). *Social Psychiatry in Practice* (Penguin Books).
34. George, H. R. and Glatt, M. M. (1967). *Brit. J. Addict.*, **62**, 147.
35. Ottenberg, D. J. and Rosen, A. (1971). *Quart. J. Stud. Al.*, **32**, 94.
36. Neumann, C. P. and Tamerin, J. S. (1971). *ibid.*, **32**, 82.
37. Connell, P. H. (1969). *Drugs and Youth* (J. R. Wittenborn, H. Brill, J. P. Smith and S. A. Wittenborn, editors) (Springfield: Charles C. Thomas).
38. Butterworth, A. T. (1971). *Quart. J. Stud. Al.*, **32**, 78.
39. Frisch, E. P. (1966). *Chlormethiazole* (Copenhagen: Munksgaard).
40. Glatt, M. M., George, H. R. and Frisch, E. P. (1965). *Brit. Med. J.*, **2**, 401.
41. Lundquist, G. (1966). *Chlormethiazole*, 20 (E. P. Frisch, editor).
42. Smart, R. G., Schmidt, W. and Moss, M. K. (1969). *Int. J. Addict.*, **4**, 543.
43. Taylor, J. A. (1964). *Bull. Los Angeles Neurol. Soc.*, **29**, 158.
44. Dent, J. Y. (1947). *Anxiety and its Treatment*, 2nd ed. (Belfast: Mullan).
45. Smart, R. G., Storm, T., Baker, E. F. W. and Solursh, L. (1968). *LSD in the Treatment of Alcoholism* (Toronto: Univ. Toronto Press).
46. Dally, P. (1967). *Chemotherapy of Psychiatric Disorders* (London: Logos Press).
47. Glatt, M. M. (1961). *Acta Psychiat. Scand.*, **37**, 143.
48. WHO Study Group (1957). *Bull. Narcot.*, **9**, 36 (3).
49. Martin, W. R. and Jasinski, D. (1969). *J. Psychiat. Res.*, **7**, 9.
50. Blachly, P. H. (1966). *Amer. J. Psychiat.*, **122**, 742.
51. Fraser, H. F. and Isbell, H. (1961). *Bull. Narcot.*, **13**, 29 (1).
52. Glatt, M. M., Lewis, D. M. and Wilson, D. T. (1970). *Brit. J. Addict.*, **65**, 237.
53. Goodman, A. (1968). *Southern Med. J.*, **61**, 313.
54. Brill, L. (1972). *The De-Addiction Process*, III (Springfield: Charles C. Thomas).
55. Goldstein, A. (1972). *Proc. 4th Nat. Conf. Methadone Treatment, San Francisco*, 27 (N.Y.: Nat. Ass. Prev. Addict.)
56. Interdepartmental Committee on Drug Addiction. Second Report (1965). (London: H.M.S.O.).
57. Blumberg, H. and Dayton, H. B. (1973). *Agonist and Antagonist*

Actions of Narcotic Analgesic Drugs, 110 (H. W. Kosterlitz, H. O. J. Collier and J. E. Villarreal, editors).

58. Cohen, S. (1969). *The Drug Dilemma*, 33 (N.Y.: McGraw Hill Book Co.)

59. Winick, C. (1962). *Bull. Narcot.*, **14**, 1 (1).

PART 7

PREVENTION

Unfortunately many alcoholics and drug addicts will fail to recover, therefore the task of prevention is most important. As the late Lord Rosenheim, President of the Royal College of Physicians, and at the time of his death Chairman of the Medical Council on Alcoholism said in 1968, 'It must increasingly be the purpose of the Medical profession and of all who work with them to aim at prevention rather than cure' [1]. Ideally such prevention should be *primary*, i.e. forestalling the development of dependence by creating favourable psychological and social conditions as a matrix in which there is no need for people to attempt to escape from reality by taking dangerous drugs. As however, complete primary prevention will always remain beyond one's means, *secondary prevention*, i.e. prevention of progression of the illness once it has set in, will also always be an important goal. This can only be achieved by as early diagnosis and intervention as possible. No-one is likely to be a better 'secondary preventer' than the family doctor [2]. We have already seen how doctors by instituting research, by setting an example to the general public in accepting the illness concept of alcohol and drug dependence, and thereby reducing the stigma, and by early detection and diagnosis (secondary prevention) can greatly contribute in this task [3].

Though prevention is of paramount importance, complete pre-occupation and reliance on the task of prevention to the exclusion of therapy, with the implication that 'mopping up operations', i.e. interest in treatment, may detract from taking prophylactic measures, is surely unrealistic. Drug addicts often claim that all their troubles stem from malaise of society, and similarly some sociologists state that the only sensible approach would be to eradicate those ills of society

271

which give rise to drug dependence [4, 5]. That social factors are of the utmost importance in the health of the community and thereby also in the prevention of drug dependence and alcoholism, is beyond doubt, and they therefore require urgent attention [6]. It is therefore right and proper to be concerned with the 'macroproblem of the society which nurtures' alcoholics and drug addicts [7], but, 'As the hope of total prevention of drug dependence (and alcoholism) seems Utopian, the community will have to go on working steadily towards perfecting its methods of rehabilitation' [6]. Like the arguments concerning 'out-patients versus in-patients' or 'psychological versus physical versus social therapies,' the question, 'Is prevention or rehabilitation the main priority?' seems mainly academic. There is an urgent need for both.

Measures of prevention will naturally cover a wide field and will have to be directed first at the host (for example by impressing on parents the need to forestall, as far as possible, emotional insecurity in their children, by giving them genuine affection, making them feel wanted and treating them in a consistent manner; by measures of mental hygiene in childhood; by helping youngsters to find an identity in activities other than by drug taking and antisocial behaviour etc.); second, at the environment (for example, attempts at influencing social attitudes and improving socio-economic conditions by correcting social injustice and economic inequality) and third at the agent (by legislative measures, as, for example, incorporated in the new Misuse of Drugs Act, 1971).*

---

* As discussed in Part 2, the spread of drug dependence from person to person resembles in certain ways and in certain cases the spread of infectious diseases. However, in the spread of infectious diseases the newly infected person is merely a passive recipient of the infection after being attacked by the infective agent. In certain cases of alcoholism and drug dependence, the host (who probably has a rather weak personality) may originally also have been a passive and unwitting recipient: e.g. the therapeutic addict who originally received the drug (the agent) whilst he was in a physically very ill state that required medication; or possibly also a minority of youngsters who were persuaded by others to try hashish, LSD or pep pills etc. at parties. The great majority of drug abusers, however, clearly evince active drug-seeking activities [8]. Unlike the individual struck by an infec-tive agent, such drug takers and alcoholics go out of their way to seek out the agent (drugs or alcohol), often in the face of considerable obstacles. This may be so even at the start of their drug-taking career; it becomes more intense the longer the addictive process continues, and it develops secondarily even in that minority of drug abusers who initially had been merely passive recipients. Later on in the drinking or drug-taking career naturally secondary processes such as the fear of the abstinence syndromes, conditioned responses etc. occur. At this stage these may be partly responsible for the alcohol and drug-seeking behaviour (see Part 2). The majority of drug abusers, however, seek out their drugs long before the onset of such secondary developments. Attempts at pre-vention and treatment of drug dependence and alcoholism must therefore keep in mind the need to cover the personal and social motivations which lead to such active drug-seeking behaviour and try to provide constructive alternatives which are acceptable to and found rewarding by the individual concerned (see Section 7.2)

In the task of prophylaxis, the improvement of social and other environmental conditions is naturally of paramount importance, although the modern affluent society has unfortunately failed to prevent a rise of alcohol and drug misuse. As regards alcohol abuse, affluence alcoholism has now taken the place of yesterday's poverty alcoholism [2]. In regard to drug dependence, Professor Martin Roth has written [9], 'If an expert in the field of drug dependence with knowledge of the international scene had been asked to predict the effects of improved living conditions on the prevalence of drug dependence he would very likely have forecast a decline in parallel with the reduction of poverty and disease and the improvement of living standards. The trends we have witnessed have proved very different. A new population of drug users drawn mainly from the 15–25 year age group and with a social class distribution close to that of the population at large has arisen'.

7.1 THE DOCTOR'S ROLE (THE RISK OF 'IATROGENIC DEPENDENCE')

In the field of prevention of drug abuse and dependence the family doctor has a very important, direct role to play. To a large extent – for example in the great majority of cases of drug abuse by the middle-aged – the condition has been *iatrogenic*, the drug concerned first prescribed by a family doctor, and then often prescribed again and again, often in increasing doses, usually at the insistent demand of the patient. If a patient comes again and again, insisting that only one special drug is of any use to him, if he keeps asking for increasing amounts etc., the greatest care is obviously necessary. In spite of this one comes across many patients who have obtained increasingly large doses of dependence-producing drugs from their own family doctor for long periods and also from doctors who did not know these individuals when they presented themselves as temporary patients. Even greater has been the responsibility of those few doctors who through gross overprescribing, whatever their motives, were largely responsible for the development of the heroin, cocaine [10, 11] and later the methylamphetamine epidemics in England in the 1960s. Obviously better instruction in medical school on the problems of drug dependence is vital.

A voluntary ban on the prescribing of amphetamines has been recommended by the British Medical Association, as – in cases of narcolepsy (and possibly hyperkinetic children*) apart – there is hardly any indication that their function cannot be equally well fulfilled by other, less harmful drugs. In particular there is no indication for their formerly so prevalent use in obesity and depression (which caused so many cases of dependence on amphetamines and phenmetrazine). In contrast to the modern tricyclic antidepressant occasionally cases of dependence have occurred after the use of certain MAO inhibitors [13] (see Section 5.1). The MAO drugs are therefore perhaps best avoided in the treatment of alcoholics and drug abusers – the more so as they potentiate or prolong the action of opiates.

Equally there seems to be no indication for the prescribing of bar-biturates to young patients, except during withdrawal from barbiturate dependence and in special circumstances such as the need for pheno-barbitone in epileptics etc. Neither should barbiturates be prescribed to temporary patients of any age group who are not on the particular doctor's list, without prior reference to their own doctor [7]. Metha-done as yet can still be prescribed to addicts by any doctor. However surely it would be preferable if newcomers who claim to be dependent on this drug but have not previously been notified to the Home Office were first referred for investigation to a Treatment Centre, rather than being supplied by the GP with methadone for a few weeks and then referred to the Centre. In the latter situation, the patient could claim that he had become dependent during those few weeks and that he quite legitimately required further, regular supplies.

There is another indirect way in which medical practitioners – in particular family doctors, but also hospital doctors – can help in the task of prophylaxis. By becoming much less generous in their prescrib-ing of CNS-affecting drugs – even considering the pressure presented by the insistent demands of too many patients clamouring for such drugs, and the insufficient time at their disposal to discuss the pros and cons with such patients in greater detail – doctors could in time begin to counteract the ever-increasing legitimate drug use in this drug age. Young drug abusers are often indignant because only their drug taking is under criticism. That of their elders who not only drink and smoke a great deal, but who also swallow all types of pills to tranquillise or pep themselves up at daytime and to put themselves to sleep at night

---

* Whilst the use of amphetamines in the case of hyperkinetic children in the UK seems uncommon, methylphenidate (an amphetamine-like substance) seems to be widely employed in the USA as an adjunct to counselling and therapy of 'Minimal Brain Dys-function', the aim being to control the purposeless hyperactivity of such children [12].

is not criticised. Some youngsters started their drug-using career by taking some of the tranquillising or stimulating tablets prescribed to their mothers by the family doctor.

In 1968 psychotropic drug prescriptions in Great Britain under the NHS made up one-sixth of all NHS prescriptions[14].Out of a total of 58·4 million prescriptions (which did not include hospital and private prescriptions) approximately 25 million were for barbiturates, 12.5 million for benzodiazepines, 6 million for phenothiazines, 5·5 million for non-barbiturate hypnotics, 5 million for tricyclic antidepressants, 4 million for amphetamines and nearly 0·5 million for MAO inhibitors. In addition to these prescriptions come another 20 million prescriptions for various analgesics. The journal 'Drugs and Society' (June 1971) comments that 6.1 million prescriptions for phenothiazine tranquillisers amount to enough tablets for a month's treatment for every tenth person in the UK. There were twice as many prescriptions for the minor tranquillisers (the benzodiazepines) and the total number of hypnotic (barbiturate and non-barbiturate) tablets prescribed amounts to enough pills 'to make every tenth night's sleep in the UK hypnotic-ally induced'.

Many of these prescriptions are for drugs which may more or less readily lead to dependence, such as the barbiturates, the non-barbiturate hypnotics and the amphetamines. Sir Derek Dunlop[14] (reporting the above figures) remarked that it looked as if, 'The overworked medical profession in this country may be unduly concerned with satisfying the public's wants rather than what we think it needs'. He also regarded the extent of drug seeking by patients and the accession to such demands by doctors, as disturbing features of modern medicine. In this connection, a great deal of responsibility rests on parents' own drinking and drug-taking habits. 'If you want your children to use illicit drugs, be a user of sedatives or tranquillisers or stimulants your-selves, or an excessive user of alcohol or tobacco' – is the warning given to parents by Dr D. B. Louria [15] (See Section 7.3). A special responsibility rests naturally on the woman who is pregnant. For ex-ample, infants born by mothers dependent on opiates may themselves show evidence of physical dependence in the shape of physical absti-nence symptoms. A recent study carried out by three New York pae-diatricians has shown that, 'The severity of withdrawal signs in the infant, the time they began, and the duration, were found to be related to the size of the heroin dosage taken by the pregnant mother, the length of her addiction and the time of her last dose' [16].

Because of the danger of a teratogenic effect of drugs (including analgesics and sedatives) during the first trimester of pregnancy, doctors prescribing for women of child-bearing age should first enquire whether they are pregnant. 'In the first eight weeks of pregnancy particularly drugs should be withheld unless they are absolutely vital' [17].

In view of the various hazards associated with the widespread use of psychotropic drugs, it is vital that doctors should exercise great restraint when prescribing them; they are not placebos and should not be the immediate, automatic answer to each and every one of the frustrations, disappointments and anxieties of everyday life [14]. In this way the medical profession may contribute towards stemming the ever-rising tide of consumption of such psychotropic drugs. It may thereby forestall not only many possible occurrences of deliberate and accidental over-dosage and habitual drug misuse and drug dependence among their patients, but also reduce the risk of a further progression of our time into a drug age, in which youngsters may be inclined not only to follow but to outdo their elders in the dangerous habit of swallowing more and more pills.

7.2 HEALTH EDUCATION

In the long run preventive public health measures aimed at reducing the demand for, and the illicit use of, drugs by making the risks generally known, and changing the attitudes of the public towards alcoholics and drug addicts – if successful – could probably be much more effective than legislation. Writing on another theme – that of the motoring offender – a recent editorial in the 'British Medical Journal' notes that, '...the really difficult task is to induce people to want to behave, and this is more likely to be achieved by parents and teacher than by all the king's horses and all the king's men' [18]. But such preventive public health measures are much more difficult to plan and to carry out. Their effectiveness may show itself only many years later and may be difficult to evaluate. Certainly this is another example indicating that research is needed to accompany and to evaluate the effects of such educational programmes. As stated in a recent WHO Working Group Report [19] there is a great need for carefully organised and controlled trials of health education programmes of different types.

Opinions differ as to the places, the value and effectiveness of mass-media presentations in the task of health education about drugs – and likewise as to the needs or advisability of educating school children about drugs. Certainly all those concerned in educating the young, such as teachers, leaders of youth clubs, clergymen etc. should be well informed about drugs, and the task should not be left to well meaning but ill-informed do-gooders. Schoolteachers should be taught about the subject of drug education; relevant questions may crop up unexpectedly in lessons in various subjects and the teacher will then be in a position to discuss such problems whenever the opportunity presents itself. This is probably preferable to the presentation of the subject by invited 'expert' guest lecturers who may unwittingly create inordinate interest and curiosity. Education at schools as of all other sections of the general public should be non-glamorising, factual and objective, rather than moralistic – although ethical considerations obviously enter into all these problems. There is no room for scare tactics in such teaching, as children who find that these 'horror stories' are not substantiated by their own experience (e.g. in the case of cannabis) may then write off any information coming from such sources. Many young drug users state that they were first attracted to drug use by reading or hearing about it in mass-media communications. Therefore, in certain youngsters the lure of excitement, accompanying the risk of taking drugs, might possibly be a greater problem than ignorance about such risks. But majority opinion probably holds that – as youngsters nowadays learn and hear about drugs anyway, and often in a manner stressing allegedly glamorous and exciting aspects – it is necessary to counteract such propaganda by non-glamorising, factual education.

All too often, to the youngster, the drug scene appears attractive, exciting, romantic and mystic; he hears and reads about pep-pills, drugs providing stimulation, energy, a 'high' and a 'buzz'; about great experiences, colours and paintings which are indescribably beautiful, and of music which cannot be perceived in its full glory without the aid of mind-expanding drugs. Without some counteracting factual (but not horror arousing) education the way would seem clear for the uncritical acceptance of such grapevine (and frequently) legends.

Other preventive measures stressed by the WHO Working Group [19] include close consultation between health authorities and those employed in mass-media communications, in order to provide accurate non-emotional information on the subject etc.; the need for adequate education of the various professional groups and moulders of opinion; and the value of social measures designed at seeking out and bringing help to the drug-dependent individuals in the community. Such social measures could include the use of professional teams, open youth-guidance clinics, routine psychiatric interviews of people who attempted suicide, clubs for drug-dependent individuals and sports clubs which offer counter-attractions and discourage drug abuse etc. To what extent such activities which may have proved helpful in certain countries can be transplanted to other countries can of course not be foreseen. For example, clubs run for drug dependents may indeed be a very helpful measure. However, it is essential that a team of mature, stable, well-informed and trained workers be closely associated with such ventures. The importance of this last point can be seen in the fact that a club opened a few years ago in London's West End under the supervision of individuals claiming to be 'recovered' drug addicts soon ran into serious trouble.

Another important point in health education refers to the need in such teaching to get away from preoccupation with drugs and the negative aspects and hazards of a particular chemical, and concentrate instead on the positive values and rewards of a dependence-free life and of more fulfilling patterns of living [20]. One aspect of such education may be the appreciation of the goals of the drug abuser – at least initially – rather than society's goals [20]. Preventive programmes should obviously aim at elucidating the nature of the psychological, social etc. problems which led to drug abuse and should try to provide the drug taker with constructive alternatives, as satisfying to him as drug use. Among such alternatives to drug use, Dr A. I. Malcolm [21] refers to the possibility of achieving a 'non-drug high' by accepting life's challenges and trying to resolve them. A 'non-drug high' occurs when an aware and responsive person experiences the variety and tension of the world through the agencies of mind and body. Such considerations are similar to the ones discussed in Section 5.3 in regard to the 'amotivational syndrome' in a youngster who regularly smokes hashish; they obviously run counter to the 'turning-on, tuning-in, opting-out philosophy' propagated by the apostles of the LSD cult. Today's youth are often attracted by the rapid, effortless achievement of a 'high' through the use of drugs, so that they miss the opportunity of achieving deeper and longer lasting satisfaction as a result of painstaking, energy consuming, persistent effort of mind and body. 'The fullest possible use of the human mind in all its rational and emotional complexity is finally the most natural, and at the same time the most civilised alternative to the use of psychoactive drugs' [21].

7.3 TARGETS OF PREVENTION PROGRAMMES; SELECTIVITY VERSUS THE SHOT-GUN APPROACH

Discussing the problem of preventing heart-disease, a recent Lancet Annotation [22] refers to the question of '. . . whether it is better to pick out specific target "high-risk" individuals. . ., or to adopt the shot-gun approach of advice and health warnings to the entire population. . .'. Do similar questions of giving priority also arise as regards the prevention of alcohol and drug abuse and dependence?

There are obviously certain sections of the population who are for some reason or other more subject to the risk of developing alcoholism or drug dependence (see Part 2), e.g. because of personality instability, occupational hazards, membership of social subcultures etc. Clearly, members of such vulnerable sections of the community should be fully informed about the special risk. This seems to be so obvious that it would seem unnecessary to single out such groups as targets for programmes of special education. Yet the continuing high incidence of alcoholic liver cirrhosis among publicans and allied occupations, or of dependence on other drugs among doctors and other members of the healing professions, and also the general lack of interest in industry towards dependency problems, all indicate the necessity to pay more attention to the special education of such 'target' groups. The need for such a programme as regards the risk of alcoholism among one group, i.e. journalists, was discussed at great length a few years ago by a relatively large number of members of this profession who all happened to be patients at the Alcoholism Unit at St. Bernard's Hospital. These men felt that in journalism there are so many opportunities and socio-occupational pressures to drink that alcoholism in the case of journalists was not merely an occupational hazard but almost an occupational necessity. They therefore regarded a preventive educational programme making newcomers to the profession aware of this risk as possibly a very valuable and health maintaining task.

How about the alternative, an attempt at preventing alcohol and drug dependence by approaches directed at the entire population? Some of the measures discussed in the preceding pages as regards under- and post-graduate training of doctors and the health education of the general public – as well as legal steps (discussed in Section 7.4) – also aim at reducing the general level of drug consumption. This could be done by asking doctors to be less forthcoming with prescribing of CNS-affecting drugs, by making the public aware that there are better ways of dealing with problems than immediate recourse to tranquillisers and pep pills, or by control measures aiming at reducing availability. Is a general reduction of the level of consumption likely to have any implications on the incidence of more definite abuse of, and dependence on drugs?

Approximately ten years ago, Dr S. Ledermann concluded from his work in France on the relationship between alcohol consumption and alcoholism that there existed a '. . . quasi-mathematical connection between reasonable consumption and unreasonable consumption'. This state of affairs, he felt, had a '. . . most direct affect on anti-alcoholic action . . .' as there was little hope of reducing alcoholism unless consumption and production could be reduced [23].

More recent studies by the Toronto research workers J. de Lint and W. Schmidt [24] produced '. . . further evidence for the apparently fixed relationship between consumption averages and alcoholism prevalence'. They pointed, for example, to the finding that in many populations the distribution of alcohol consumption levels approximated closely to '. . . a smooth skewed curve known as the logarithmic normal curve'. In a log normal distribution moderate consumers are common, heavy drinkers less common, and very heavy drinkers, including alcoholics, least common. However the transition from moderate to excessive quantities is very gradual and, therefore, a definition of alcoholism on the basis of consumption levels is inevitably arbitrary. Whatever arbitrary definition of alcoholism is employed, the distribution of individuals according to consumption quantities clearly illustrates that the prevalence of alcoholism is invariably determined by the overall level of consumption.

Discussing the implications of such findings for preventive programmes in alcoholism, de Lint and Schmidt point out that preventive programmes reflect a duality observable also in epidemiological research. One group of workers regard the overall level of consumption as crucial, studying the relationship between consumption averages and alcoholism prevalence, and such socio-cultural factors that may affect *per capita* consumption. Preventive programmes based on such views aim at suppressing or reducing the use of alcoholic drink, whether beer, wine or spirits. Other epidemiological studies tend to ignore the aetiological importance of the overall level of alcohol consumption in a population. Their preventive programmes attempt to alter drinking practices, by measures such as encouraging the use of less concentrated drinks (beer, wine) as against spirits or encouraging less dangerous drinking habits (such as drinking with meals) – independent of the effect of such measures on the overall level of alcohol consumption. De Lint and Schmidt conclude from their research findings that '. . . a reduction in the *per capita* alcohol consumption must lead to lower rates of alcoholism'. They therefore regard steps such as taxation of alcoholic drinks and all control measures which would reduce accessibility as likely to be effective. In particular, the public health value of such controls is generally accepted. On the other hand, they question the wisdom of those preventive programmes aimed at popularising desirable drinking habits, such as reducing spirit consumption in favour of less concentrated drinks, or drinking with meals etc. Such measures and altered drinking patterns might possibly reduce the rate of intoxication relative to all drinking occasions, but are also likely to '. . . lead to high overall levels of consumption and to higher rates of alcoholism' [24].

Do similar considerations also apply to drugs other than alcohol? Less research has been carried out in this field but another group of Ontario research workers – Smart, Whitehead and Laforest – have found a log normal distribution in a number of large scale surveys in Canadian cities [8].

Infrequent drug users were found to be most numerous, moderate users less numerous, and heavy users least numerous. No clear differentiation was found between users and abusers in terms of frequency of use. Studies of distribution of use of each of seven types of drugs (marihuana, LSD, solvents, barbiturates, tranquillisers, speed and stimulants other than 'speed') among three different high school populations in three Canadian areas, indicated that the log normal distribution, in general, describes psychoactive and hallucinogenic drug use of many types. Similar to their colleagues in the field of alcohol prevention, Smart and Whitehead feel that '. . . to reduce the abuse of drugs for which consumption is log normal it will be necessary to reduce *per capita* drug consumption', and '. . . any legal or social measures which reduce drug consumption by large numbers of persons will lower average drug use and eventually reduce heavy use'. Among such measures, they mention, for example, removal of some drugs from the 'Pharmacopoeia', limiting prescriptions for psychoactive drugs, and a reduction of illicit drug use by campaigns aimed at information and persuasion of the drug abuser population, '. . . supported by more strict enforcement' [8].

In a very recent report Smart and Whitehead [25] expanded the data base for their theories which were originally based on their studies among Canadian High School students (1968–1970). They now include more recent data obtained from studies with Toronto adults (1971) and British university students. With these selected samples the same sort of unimodal distribution of drug use was observed as in the original investigations.

Nevertheless, the Canadian researchers are cautious in their conclusions. Unlike the studies of De Lint and Schmidt [24] – which indicated a correlation between hazardous alcohol consumption and *per capita* consumption existing across a wide variety of countries – in the studies of the use of other drugs so far only a few samples from two countries are involved. Therefore it is necessary to obtain further cross-national data on drug use from further samples from more countries, though it is '. . . becoming more probable that drug use may show the same generality as alcohol consumption'. Smart and Whitehead conclude again that, 'Many people in the population may have to use fewer drugs in order to have fewer drug abusers or heavy users in the next generation'. They point out the need for research experiments during which drug use in a population is reduced and the corresponding changes in the proportions of heavy drug use are examined. They hope that it may be possible to reduce such general drug use, '. . . by a variety of legal, educational or preventive approaches'.

Clearly these Canadian findings, conclusions and recommendations are of the greatest importance, and further research in this field is urgently required. In such complex conditions as alcohol and drug abuse and dependence, with so many various factors involved in their aetiology, views as to the best methods of prevention must obviously differ a great deal. Many would probably agree that, in principle, the reduction of *per capita* consumption of alcohol and other drugs is highly desirable. Also, there may be some correlation between the presence of a high number of heavy drinkers and heavy users of a particular drug (some points with some bearing on this question have been discussed in Part 2). However, not unexpectedly, the views of the Canadian researchers have come in for some criticism. For example, Ole-Jorgen Skog of the National Institute for Alcohol Research in Oslo, believes that, 'The existing data are not sufficient to prove that a change in average consumption is the instrument of choice in the fight against alcoholism'. In his view, 'The causal relationships relevant to the problem of alcoholism are much too complicated for that to be the case' [26].

Some further Canadian research work in this field refers to the possible relationship between the drug use of adolescents and of their parents [27]. As described in Part 2, alienation of youngsters from the habits and attitudes of their parents, and the generation gap, are seen by many observers as one important contributory reason for the world-wide emergence of drug abuse problems among youth. Smart and Fejer [27], in their questionnaire – drug-use surveys of approx. 9000 Toronto students in 1970 – found, however, a positive association between the parental use of psychoactive drugs, alcohol and tobacco (as reported by the students) and the use of psychoactive and hallucinogenic drugs by the students themselves. The relationship between reported parental and student drug-use was found to be statistically significant. For every drug examined, in cases where parents were frequent users, children were also likely to be frequent users; when parents were infrequent users or non-users, the children too were infrequent or non-users. These relationships between parental use and children's use applied for psychoactive drugs, tranquillisers, barbiturates, stimulants, marihuana and LSD, but only to a lesser extent for alcohol and tobacco. There was a closer relationship between the mother's use of alcohol and/or tobacco and student use than such use by the father. The proportion of students using tobacco, marihuana, barbiturates, opiates, stimulants, tranquillisers and LSD was at its lowest when the mother neither smoked nor drank; student use was highest when mother used both alcohol and tobacco. Similarly, mothers taking tranquillisers were more likely to have children taking all types of drugs, such as marihuana, opiates, stimulants, tranquillisers, hallucinogens, barbiturates etc. The heavier the mother's tranquilliser use, the more likely was the child to use such drugs. In cases where the mothers used tranquillisers daily, approx. 31 % of their children used tranquillisers, 29 % used marihuana, 25 % used stimulating drugs, 30 % used LSD or other hallucinogens, 13 % used barbiturates, 11 % used opiates and 10 % used glue. The proportion of students using a given psychoactive drug was highest in cases where their parents were daily users of the same drug; e.g. 31 % of students having a mother taking tranquillisers daily, took tranquillisers, but only 4·4 % did so when the mother never took tranquillisers. In cases where the father took tranquillisers daily, 36 % of students took them; in cases where the father never took tranquillisers only just over 5 % of the students took them. There was a closer relationship between male and female student use of tranquillisers and parental use of tranquillisers, barbiturates and stimulants, than in the case of marihuana. Over 50 % of male student users of tranquillisers and over two-thirds of the female users reported tranquilliser use by one or both parents. The child's sex did not make any difference to the relationship between child and parental drug use.

A similar study carried out by the same authors in 1970 on a sample of students in Southern Ontario obtained similar findings [28]. The authors discussed some possible criticisms and drawbacks of their methodology. They concluded that a causal connection cannot be clearly drawn between drug use by parents and their children; however, there seems to be some evidence that students model their drug use after their parents'. In particular, they tend to use the same drug as their parents. Much drug use by adolescents seems to occur in families where parents take pills freely. It may therefore not be possible to reduce drug use or abuse by adolescents without also reducing the parents' consumption.

The authors stress that the association between drug use of parents and adolescents requires much further research. The Canadian studies and conclusions on the association between *per capita* alcohol use, alcohol abuse and related damage were based on statistics obtained from a variety of countries, those between average drug use in a population and heavy drug use [8, 25] on a few selected samples in two countries. The suggestions and tentative conclusions relating to the association between parental and adolescent's drug use and frequent use [27] are derived from two studies in one Canadian County only, and they obviously need confirmation by studies elsewhere. Nevertheless they appear very striking and are possibly of high significance. The present section opened with the question concerning the feasibility of prevention by selective approach to high-risk groups or by a shot-gun approach to the whole population. Smart and Fejer conclude from their studies that in the treatment of drug abusers there is a need to consider not just the individual but the whole family; also, 'The target populations for drug education should not be students but entire families' [27]. Surely everyone would agree with a preventive approach directed at known, vulnerable target groups of people specially prone to alcohol or drug misuse. Now, however, it would seem possible, or indeed likely – if the Ontario findings are confirmedy by further research – that one such special target group includes parents and the whole family, including of course adolescents. That makes practically the entire population one of the special targets at which to beam one's programme of drug education. In this section, we certainly seem to have come full circle. There obviously remains the necessity for preventive programmes directed at special high-risk groups with research elucidating the best way to 'get through' to such groups, which may vary from group to group. Beyond this, there is a need for programmes aiming at such large target groups as parents and adolescents – in the case of the latter not only at such vulnerable sections as the emotionally disturbed and maladjusted: adolescence may be for many ordinary youngsters a time of special strain and stress, uncertainty about their identity and role, anxiety about their sexual role and choice of occupation etc. At this intermediate stage of growing towards adulthood alcohol and 'other drugs' may all too readily offer a temporary respite from nagging doubts. As far as possible the development of prevention policies and programmes should be accompanied by methods designed to evaluate the success or otherwise of such programmes. Beyond such smaller or larger 'target' groups the findings of the Ontario research workers clearly highlight the need for educational programmes designed to educate the population as a whole about the risks arising from a too liberal use of alcohol and other drugs – 'legal' or illicit ones – and to encourage a general reduction of consumption.

7.4 INTERNATIONAL AND NATIONAL CONTROL OF DRUGS*

In discussing the task of preventing drug abuse and dependence we have in the foregoing briefly outlined the importance of attempting to influence social and professional attitudes. It is equally important to reduce the demand for and the prescribing of drugs by public and professional education and to understand the needs for mental hygiene measures, for improving socio-economic conditions, for earlier diagnosis and earlier treatment and research.. In the long run such steps may be of much greater importance than control and legislative measures, which however, remain indispensible.

* This section is largely based on a talk given at the British Pharmaceutical Conference in Belfast in 1969 and published in the 'Pharmaceutical Journal' (1969, **203,** 393) and (in an abbreviated form) in the 'WHO Chronicle' (1971, **29,** 189)

In the past such legislative approach to alcoholism and drug dependence consisted in the main in deprivation and punishment: prohibiting or restricting the sale of drinks, limiting opening hours of public houses, punishing and imprisoning the drunkard and the addict found 'in possession'. Punishment does not deter the alcoholic and drug addict from repeating over and over again their self-destructive behaviour – which often seems almost designed to invite punitive measures. However, in an overall preventive programme attempts – by law – at eliminating or reducing the influence of the causative agent by approaches aiming at control can make an important and essential contribution. Such measures may be taken by local and regional authorities or on a national basis, but at a time of international co-operation, of easy travel and of youngsters in one country rapidly learning about new drugs fashionable and more easily available in other countries, of 'refugees' from oppressive, punitive drug laws in their home country going to countries with more permissive drug policies, etc., there is clearly a need for taking international as well as local and national control measures. Indeed in order to be really successful, it is necessary to establish a control system which is world wide, universally accepted and receiving the full co-operation of governments, a goal which has not yet been achieved. What are the criteria for subjecting a substance to drug control, i.e. 'National law or international agreement governing and restricting production, movement and use of a drug to medical and scientific needs in the interests of public health and for the prevention of drug abuse'? [29]. There are – according to a 1969 WHO Report [29] – two main conditions of which at least one must be present for the drug to come under consideration for control; if neither condition exists there is no need for the drug to be considered for control:

(a) The drug is known to be abused other than sporadically or in a local area and the effects of its abuse extend beyond the drug taker; in addition its mode of spread involves communication between existing and sporadic drug takers, and illicit traffic in it is developing.

(b) It is planned to use the drug in medicine and experimental data show that there is a significant psychic or physical dependence liability; the drug is commercially available or may become so.

The need to control narcotic and other dangerous drugs affects all countries in the world and, in order to protect the individual and society against drug abuse, national and international control must go hand in hand. Sixty years ago, when the first steps towards international control were taken, it was mainly the menace of misuse of the natural narcotic drugs stemming from the underdeveloped countries which aroused international disquiet. In modern times more danger possibly results from the ready availability in the highly industrialised states of synthetic narcotic and psychotropic drugs that depress or stimulate the central nervous system, than from the illicit import of drugs emanating from the East and finding their way towards widespread abuse by Western addicts. That the drug situation in one country is of more than academic interest to others can be illustrated by many recent examples. For instance, the heated arguments in the UK 15 years ago when Britain refused to outlaw the medical use of heroin; the comparisons and contrasts made continually between the American and British systems of narcotic control, leading to an influx of North American refugees from their strict home laws to the more permissive British drug climate [10, 30] and the disquiet of the Swedes about the production in other European countries of the stimulant phenmetrazine, which created a great problem amongst Swedish youth [31].

Situation before international control
According to Lewin [32], capsules of poppies were found among relics from the Stone Age in the Swiss Lakes. These were apparently obtained by cultivation, possibly in order to extract the narcotic juice. Lewin also quotes from Homer's description in the Odyssey, of nepenthes, '. . . the drug of forgetfulness', which in his view was a preparation of opium. Opium cultivation and use probably spread from Asia Minor to neighbouring regions long before reaching China, involving many other peoples such as the Egyptians, the Assyrians, the Greeks and the Romans. There are reports of the widespread abuse of opium among the Turks in the sixteenth century. The importation of opium into Europe from the East led to much abuse of the drug in countries such as Germany and England.

In the eighth century, Arab traders brought opium, by way of Persia, to India and China where official mention of it was made in about the year 1000 and where an important opium traffic, imported as well as home-produced, existed in the fifteenth century. Widespread opium smoking did not start until the seventeenth century at the time when tobacco smoking was temporarily prohibited. Early in the eighteenth century, a Chinese Emperor strictly forbade the sale and smoking of opium in a vain attempt to stem increasing import and consumption. There was another attempt made at prohibiting the import of opium into China in 1820, but some years later the Treaty of Tientsin (1858), at the end of the Opium Wars forced the Chinese to legalise opium traffic. At the same time, the cultivation of the poppy itself (at the expense of the cultivation of foodstuffs) became widespread and the number of opium smokers increased. In China, as well as in the British colony of Hong Kong, opium revenue became important for the economy and the imports from India to China provided a high proportion of India's income. However in 1906, China decided to gradually reduce the cultivation of opium; correspondingly, according to the Ten Years Agreement with India, the import of opium from India into China was likewise to be reduced and to terminate within ten years. Anti-opium sentiments had grown not only among Chinese reformers, but also in England [33].

The treaty system up to the Second World War [34, 35].
The growing realisation of the seriousness of the risk involved in the opium traffic in China and abroad led to calls for concerted international action. Following a suggestion made by President Theodore Roosevelt in 1909, the first international conference to deal with opium, at which thirteen states were represented, took place in Shanghai. The representatives had no power to sign an international treaty; nevertheless the nine resolutions adopted in Shanghai became the basis for the work of the First Opium Conference in the Hague three years later and all the following agreements and conventions. Briefly, the resolutions urged states progressively to restrict opium to medical use only; to prohibit opium exports to countries in which its import was forbidden; gradually to suppress the smoking of opium; and to establish national control of the manufacture, sale, and distribution of morphine and other dangerous opium derivatives.

In 1912, the International Opium Convention was signed at The Hague. It formulated the fundamental principles for the international control of drugs, which have since retained their validity. Manufacture and trade in medicinal opium, morphine and other opium alkaloids, as well as cocaine and other salts, were only justified by medical and scientific needs; production and distribution of raw opium was to be controlled, and the manufacture and use of prepared opium gradually suppressed; and governments were to establish national control of the manufacture and distribution of opium derivatives. Because of the First World War, The Hague Convention did not come into effect until the ratification of the peace treaties in 1919–1920.

After the war, the duty of supervising the execution of the agreements regarding the traffic in opium and other drugs fell upon the League of Nations, which established an Advisory Committee on Traffic in Opium and Dangerous Drugs. The Committee met regularly during the inter-war years until 1939. After the Second World War its functions were taken over in 1946 by the Commission of Narcotic Drugs of the United Nations [36]. Among several projects initially suggested by the Advisory Committee, and later taken up by the new Commission, was the Single Convention (see below).

With the main aim of organising international control over the international trade in drugs another Opium Conference took place in 1925 in Geneva, resulting in the International Opium Convention of 1925 (which came into force in 1928). This Convention introduced a system of licensing and recording of all transactions involving narcotic drugs, governments being requested to provide detailed statistical information.

The task of watching over the functioning of this system was given to the newly created Permanent Central Board, the first international organisation of narcotics control to be given wide powers. It later became the Permanent Central Opium Board (PCOB), then the Permanent Central Narcotic Board (PCNB), and finally, after the Single Convention was adopted, the International Narcotics Control Board (INCB) [37, 38]. Functions allotted to the board included watching over the international trade in narcotics, seeing to it that treaties were observed and so on.

Despite these attempts at control, both illicit traffic and drug addiction continued to spread. This led to another conference (held in Geneva) which resulted in the 1931 Convention for Limiting the Manufacture and Regulating the Distribution of Narcotic Drugs. In order to achieve its aim, the Convention introduced the compulsory estimates system, countries being requested to provide in advance yearly estimates of the narcotic drugs needed for medical and scientific purposes. These estimates constituted the maximum amount that could be manufactured or imported in any given year. A newly created Drug Supervisory Body (DSB) [37, 38] was to examine these estimates and publish an annual statement. The DSB was also authorised to establish estimates for countries which had not furnished them, irrespective of their being parties to the 1931 Convention or not. As P. Reuter [34], a member of the INCB, has observed, the 1925 and 1931 Conventions (the latter coming into force in 1933) and the work of the national and international controls prevented authorised factories from continuing to provide narcotic drugs for non-medical purposes. Less satisfactory was the outcome of the 1936 Convention for the Suppression of the Illicit Traffic in Dangerous Drugs which, in view of many differences between the various countries, finished with laying down no more than general principles only.

Situation at the beginning of the post-war period

After an interval brought about by the Second World War, the work was resumed in 1948, when the Economic and Social Council of the United Nations established the Commission on Narcotic Drugs [36]. This was composed of fifteen members representing the important narcotic drug producing or manufacturing countries and countries with a serious illicit traffic in narcotics. The Protocol of 1946 (which came into force in 1948) amended the previous agreement and Conventions on narcotics concluded in 1912, 1925, 1931, and 1936. In 1968, the Commission's membership was increased to twenty-four countries, including from then on countries with a serious drug addiction problem. In addition, it became possible for the first time to elect non-members of the United Nations to the Commission.

Gradually the work of the Commission had become more complex. For example, about twenty drugs were under international control in 1946 when it began its work. Twenty years later ninety drugs were under international control. However a review of the Commission's work in its first 20 years [36] pointed out the fundamental difference between its approach and that of the pre-war League of Nations Advisory Committee from which it took over. The Advisory Committee had acted mainly as an enforcement body, implementing the Convention and controls. The new post-war Commission continued this supervisory task, but it also became a policy-making body, giving much time to problems that could not be solved by a purely legal approach. In this way problems connected with research, drug abuse, social and economic aspects, etc., were considered. At its seventeenth session, the Commission decided to deal also with substances with dangerous properties similar to those drugs already under international control (but not themselves under such control). In its work the Commission collaborates closely with a greater number of other bodies, keeping close contact not only with the INCB, but also with such bodies as FAO – which advises on the question of crop substitution for the opium poppy, the coca bush and the cannabis plant – and Interpol (International Criminal Police Organisation), for example, regarding dossiers of known or suspected international narcotic drug traffickers. There is close contact with WHO, in particular regarding problems connected with putting drugs under control or exempting them from it, WHO being asked to prepare documents and a WHO representative attending the Commission's meeting etc. Through its expert committees, study groups, conferences, regional seminars, etc., WHO can provide technical assistance, expert information, and specific recommendations.

The treaties concluded between 1912 and 1936 left many loopholes. For example, they made no provision for controlling production of, and domestic trade in, the vegetable products (opium, coca leaves and cannabis) which, with poppy straw, provide the raw materials for all natural narcotic drugs, and they failed to prohibit the non-medical use of opium, cannabis and coca leaves. There was also the new problem of the synthetic narcotic drugs, the first of which – pethidine – had appeared in 1939.

Among the problems tackled by the Commission were:

(a) The prohibition of opium smoking, a practice which by 1959 had been made illegal virtually throughout the world.

(b) The subjection to control of the new synthetic narcotic drugs. This entails new problems because such drugs are made from chemicals used in industry which are not readily controllable. This is quite different from the case of naturally-manufactured narcotics made from the narcotic substances (opium, poppy straw, coca leaves, cannabis resin), which are obviously themselves subject to control. The 1948 Protocol (Paris), however, brought under international control drugs outside the 1931 Convention for Limiting the Manufacture and Regulating the Distribution of Narcotic Drugs. Thus each country had to inform the Secretary-General of any drugs which could be used medically or for scientific purposes and which could be abused. It was then taken up to WHO to decide whether a drug was addiction producing or could be converted into an addiction-producing product. Meanwhile, it could be placed by the Commission under provisional control.

(c) The limitation of the production of raw materials. Partly because agricultural processes are more difficult to bring under control than manufacturing processes, the raw materials needed to manufacture narcotics were not effectively controlled by the pre-war treaties. As opium was the most important raw material in the manufacture of illicit traffic narcotics, a Protocol was adopted in 1953 for limiting and regulating the cultivation of the poppy plant, the production of opium, and international and wholesale trade in, and use of, opium. The Protocol did not come into force until ten years later. Non-medical opium consumption was prohibited; the number of countries permitted to produce opium for export was restricted to seven (Bulgaria, Greece, India, Iran, Turkey, the USSR, and Yugoslavia); an annual system of estimates of opium production requirements and of statistical returns was introduced; and the PCOB was made the main implementing organisation of the 1953 Protocol, which was the first international treaty aiming at the limitation of production.

The Single Convention on Narcotic Drugs (1961) [34, 39]

The Single Convention of 1961 – which came into force in 1964 – was the culminating point of the efforts at establishing, strengthening, consolidating and integrating international control which had started in 1909. It aims at bringing under national and international control all narcotic substances. At the national level, it provides for control of production, manufacture, distribution, and possession of drugs, of internal trade in drugs, and of violations. At the international level it provides for control of the import of, and international trade in, narcotics, transmission of estimates and statistical returns to the INCB, provision of information to the United Nations Secretary-General and mutual assistance of states for control purposes. As in the past, the main instruments of international control are the regular statistical returns to the INCB and the estimates of future drug requirements, which make it possible to limit manufacture, import, and export.

Satisfactory international control is based on the return of data obtained by adequate control at the national level. Under the Convention, states are to take steps against illicit traffic and to provide for treatment of addicts. While it imposes many stringent obligations on states, it also makes a number of recommendations couched in more flexible terms.

The Single Convention lays down that the consumption of narcotic drugs is allowed on medical prescription only, and outlaws the non-medical use of narcotic substances, including opium, coca leaves, and cannabis (pharmacologically coca leaves and cannabis are not narcotics), and their preparations. Their possession is permitted to authorised persons and trade, distribution, import, export, manufacture, and possibly cultivation can only be carried out by states or state-licensed private enterprises. States are obliged to supervise constantly all activities related to narcotic drugs and to keep precise records.

Thus a comprehensive system closely integrating international and national attempts at control of narcotics has finally superseded the former piecemeal provisions which have been prepared gradually over more than half a century. Beyond the control aspect, the Single Convention contains recommendations referring to other matters, such as the provision of facilities for the treatment, care and rehabilitation of addicts.

With the coming into force of the Single Convention the PCNB and DSB were replaced by a single organisation, the International Narcotics Control Board, (INCB) which started its work in 1968 [37, 38]. Looking back in 1968 on the work of the older bodies, extending over four decades, Sir Harry Greenfield [38], President of the PCNB for 15 years and of the new INCB from its inception, recalled '. . . the dramatic reduction, following the introduction of international control, in the flow of illicit narcotic substances', though it remained distressingly high. The quantity of opium annually available for illicit purposes dropped from 4000 tons in the early 1930s to 1200 tons in the mid-1960s, as a consequence of the implementation of the 1925 and 1931 Conventions. In the late 1920s about 300 tons of legally manufactured morphine (and similar conditions prevailed for heroin and cocaine) had gone into the illicit traffic. Forty years later, narcotic drug manufacture – as a consequence of applying the treaties – no longer exceeded the quantities needed for legitimate medical and scientific needs, and little of the manufactured narcotic drugs passed into the illicit market. Seen in relation to the rising world population, the incidence of drug dependence to manufactured drugs had diminished since the treaty system was started, and the permitted non-medical consumption of opium – amounting to 1600 tons in 1929 – has been greatly reduced and, it was hoped, would soon vanish altogether [38].

Development of international control of cannabis

In view of the current controversy in various countries regarding the bracketing by the law of cannabis with the opiates and cocaine as a supposedly equally dangerous and prohibited drug, a brief account of this subject may be of some interest.

The question of the need for study of Indian hemp was brought up at the First Opium Conference in 1912. In 1923, South Africa suggested the inclusion of Indian hemp as a habit-forming drug in the International Convention. At the 1925 Opium Conference, the Egyptian and Turkish delegates proposed the inclusion of hashish among the narcotics to be dealt with. After some discussion the proposal was accepted, and the 1925 Convention asked the parties to impose national control over extracts and tinctures of Indian hemp and of resin prepared from it. An inquiry carried out in 1925 on behalf of the Advisory Committee on Traffic in Opium and Dangerous Drugs showed that out of twenty-one governments sending replies, nineteen regarded Indian hemp as harmful.

In 1935, the Advisory Committee reviewed the Indian hemp situation. A US memorandum reported widespread habitual marijuana use and '. . . the alarming influence of addiction to Indian hemp on the development of criminality'. In view of the lack of thorough medical and scientific studies, the Committee set up a subcommittee which was to study the whole problem of Indian hemp. It met first in 1935, and the last time in 1938, when it concluded that '. . . certain points still require clarification'. The newly formed United Nations Commission in 1946 did not reappoint a subcommittee on Indian hemp, representatives of various countries disagreeing strongly about its dangers.

In 1948, the Commission decided to provide in the planned Single Convention for the prohibition of hashish. In 1954 it urged governments to consider the discontinuation of cannabis use, after WHO had stated that cannabis preparations were no longer medically useful. A 1957 resolution of the Commission requested the abolition of legal consumption of the drug and the promotion of research. In view of the statements in the Dutch Press that cannabis addiction was no worse than alcoholism, the Commission reiterated in 1961 – in line with the WHO opinion – that cannabis abuse was a form of drug addiction. Alcohol, too, is of course regarded by WHO as a dependence-producing drug. At present there is a renewed clamour in many quarters for the legalisation of 'pot', based partly on a comparison between cannabis and legally available alcohol – a comparison which appears to be no more than a red herring' 'The fact that so many middle-aged addicts nowadays choose two potential poisons as their daily fare is in itself no good argument to encourage youngsters to add to these a third one on top of alcohol and nicotine' [40].

In 1961 the United Nations Conference for the Adoption of the

Single Convention on Narcotic Drugs decided to include cannabis
and cannabis resin (like heroin) in Schedule IV (i.e. complete prohibition), deeming the drug '. . . particularly liable to abuse and to produce
ill effects and . . . such liability is not offset by substantial therapeutic
advantages not possessed by substances other than drugs in Schedule
IV'. (Schedule IV substances are described as having '. . . strong
addiction-producing properties or a liability to abuse . . .' However, in
the case of cannabis only the term '. . . liable to abuse' is given). The
UK and France had indicated in the plenary discussions that (at the time)
the cannabis problem was of little concern in their countries! They
requested that it should be left to individual governments to decide –
if they so wished – on complete prohibition, in line with the WHO
suggestion to recommend prohibition or restriction of the medical use
of cannabis without making it mandatory. But in 1963 the Commission, whilst agreeing that '. . . there might be some variations in the
type of national control', stressed that '. . . the principle (of subjecting
cannabis to the strictest regime of control) as such could not be called
into question'. Again, in 1968 the Commission recommended that
governments should increase their efforts to eradicate the abuse of and
illicit traffic in cannabis, should promote research and advance
additional medical and sociological information, and take steps to deal
with publicity advocating legalisation or tolerance of the non-medical
use of cannabis as a harmless drug. In its final report in 1967, the
Permanent Central Narcotics Board [37] whilst stating that it has less
information about cannabis than about any other substance under
international control, reiterated its adherence to the decision of the
1961 conference when drafting the Single Convention to prohibit the
production, distribution and consumption of cannabis, even for medical
purposes.

The international control of psychotropic substances [41, 42]

The drugs to be discussed now – stimulants, sedatives, tranquillisers
and hallucinogens – have, with the exception of some of the hallucinogens, only recently come into use. Attempts at controlling them
internationally began only over the past 20 years – i.e. half a century
after the start of the treaty system aimed at control of the opiates. It
may be of some interest to note here that the synthesis of the first
barbiturate practically coincided with the start of negotiations for
instituting international control over the opiates; amphetamines came

on the scene a quarter of a century later, followed by the tranquillisers in the 1950s. Of these psychotropic substances the most recent ones to arouse public disquiet are the hallucinogens. The hallucinogenic properties of LSD were discovered by Hoffman in 1943, though long before that, in the 1880s, Louis Lewin came across Peyotl, the mescaline-containing cactus (which became known as *Anhalonium lewinii*) and described its active principles [32] (see Section 5.3).

These substances are outside the scope of the Single Convention on Narcotic Drugs, 1961, although from time to time certain countries felt that they could be brought under it. The United Nations Commission on Narcotic Drugs first raised the question of the desirability of international control of members of this group – i.e. the amphetamines – in 1955. WHO Expert Committees had been regularly concerned with the abuse of these substances since 1949 when an Expert Committee on Habit-Forming Drugs referred to amphetamine abuse. Later WHO Expert Committees pointed to the risks stemming from misuse of the barbiturates (1950), tranquillisers (1956) and hallucinogens (1963), and recommendations for their control were made regularly during subsequent meetings. The United Nations Commission on Narcotic Drugs having discussed amphetamine problems first in 1955, turned its attention to the barbiturates and tranquillisers in 1957, and LSD in 1963. In most instances, the observations of the WHO Expert Committees preceded discussion of the matter at the United Nations Commission.

At these earlier meetings emphasis was laid on the need for strict control at the national level. For example, in 1957 the Commission recommended control measures in order to prevent barbiturate abuse, and close watch on any developing abuse of tranquillisers. In the following years growing barbiturate abuse aroused increasing concern. Meanwhile, the addiction-producing potentialities of the barbiturates had been generally recognised, but in 1962 a move by three countries (Turkey, The United Arab Republic and Yugoslavia) to consider international control was rejected in favour of a recommendation for strict national control of production, distribution and use. However, in the following years, it became clear that these recommendations had failed to stem the growing tide of abuse of amphetamines, barbiturates (especially among the young) and tranquillisers.

The Commission, therefore, established a Special Committee which was to consider the question of control over psychotropic substances not under international control. By the time this committee met in

August 1966, the abuse of LSD in North America and certain European countries had made these substances, in the committee's view, the most urgent problem. In view of the ever-growing abuse of all such substances, the committee suggested establishing a measure of international control as soon as possible.

The Commission accepted the recommendations of its special committee and, like it, was doubtful whether it would be possible to include the new psychotropic substances under Article 3 of the Single Convention – i.e. the Article dealing with changes in the scope of control [39]. It stressed the need to apply common criteria to these substances as regards their control, and recommended strict national measures as the first step towards international control. Governments were urged to control not only their production and distribution but also their import and export, and to restrict their use of scientific research and medical purposes. Priority was to be given to control of LSD, and at the next (22nd) session of the United Nations Commission on Narcotic Drugs in January 1968, 22 states reported having taken such control measures [43].

In view of the likelihood that the application of control measures in one country but not in another, might lead to import of a drug from one to the other, it was decided to research for the best form of treaty action of applying national control by international agreement, as well as some degree of international control. National control measures for the psychotropic substances were to include: availability on medical prescription only, supervision of all transactions from production to distribution, licensing procedures limiting trade to authorised people and prohibition of non-authorised possession for distribution. In view of the great differences between the four groups of substances and between the individual substances in each of the groups, control measures would have to be decided individually in the case of each substance. Responsibility to select the substances to be controlled was to rest with WHO. A draft international agreement containing these recommended controls was to be drawn up for discussion at the next Commission session. In a resolution, governments were urged to prohibit the use of hallucinogens except in special medical or scientific institutions and for approved medical or scientific purpose, and to prohibit all import and export except between governments or specially government-approved organisations.

At a further meeting of the Commission, concern was expressed at amphetamine abuse in Sweden, and a draft resolution submitted by that country asked governments to apply to the amphetamines provisional control under Schedule I (of the Single Convention) which would be immediately binding on states. However, in view of the doubts as to the applicability of the Single Convention, another draft resolution (proposed by the UK, USA, France and Canada) was adopted instead. This recommended the application to amphetamines of national control measures closely resembling those provided by the Single Convention for Schedule I Substances* and the mutual assistance of governments in the regulation of the movement of these substances so as to safeguard against their misuse.

After working on it for several years, the Commission on Narcotic Drugs prepared a revised draft Protocol on Psychotropic Substances. Under the name, 'Convention on Psychotropic Substances', the draft–having undergone many alterations – was adopted by a United Nations Conference held in Vienna in January and February 1971 [44]. Hallucinogenic drugs (including the tetrahydrocannabinols) were put into Schedule I (prohibiting all use except for scientific and very limited medical purposes, and requiring that manufacture, trade, distribution and possession be under a special licence or prior authorisation etc.). Amphetamines, drugs related to them, and phencycladine were put under Schedule II. Most barbiturates and glutethimide were put under Schedule III and a mixed bag, comprising a number of barbiturates, non-barbiturate hypnotics, meprobamate etc. under Schedule IV (Substances under Schedules II, III, and IV are available on medical prescriptions only). Among the changes which the Convention shows compared to the draft Protocol (which had followed recommendations made by WHO) was the deletion of certain drugs from Schedule IV, including chlordiazepoxide, diazepam, chloral hydrate, paraldehyde etc.

Half a century ago, on the last page of his authoritative book on the 'Phantastica', Louis Lewin concluded that '. . . the fatalist . . . cannot shut his eyes to the fact that if the abuse of narcotic substances continues to increase at the same rate as during the last 50 years it would represent a calamity, which in the consequences would concern in some way or other every one of us . . .' [32]. One year earlier, a writer, in the 'British Journal of Inebriety' had uttered a warning that '. . . few realise how perilous (the world) traffic (in dangerous drugs) is becoming . . .',

---

* Schedule I drugs are subject to all control measures applicable to drugs under the Single Convention

and that '. . . the Western world has hardly yet begun to awaken to the seriousness of the menace of itself. . .' [45].

Now another half century has passed, and the fact that the situation as regards control of the narcotics has not only not deteriorated but, on the whole, greatly improved, illustrates the value of the coordinated painstaking attempts at international and national control. Such efforts have been made over the past 60 years by a large number of dedicated men of all nations, under the leadership of international organisations, such as the Advisory Committee on Traffic in Opium and Dangerous Drugs of the League of Nations up to the Second World War and the United Nations Commission on Narcotic Drugs since. Much has been achieved, but one only has to remember the large number of new potentially dangerous and dependence-producing substances which are being produced constantly or the emergence of the new drug epidemics among youngsters during the last decade, to realise how much there remains to be done. Therefore, there is still a necessity for constant vigilance on the part of international and national organisations of control of dangerous drugs. Moreover, although by the beginning of 1972 the number of countries who were parties to the 1961 Convention had risen to 85, the 1971 Report of the International Control Board regretfully noted that among those which had not become Party to the treaty were some important producing and manufacturing countries [46].

Yet, by themselves, the passing of laws, however wise, the restriction and control of the production, distribution, import and export of drugs, and the punishment of illicit manufacturers, smugglers, and pushers cannot solve the problem of preventing drug abuse and dependence, any more than picking up and treating the casualties – the drug addicts. In the aetiology of drug dependence, apart from the agent (the drug), the personality make-up of the user (the host) and the environment play an essential role (see Part 2). Attention has therefore to be given to all these various factors in the task of preventing drug abuse [47]. The international organisations are well aware of the comprehensive nature of the measures needed. In view of this they have widened the composition of the WHO Expert Committee on Drug Dependence to include members from many disciplines. They have also extended the work of the United Nations Commission on Narcotic Drugs far beyond the original task of its predecessor, the Advisory Committee on Traffic in Opium and Dangerous Drugs of the League of Nations (which served merely as an enforcement body), so as to deal also with problems affecting host and environment and not only those directed at control of the agent.

Drug control in the UK [10]

The rise of the narcotic drug problem is perhaps better documented in the UK than in many other countries (see Sections 5.4 and 6.2). Although until 1968 there was no official registration or rather notification system in the UK, the Home Office was able to keep track of at least a high proportion of narcotic addicts because doctors in contact with them usually informed the Home Office. Whilst the number of black market addicts was of course unknown, the general trend indicated by the number of known addicts was extremely instructive. Since 1968, doctors have been obliged by law to inform the authorities about any new person whom they know or suspect of using a narcotic drug. The Inspectors of the Home Office Drug Department have for years taken a very constructive interest in the problems of drug abuse (greatly beyond the calls of duty) and their help has been much appreciated by doctors working in the field, as well as by drug addicts.

Tables 4a and 4b in the Appendix are reprinted from an article written a few years ago by Home Office Deputy Inspector, H. B. Spear [48]. They indicate that the number of known narcotic drug addicts (including here the users of the stimulant cocaine) was fairly steady prior to the 1960s but was then followed by a clear rise throughout the sixties. This rise has been characterised by a gradual increase of the proportion of the non-therapeutic, at the expense of the therapeutic addicts and, to a lesser extent, of the professional addicts. Heroin has assumed the role of the most popular drug and methadone abuse shows a rise (much less than heroin) since 1966. The number of the very young addicts gradually rises in the under twenties as well as the 20–34 age group. The 'H' (and 'C') rise was virtually limited to the younger age groups. Also shown in Tables 4a and 5a in the Appendix is the gradual substitution of methadone for heroin as a consequence of the Treatment Centres prescribing policy. Therefore, in 1969, methadone became the most popular known narcotic drug used by British addicts. The prevalence of misuse of Chinese 'H', increasingly used on the British black market since the late 1960s cannot be estimated [10, 49].

By and large legal measures taken in this country followed the advice given by the UN. An obvious exception is the fact that British doctors have the right to prescribe heroin to addicts (although since

1968, it is only the doctors in the Treatment Centres who can do so). This has led to many arguments as to whether the permissive British approach in the past had been responsible for preventing the emergence of a large-scale epidemic, unlike the punitive approach in the USA. However, as already touched upon, there were probably quite a number of factors involved [10].

Controls on narcotic drugs were first imposed in Great Britain by the Dangerous Drugs Act of 1920. In view of certain ambiguities in this Act, a few years later the Departmental Committee on Morphine and Heroin Addicts published in 1926 the Rolleston Report which distinguished between providing drugs to addicts under suitable controls, and supplying them merely for the gratification of addicts. Indications were outlined as to when morphine or heroin could be given properly. The Rolleston Report dealt mainly with morphine and heroin addiction.

In the following years many new (e.g. synthetic) preparations were put on the market which themselves could lead to dependence, and in view of these and other developments an Interdepartmental Committee on Drug Addiction was appointed in 1958. Its report published in 1961 found that there was little cause for concern regarding the drug situation and no need for radical changes; illicit traffic was regarded as negligible. The few doctors (and Home Office officials) actively interested in the problem were much less optimistic, mainly in view of the patterns of prescribing adopted by several medical practitioners who seemed willing to prescribe large amounts of heroin and cocaine to people presenting themselves as in need of these drugs – whether or not these doctors were able to check such claims[10].Largely as a result of such indiscriminate overprescribing, there was a rising incidence of abusers of 'H' and 'C' chiefly among the young.The Second Report of the Interdepartmental Committee, published in 1965 [11] felt compelled to suggest certain alterations – such as removing the GP's right to prescribe 'H' and 'C' to addicts, the establishment of Treatment Centres, compulsory notification – whilst still avoiding a punitive approach and emphasising the addicts' need for medico-social treatment. Most of the Committee's recommendations were incorporated into the Dangerous Drugs Act of 1967, and following the establishment of Treatment Centres in two London teaching hospitals in 1967, many more came into being in 1968, mostly in London.

It was, however, widely felt that the drug legislation was uncoordinated, clumsy and not sufficiently flexible (the latter obstacle proved a great handicap, for example, in attempts to stop the over-prescribing of methylamphetamine in 1967/68 – which would apparently have required a new Law). The Dangerous Drug Acts of 1965 and 1967 applied only to drugs controlled by the Single Convention on Narcotic Drugs, 1961, i.e. opiates, cocaine (which of course has no narcotic effects but has stimulating effects), cannabis (which is not a narcotic) and some synthetic narcotics (methadone was not affected by the DDA of 1967; it can still be prescribed by GPs to addicts, and in a few instances this has given rise to concern due to overprescribing). Amphetamines and LSD were affected by the Drugs (Prevention of Misuse) Act of 1964 which controls possession and importation but not production, distribution or export. Retail sale by pharmacists was controlled by the Pharmacy and Poisons Act 1933. In an attempt to make new, extensive and flexible provisions for the control of drugs the new Misuse of Drugs Act 1971 (which after some delay came into force in 1973) aims at replacing the various Acts previously in use, by a single Act. Wide powers are given to the Home Secretary to make regulations preventing the misuse of controlled drugs. The power given to Police to make searches and the wide discretion left to Courts has come in for some criticism [50]. On the other hand, the Act clearly recognises the need for research, educational, treatment and rehabilitation measures, and the law is to be relaxed in allowing serious research into cannabis (though the Act largely ignored the recommendations contained in the Wootton Report published in 1968 [51]. No mention is made in the bill of barbiturates. If employed judiciously and under medical control the barbiturates have a number of indications and therefore control measures are more difficult to establish than in the case of amphetamines. However, in view of their widespread abuse by the middle-aged and recently also by the young [49], additional control measures clearly seem necessary.

The Misuse of Drugs Act divides the controlled drugs into three classes, A, B, and C, according to the degree to which they are deemed harmful, and provides for penalties accordingly. Briefly, class A drugs include opiates as well as pethidine and methadone, cocaine, LSD, other hallucinogenics and also THC. Class B drugs include cannabis and its resin and the amphetamines. Class C drugs include methaqualone and benzphetamine.

The new Misuse of Drugs Act [52] also provides for the establishment of an Advisory Council on the Misuse of Drugs which is to keep the drug situation under constant review, to advise on matters such as treatment facilities and rehabilitation, and on promoting education and research. The importance of research is reflected in the setting up of three working parties by the Medical Research Council. The importance of education has been stressed before in this text. There is evidence of abuse of drugs in English schools although its extent in unknown.

Apart from the efforts of the official Treatment Centres and a few in-patient units, great efforts are being made by a large number of voluntary bodies in the fields of prevention and rehabilitation. There is an obvious need for closely correlating the various official and voluntary efforts.

Since the introduction of the Treatment Centres in 1968, the British drug scene has continued to change, and opinions vary as to their impact. However, the former steadily uphill trend in narcotic abuse has been stopped and the abuse of narcotics contained. The British drug problem is, therefore, much more an alcohol and soft drug problem than a hard drug problem. Nevertheless, vigilance is needed throughout. In regard to narcotics, for example, the past few years have witnessed the emergence of methadone (in ampoule form) and of Chinese heroin as easily available and widely sold and bought illicit drugs. In spite of this, the altered British approach seems – with all its imperfections – greatly superior to the former overpermissive approach. Much, one may hope, will be learned from close observation of the various therapeutic and rehabilitation techniques employed under widely differing and legal conditions, by means of built-in facilities for research, and by comparison of results obtained by variants of the approaches now used on both sides of the Atlantic [52].

REFERENCES

1. Lord Rosenheim (1968). *Lancet*, **ii**, 821.
2. *Aspects of Alcoholism*, 60 (1966) (Philadelphia: J. B. Lippincott Co.).
3. Glatt, M. M. (1972). *The Alcoholic and the Help He Needs*, 2nd ed. (London: Priory Press).
4. Young, J. (1971). *The Drugtakers* (London: MacGibbon and Kee).
5. Cohen, S. (ed.) (1971). *Images of Deviance* (London: Penguin Books).
6. Glatt, M. M. (1969). *Brit. J. Addict.*, **64**, 109.
7. Wiener, R. S. P. (1970). *Drugs and Schoolchildren*, 165 (London: Longman).

8. Smart, R. G., Whitehead, P. and Laforest, L. (1971). *Bull. Narcot.*, 23 (2).
9. Roth, M. (1970). Foreword to Bejerot, N. (1972). *Addiction and Society*, 5 (Springfield, Illinois: Charles C. Thomas).
10. Glatt, M. M., Pittman, D. J., Gillespie, D. G. and Hills, D. R. (1969). *The Drug Scene in Great Britain* (Revised reprint) (London: Edward Arnold).
11. Interdepartmental Commission on Drug Addiction (1965). *2nd Report* (London: H.M.S.O.).
12. Eisenberg, L. (1972). *New Engl. J. Med.*, **287**, 249.
13. Glatt, M. M. (1970). *Lancet*, **i**, 889.
14. Dunlop, Sir D. (1970). *Proc. Roy. Soc. Med.*, **63**, 1279.
15. Louria, D. B. (1971). *Overcoming Drugs* (New York: McGraw-Hill Book Co.).
16. U.N. Inform. Letter Div. Narcot. Drugs (1971). *Paediatrics.*
17. Davis, P. A. (1972). *Mod. Med.*, 387.
18. *Brit. Med. J.* (1973). Editorial, **2**, 371.
19. Glatt, M. M. (1971). *WHO Chron..* **24**, 189.
20. Einstein, S. (1973). *Caveat* **1**, No. *3 (Nov.)*, 4.
21. Malcolm, A. I. (1971). *Inventory* **20**, No. *3*, 5.
22. *The Lancet*, (1973). Annot, **11**, 1135.
23. Ledermann, S. Quoted from Ref. 24.
24. De Lint, J. and Schmidt, W. (1971). *Brit. J. Addict.*, **66**, 97.
25. Smart, R. G. and Whitehead, P. C. (1973). *Bull. Narcot.*, **25**, No. 4, 49.
26. Skog, O. J. (1973). *The Drinking and Drug Practices Surveyor (Calif.)*.
27. Smart, R. G. and Fejer, D. (1972). *J. Abnorm. Psychol.*, **79**, 153.
28. Smart, R. G., Fejer, D. and Alexander, E. (1970). quoted from Ref. 27.
29. WHO (1969). *Tech. Rep. Ser.*, **40**, 7.
30. Spear, H. B. and Glatt, M. M. (1971). *Brit. J. Addict.*, **66**, 141.
31. Bejerot, N. (1970). *Addiction and Society* (Springfield, Illinois: Charles C. Thomas).
32. Lewin, L. (1964). *Phantastica* (London: Routledge & Kegan Paul).
33. Hess, A. G. (1965). *Chasing the Dragon* (Amsterdam: North-Holland Publish. Co.).
34. Reuter, P. (1968). *Bull. Narcot.*, **20**, 3 (4).
35. Steinig, L. (1968). *Bull. Narcot.*, **20**, 1 (3).

36. U.N. Econ. Soc. Ccl. Comm. Narcot. Drugs (1965). *Review of the Commission's Work during its first 20 Years,* E/CN 7/471 (New York: U.N.).
37. U.N. Permanent Central Narcotic Board and Drug Supervisory Body *Final Report* (1967). E/OB/23 E/DSB/25 (New York: U.N.).
38. Greenfield, H. (1968). *Bull. Narcot.,* **20,** 1 (2).
39. U.N. Conf. for Adoption of Single Convention Narcotic Drugs. *Final Act* (1961). (New York: U.N.).
40. Glatt, M. M. (1969). *Brit. J. Addict.,* **64,** 109.
41. *Bull. Narcot.* (1967). **19,** 15 (1).
42. WHO (1969). *Handbook resolutions and decisions of the World Health Assembly and Executive Board,* 10th ed., Resol. WHA21.42 (Geneva).
43. *Bull. Narcot.* (1968). **20,** 37 (2).
44. *Bull. Narcot.* (1971). **23** (3) 1.
45. Matthews, B. (1923). *Brit. J. Inebr.,* **21,** 46.
46. *Bull. Narcot.* (1972), **24,** 29 (2).
47. Halbach, H. (1959). *Brit. J. Addict.,* **56,** 27.
48. Spear, H. B. (1969). *Brit. J. Addict.,* **64,** 245.
49. Glatt, M. M. (1969). *Lancet,* **ii,** 429.
50. Simons, B. and Mansfield, M. (1973). *Drugs and Society,* **2,** (10), 5.
51. *Advisory Committee on Drug Dependence (Wootton Committee)* (1968) (London: H.M.S.O.).
52. Glatt, M. M. (1972). *Drug Forum,* **1** (3), 291.

PART 8

CONCLUSIONS:
SOCIETY, HOST, AGENT

'Of the innumerable chemical substances other than foodstuffs which the world contains', wrote Louis Lewin [1] half a century ago 'none have a more intimate connection with human life than the narcotic and stimulating drugs'. These he describes in his book 'Phantastica' as '. . . substances of no nutritive value, but taken for the sole purpose of producing for a certain time a feeling of contentment, ease and comfort', and as '. . . worldwide in the good and evil results they produce'. Over the centuries quite a number of these natural substances and more recently also their synthetic substitutes have from time to time enjoyed a great vogue as highly effective therapeutic agents for a wide range of illnesses. Nowadays some of these drugs are generally held to be of no or very limited therapeutic value. Just 100 years ago, a medical journal gravely warned doctors that the '. . . rash attempt to treat disease without alcohol might result in conviction for manslaughter'. Today on the rare occasions when a practitioner prescribes alcoholic drink for a patient, under the NHS, his prescription is usually ruled unnecessary by the medical 'Referee'. A Chinese pharmacopoiea of 2737 BC described marijuana as an important medicine, but in recent times the WHO has declared cannabis to be void of medicinal value. Practitioners in the UK have been informed by the British Medical Association that there were no more than one or two indications for the prescribing of amphetamines. The indications for the use of LSD have been narrowed down progressively over the past few years. The barbiturates, in spite of their efficacy have, because of their risks, gradually been replaced by somewhat less dangerous tranquillisers and non-barbiturates. There are continued attempts to replace the opiates, despite their undoubted

309

analgesic properties, by less addictive drugs. The cocaine 'epidemic' came to an end when the advent of the Treatment Centre halted the more or less indiscriminate prescribing of this drug (by a few GPs) to drug abusers and addicts. 'Many kinds of alcohol, opium, purple hearts, cocaine and the fantasticants beloved of Aldous Huxley' – writes Dr C. R. B. Joyce [2] –'are all drugs for none of which, in my view, are there any therapeutic indications whatsoever'.

Clearly, it is not the physiological effects of these drugs that have altered over the years but rather society's perception of them due to changing attitudes and judgment [3]. It may take hundreds of years before unsuspected risks come to light. Over 400 years after tobacco had become fashionable in Europe, an English doctor pronounced that, 'It may be unhesitatingly affirmed that of all forms of self-indulgence to which frail humanity is addicted, that of tobacco smoking is most general and least harmful' [4]. In the case of alcohol, in spite of its manifold and well-known dangers, its use had remained widely accepted and the majority of people have learned to live with it. There are of course other widely accepted forms of dependence on mild psychotropic drugs. In Anglo-Saxon countries there are few people who go through the day without making use of the stimulating action of caffeine contained in coffee and tea, and more and more individuals nowadays avail themselves of the tranquillising effects of modern drugs on the slightest or no provocation.

The present review of drug dependence started off with a discussion of its multifactorial causation (see Part 2). Multifactorial causation, social contagiousness of drug dependence, the importance of exposure in determining vulnerability etc. are all factors which are given by D. V. Hawks [5] as recommending the application of the epidemiological method to the problem of drug dependence [6].(Epidemiology is 'the study of the distribution of a disease or condition in a population and the factors that influence that distribution'.). In subsequent chapters the triad, host, environment and agent was found to be of importance not only in aetiology (although the host in drug dependence often exhibits an actively agent-seeking behaviour not shown by the host in infectious diseases), but also in many other aspects of drug dependence: e.g. in the pace of its development 'including the remote chance of a few alcoholics' or drug addicts' stabilisation on a given, low dosage, or in arranging programmes of treatment, rehabilitation and prevention, and in assessing prognosis in individual patients. In prevention, for example, efforts must be directed at improvements of 'host' and society as well as at controlling the agent.

At present the use of psychoactive substances is increasing. This includes the ones generally accepted by society as well as the illicit substances. The study of drug dependence must be broadened to include both these types: there is no basic difference between licit and illicit drugs, between those prescribed by doctor and those not prescribed, between the ones traditionally accepted by society and those not accepted; they all can – under certain circumstances and when taken to excess – be highly dangerous. Although some drugs are widely accepted by society and others rejected, there is no clear dividing line. What is regarded as 'deviant' behaviour today by some societies and groups, may be considered quite normal behaviour somewhere else; and what is stated to be deviant behaviour, very often depends, after all, on the views of the majority and the current Law which is subject to frequent modifications. The abuse of alcohol and tobacco does not become less dangerous merely because these are legally available. The educational programmes, dealing with drugs, aimed at schoolchildren, teachers, the general public etc. must not be restricted to the condemnation of illicit drugs but must deal with all types of psychoactive drugs: the legally accepted alcohol and tobacco and those often prescribed by doctors, such as barbiturates and tranquillisers, as well as the illicit heroin, LSD and cannabis.

In today's smoking, drinking and pill-taking society, the prevailing social climate directly and indirectly encourages drug taking by adults and youngsters. Disillusionment amongst youngsters with adult society as a whole and with the attitudes and outlook of their parents in particular has often been regarded – and probably rightly so – as one important reason for the misuse of drugs by youngsters. It is interesting therefore to learn from the recent Canadian studies (see Section 7.3) that, at the same time, many youngsters seem to take the generous consumption of alcohol, tobacco and tranquillisers by their parents as a model and cue for their own drug-taking habits. Canadian studies have also indicated that the use of psychoactive substances as a whole – including alcohol and legitimate tranquillisers – may have to be drastically reduced before many inroads can be made into the numbers of those who come to grief as a consequence of excessive alcohol and drug use. Therefore attempts to curb and control drug abuse cannot be left merely to law-enforcement agencies, the police, doctors, teachers and youth leaders. In coping with the problem of drug dependence, it is clearly not enough to study and control the individual drugs. One's main concern has to be not only the addict but practically the entire population (nearly everyone consumes CNS-affecting drugs in one form or another) and its dynamic interaction with their socioeconomic environment. Today's typical drug abuser is no longer the person attracted by one individual drug: he is a polydrug abuser for whom 'everything goes'. As Dr George Birdwood put it [7], 'Their dependence . . . is not on a particular drug, but on drugs in general, on being stoned out of their minds, on injecting, and even on the life-style of their particular drug subculture'.

This volume is thought of as a plea for a middle-of-the-road, comprehensive, co-ordinated multi- and interdisciplinary approach to the complex problems of drug dependence. The rather pretentious title 'Guide to Drug Addiction' is obviously not thought of as providing instant solutions – which do not exist – but rather as pointing out some of the snags involved in the search for easy, immediate, ready-made answers. The term 'addiction' in itself raises many questions, and in many ways the term 'dependence', as suggested by WHO, is preferable. At the same time, there remains the question as to the role and importance of physical dependence as indicated by the development of physical abstinence symptoms. Physical dependence was formerly regarded as the characteristic feature of 'addiction'. Yet it can occur without any drug-seeking behaviour and compulsion on the side of the sufferer, as illustrated by the physical abstinence syndrome seen in newborn children of heroin-taking mothers (see Part 2). Moreover such 'physical dependence' can develop fairly rapidly, as shown by Ontario research workers in the case of alcohol not necessitating years of heavy drinking; and physical abstinence symptoms can certainly develop without psychic dependence, as for example in publicans as a consequence of (withdrawal from) habitual (but not necessarily compulsive) heavy alcohol intake. Possibly it should also be stressed more clearly that drug dependence is only one of quite a number of possible hazards of drug abuse (or rather misuse). The emphasis on 'dependence' – as Birdwood [7] points out – '. . . excludes the experimenter and the LSD tripper. . ., overdosing and the haphazard but habitual consumption of a variety of drugs'. Definite mental and physical complications may follow excess alcohol intake even in the absence of dependence: the liver does not distinguish between alcohol excess consumed as a consequence of dependence or of self-indulgent habitual heavy drinking. For all these reasons, in education on the risks of heavy alcohol and 'other drugs' intake, it should be made clear that lack of 'addictive' properties in itself does not necessarily make it a safe drug; and that in the long run it is psychic (and possibly social) dependence which is much more important than physical dependence.

Everyone working with drug addicts and alcoholics is aware of the need for patience, tolerance and the maintaining of communications. What, however, is sometimes overlooked is the importance of good communications between members of the various professional disciplines working in this field who may be speaking a somewhat different language. There is in this field an absolute need for inter-disciplinary and international co-operation, free from narrow professional and national blinkers.

In recent years it has become fashionable in certain sociological and psychological quarters to attack the so-called 'medical model' and the 'disease concept' of alcoholism and drug dependence. In many ways these attacks seem to be based on misconceptions and misunder-standings, and the setting up of a 'straw man' [8]. These critics when attacking the 'medical model' and the 'disease concept' equate 'medical' with 'physical' or 'physiological', and 'disease' with a purely physical illness. But medical men – whether the modern family doctor, the community physician, the social psychiatrist etc. – have for a long time been concerned with the 'whole' man and his interaction with society, with psychosomatic and psychosocial aspects [8]. Certainly those psychiatrists who over many years have participated in the regular meetings arranged throughout the world by the International Council on Alcohol and Addictions have always been actively interested in the psychological and social aspects of alcohol and drug abuse, lecturing on such themes in plenary or other sessions and discussing them in interdisciplinary sessions with leading international sociologists, as e.g. Professor Kettil Bruun from Finland or Professor David Pittman from the U.S.A. The willingness of members of various professional disciplines to look at problems not only from their own narrow professional viewpoint has indeed always been one of the most attractive features of such international conferences. The absolute need to become interested in sister disciplines and the opportunity given for doing so, adds to the fascination which the subject of alcoholism and drug dependence exerts on its students. To take another example, this time from England: when the first National Health Service Unit for alcoholics was set up in 1952 it functioned from the beginnings as a therapeutic community with the emphasis on group therapy and on psychosocial aftercare, with drugs being employed as no more than adjuncts to the psychological and social core of treatment [9]. The acceptance of the 'disease' or 'illness' concept of alcoholism or drug dependence does not mean treating it exclusively or even mainly by physical therapies. By no means has the term 'disease' to be restricted to physical abnormalities and suffering.* Critics of the 'disease concept' of alcoholism tend to refer to the occasionally described cases of alcoholics who have learnt to drink in moderation, as indicating that alcoholism and 'loss of control' are not diseases: the possibility of reverting to moderate drinking is taken as evidence of the lack of a biochemical change. But as discussed in Part 2, such exceptional occurrences by no means preclude the activity of factors pertaining to 'host' and society as well as to the 'agent' alcohol and any biochemical changes produced by interaction between agent and host [8]. Thus, if 'medical model' is indeed equated with 'physical model', and 'disease' with 'physical disease' – as done by the critics – the application of such terms to alcoholism and drug dependence would be wrong. However, no medical man actively interested in these conditions would define medical model and disease in this way. For him the term 'medical model' as applied in this context, means an interdisciplinary model, concerned not only with the psychological and physiological aspects of the host but also with the society and 'agent'. Not surprisingly, therefore, at the recent First International Medical Conference on Alcoholism in London (1973) practically all doctors speaking on this subject came out in favour of the 'medical model' and the 'disease concept' [11, 12].

In the fields of alcohol and drug abuse and dependence all too many questions remain unanswered but progress is being made slowly and steadily by painstaking research in many parts of the globe. There seems little genuine purpose or hope in the many claims poured forth from time to time that 'the' answer to the whole of the problem lies in yet another infallible wonder drug, or alternatively one or the other types of psychotherapy applicable to all sufferers, or perhaps an

---

* According to an article in the January 1974 issue of the 'Journal of the Royal College of Physicians of London' (by G. M. Howe), health—described by the World Health Organisation as, '. . . a state of complete physical, mental and social well-being and not merely the absence of disease or infirmity'—represents, '. . . a balanced relationship of body, mind and environment. . . Disease, on the other hand, represents imbalance, a lack of harmony between the body–mind complex and its external environment'. The term 'environment' is described in the article as embracing, '. . . the totality of external influences, natural and man-made, that impinge on man and affect his well-being'. Among such environmental influences is the '. . . human, or socio-cultural, environment (which) is essentially man-made and relates to the density, geographical distribution and mobility of populations, to occupations, to socio-economic states, to housing, to diets, to habits and to customs' (10)

abolition of present-day society (or the various types of society). Everyone surely agrees that the best answer would be if societies were such that the need for some of their members to escape into psychotropic drugs would disappear. But, as far as is known, there is no society in the world today without a drug-taking problem – if one includes alcohol. The Iron Curtain countries, for example, by and large, seem to have little trouble from the abuse of other drugs, but they certainly have many problems arising out of the excessive consumption of alcohol by a great many of their young and middle-aged (and in fact they take very active steps to overcome such problems). They also have their problems with delinquent youth and their student revolts. Throughout recorded history there has never been – as far as one knows – a period where people did not make use of psychotropic substances – and not only the unstable and inadequate members of society. The general acceptance and use of relatively harmless psychoactive substances – such as tea and coffee – shows that there must be widespread need for them. This need is also reflected in the fact that in spite of all propaganda and information making the dangers of cigarette smoking clear to everyone, relatively little inroad has been made into such a pernicious and widespread habit. This probably means that society will go on using psychotropic drugs. In addition in non-utopian societies which use non-utopian, pharmacologically-effective, therapeutic agents there will always be personalities who – in spite of the best of psychological and social methods of personal and social hygiene in childhood – are inadequate, insecure or unhappy enough to feel in need of artificially-induced relaxation, sedation or stimulation. Therefore in many cases the goals of preventive and rehabilitation programmes whilst naturally aiming at the best possible results will have to be limited and realistic.

Apart from work towards improvement of society there will therefore always be a necessity for more effective psychotherapeutic approaches and for potent but less dangerous psychoactive substances. The fact that so many new drugs are synthesised almost day by day means of course that by itself legislation cannot hope to forestall and to cope with all the possible ill-effects arising out of interaction of hitherto unknown substances with vulnerable personalities under imperfect social conditions. Yet again this does not mean that the law can be of no help whatsoever. On the one hand, society, professionals, the lay public and the police etc., should certainly take care that inopportune or exaggerated concern, unduly harsh interference, and

2 2

panic measures do not lead to an amplification of the 'deviant' behaviour. On the other hand, however, passive standing by should not degenerate into a social reinforcement of behaviour which may have disastrous consequences for the individual concerned as well as for society. It should not be forgotten that whatever psychosocial circumstances may have initiated drug abuse, pharmacological factors may progressively take over during the course of the drug-taking career. These bring a new risk not usually calculated but carelessly shrugged aside when people start to take drugs. Few would claim nowadays that the social problem of drug misuse would be solved by sending addicts to prison. However, the cry that no drug abuser should be sent to prison whatever his offence seems as unrealistic as the opposite one that all belong there. Likewise the argument sometimes heard that all antisocial and criminal acts arise on a fundament of psychiatric illness is unrealistic and only serves to bring psychiatry into disrepute.

In view of so many questions remaining unanswered, there is an urgent need for inter- and multidisciplinary research. However, the present lack of information should not become an excuse and a smoke-screen for inactivity; doing nothing at all is surely more harmful by and large than making use of whatever is already known. Prevention is certainly better than cure. But that does not mean that all efforts and funds should be channelled off in the direction of prophylaxis – there are always people in dire need of help here and now.

People drink or take pills to excess for so many different reasons that there cannot be one and the same preventive, therapeutic or rehabilitation technique which is the best for each and every one abuser. Instead (a combination of) such methods should be chosen after an evaluation of the method best suited to the given individual. Nor should such techniques be selected on the basis of a preconceived bias. The question is not psychological therapy, or social therapy, or pharmacological therapy, but rather a judicious combination of the various techniques. 'Heads' of patients should not be squeezed in a previously conceived and manufactured therapeutic cap, but the caps should be chosen so as to befit the particular 'head'. It's not a question, for example, of 'Pavlov or Freud', out-patient or in-patient therapy, or of chemical therapy versus self-help. One method may be more suitable for one, another method for another patient. For example, AA is probably the best individual agency known today to help alcoholics, but not every alcoholic can be induced to go to AA, and alternative or additional methods should then be made available.

A world and society cannot be an ideal one in which – according to a recent estimate [13] – there may be thirty million addicts, including six million on opium and heroin, four million on coca leaves and cocaine (about 38 tons of coca leaf are produced annually, of which medicine needs only 1 %), and at least twenty million on cannabis, and this estimate obviously leaves out the millions who consume excessive amounts of alcohol. Clearly youngsters have some justification in complaining about 'sick society', questioning long-established values and clamouring for all-round improvement. It hardly behoves adults, parents and teachers today – when drinking, smoking and consuming tons of often unnecessary tranquillisers and antidepressants – to adopt a morally superior attitude to their children and pupils who after all have learnt to take their drugs from the habits prevalent in a drinking, smoking and pill-taking society, created by adults. But surely it is unfair, untrue and unwise if the young, in their '. . . challenge to the underlying, all-pervasive values of the acquisitive, materialistic, competitive technological society' [14] put all the blame on 'sick society'. Among those who look for improvement in society it is fortunately only a minority whose search for alternative values extends to habitual misuse of drugs. The finding that in spite of all availability and temptation the majority do not abuse drugs, indicates the presence of psychological problems in a certain proportion of the drug abusers. Once having embarked on habitual drug misuse, there is added to the original problems – whether arising from defects mainly of society or mainly from personality make-up – the risk produced by the interaction of pharmacological effects with the individual's physical and mental make-up. It is therefore not enough to limit one's attack on the drug problem to curing the maladies of society, or attempting to reduce to a minimum the numbers of clearly maladjusted personalities, or to produce better and better drugs with all the advantages of the available ones but without any of their drawbacks. Society, host and agent – they are all involved in producing and maintaining the drug problem – and there is need for a comprehensive approach and simultaneous attack on all these fronts.

REFERENCES

1. Lewin, L. (1964) *Phantastica* (London: Routledge and Kegan Paul).

2. Joyce, C. R. B. (1966). *New Horizons in Psychology*, 271. (B. M Foss, editor) (Penguin Books).
3. Emboden, W. (1972). *Narcotic Plants* (London: Studio Vista).
4. Hillier, S. (1909). *Popular Drugs*, 133 (London: T. Werner Laurie).
5. Hawks, D. V. (1970). *Bull. Narcot.*, **22** (3), 15.
6. World Health Organisation (1973). *WHO Tech. Rep. Ser.*, **526**, 17.
7. Birdwood, G. (1973). *Drugs and Society*, **3**, (3), 3.
8. Glatt, M. M. (1973). *1st Int. Med. Conf. Alcoholism* (London: Medical Council on Alcoholism).
9. Glatt, M. M. (1955). *Brit. J. Addict.* **52**, 55.
10. Howe, G. M. (1974). *J. Roy. Coll. Phycns.*, *London*, **8**, 127.
11. Van Dijk, W. K. (1973). *1st Int. Med. Conf. Alcoholism* (London: Medical Council on Alcoholism).
12. *Lancet* (1973). Annot. **ii.**
12. *World Med.* (1971). July 14, p. 12.
14. Carstairs, G. M. (1973): quoted from *Pulse* (May 26).

APPENDIX

Table 1 CNS-affecting drugs in popular and medical use. (From 'Behind the Drug Scene' by C. R. B. Joyce (Family Doctor Booklet) by courtesy of Brit. Med. Assoc.)

Group	Examples	Approx. number of forms available	Major medical uses	Death by overdose due to	Other (unwanted) immediate effects	Undesirable effects of prolonged use
1. *Caffeine*	Coffee, tea, cocoa, cola drinks	100s	Stimulant; diuretic	Does not occur	Sleeplessness	?
2. *Tobacco*	Cigarettes, cigars, pipe tobacco, snuff	100s	None	Does not occur	Impairment of taste	Cancer, coronary disease; bronchitis
3. *Alcohol*	Beer, wine, spirits, 'meths'	100s	Disinfectant	Respiratory failure; inhalation of vomit	Gastritis; dehydration; vomiting; aggressiveness	Malnutrition; cirrhosis; neuritis; psychosis
4. *Hypnotics*	Chloral, barbiturates, anti-histamines	100	Sedation; sleep	Respiratory failure	Misjudgments; slowing of reactions	Inco-ordination; lethargy; confusion
5. *Stimulants*	Amphetamines, cocaine methylamphetamine (Methedrine), phenmetrazine	50	Neurological disorders	Heart failure; stroke	Sleeplessness	Psychosis (paranoid)
6. *Analgesics*	Morphine, heroin, pethidine, methadone	50	Pain relief	Respiratory failure	Constipation	Infections; mental and social deterioration, withdrawal
7. *Fantasticants*	LSD, marihuana (cannabis), STP	0	Psychiatric disorders	?	Confusion; psychosis; possible effects on foetus	Lethargy; delusions; withdrawal

continued overleaf

Table 1 *continued*

Group	Nature of dependence: psychological (Ps) or physiological (Ph)	Effects of withdrawal (untreated)	Relative importance of drug (D) personality (P) and setting (S) in dependence 1 2 3	Population having had experience (conjecture)	Population dependent % (conjecture)	Use increasing	Rate of increase in use	Medical (M) or social (S) problem	Access
1. *Caffeine*	Ps	?	S P D	95	?	?	?	No	Open
2. *Tobacco*	Ps; Ph	Craving	S P D	75	10	Yes	Small	M	Open
3. *Alcohol*	Ps; Ph	Delirium; convulsions; death	S P D	75	0·5	Yes	Small	M, S	Open
4. *Hypnotics*	Ps; Ph	Delirium; convulsions; death	D P S	10	0·2	Yes	Medium	M, S	Open, medical or illicit
5. *Stimulants*	Ps	Intense craving &	S P D	5	0·1	Yes	Medium–large	M, S	Medical or illicit
6. *Analgesics*	Ps; Ph	Diarrhoea; cramps; excessive secretions	D P S	1	0·01	Yes	Large	M, S	Medical, or illicit
7. *Fantasticants*	Ps	?	S P D	0·1	0·001	Yes	Large	S	Illicit only

Table 2 Estimated total number of NHS prescriptions (millions) in England and Wales in 1961 and 1967–1971. (From Annual Reports of Mental Health, by courtesy of H.M.S.O.)

Broad therapeutic group	Number of prescriptions 1961	Number of prescriptions 1967	Number of prescriptions 1968	1969	Number of prescriptions 1970	1971
	Millions		Millions		Millions	
All groups		251·9	248·4	245·5	247·7	247·5
Preparations acting on the alimentary system		21·6	20·2	19·4	20·0	19·8
Antacids and antispasmodics		10·6	9·7	9·2	9·5	9·4
Bitters, tonics and gastro-intestinal sedatives		4·9	4·2	3·9	3·4	3·1
Laxatives and purgatives, evacuant enemas and suppositories, other preparations acting locally on the rectum and anti-infective agents acting locally on the gastro-intestinal tract		6·1	6·3	6·3	7·2	7·3
Preparations acting on the cardiovascular system and diuretics		19·0	18·7	19·6	20·8	23·3
Preparations acting on the heart		4·9	4·3	4·5	4·1	5·4
Diuretics		5·3	5·8	6·4	6·9	8·0
Antihypertensives		3·9	4·1	4·3	5·2	5·2
Vasodilators, vasoconstrictors		4·5	3·9	4·0	4·1	4·2
Anticoagulants and other preparations acting on the vascular system		0·5	0·6	0·5	0·5	0·6

continued overleaf

Table 2 continued

Broad therapeutic group	Number of prescriptions		Number of prescriptions		Number of prescriptions	
	1961	1967	1968	1969	1970	1971
	Millions		Millions		Millions	
Preparations acting on the lower respiratory system		27·0	27·1	27·1	26·1	24·2
Expectorants and cough suppressants		19·2	19·5	19·3	17·6	19·5
Preparations relaxing bronchial spasm		7·7	7·4	7·2	7·4	7·4
Other preparations acting locally on the lower respiratory tract, respiratory stimulants and others		0·1	0·2	0·6	1·1	1·3
Preparations acting on the nervous system		69·6	69·2	67·9	68·3	67·9
Addictive analgesics	0·9	0·9	0·9	0·8	0·9	0·7
Antipyretic analgesics	15·0	18·9	17·5	16·8	16·2	15·6
Hypnotics (barbiturate)	15·2	15·0	14·2	13·1	12·2	10·9
Hypnotics (non-barbiturate)	5·4	4·5	5·4	5·9	6·6	7·1
Tranquillisers	6·2	13·6	14·9	15·4	16·0	17·1
Antidepressants	1·4	4·6	5·0	5·4	6·0	6·6
Stimulants and appetite suppressants	6·0	4·4	3·6	3·3	3·1	2·7
Anticonvulsants, preparations used in Parkinsonism, cholinergic and neuro-muscular-blocking drugs		2·2	3·0	3·0	3·1	3·4
Local anaesthetics and counter-irritants		4·3	3·6	2·9	2·9	2·5
Antiemetics (other than preparations of unadmixed hyoscine salts)	1·2	1·2	1·2	1·1	1·2	1·3

Table 3a Suicide rates (per 100 000) in England and Wales from 1961–1971. (From Registrar General's Statistical Review of England and Wales, 1971, Part 1, Tables Medical by courtesy of H.M.S.O.)

Cause of Death		1961	1962	1963	1964	1965	1966	1967	1968	1969	1970	1971
Accidental poisoning by drugs and medicaments	M	4	5	6	5	6	6	7	7	8	9	9
	F	5	6	7	8	8	9	10	9	11	13	13
	P	4	6	6	7	7	8	8	8	9	11	11
Accidental poisoning by gases and vapours	M	15	19	20	15	14	14	11	9	8	8	7
	F	20	24	27	19	17	17	13	12	9	7	5
	P	17	21	24	17	15	15	12	11	9	7	6
Gas distributed by pipe-line	M	—	—	—	—	—	—	9	7	5	5	3
	F	—	—	—	—	—	—	11	11	7	5	4
	P	—	—	—	—	—	—	10	9	6	5	4
Suicide and self-inflicted injury	M	133	142	143	136	125	119	115	114	106	95	95
	F	90	96	98	97	89	87	79	76	72	66	67
	P	111	118	120	116	107	103	97	94	89	80	81
Poisoning by solid or liquid substances	M	21	27	34	36	34	31	32	33	34	29	32
	F	28	34	42	45	45	44	43	46	44	43	44
	P	24	31	39	40	40	38	38	40	39	37	38
Poisoning by gases in domestic use	M	59	62	60	52	43	40	35	27	20	15	9
	F	44	44	41	37	29	27	21	14	13	6	5
	P	51	53	50	44	36	33	28	20	16	10	7
Poisoning by other gases	M	4	4	4	5	5	6	5	8	8	6	10
	F	0	0	0	0	0	0	0	1	0	1	1
	P	2	2	2	2	3	3	3	4	4	4	5
Hanging, strangulation and suffocation	M	20	20	19	20	17	18	18	19	20	22	20
	F	6	6	4	5	5	5	4	5	5	6	7
	P	13	13	12	12	11	11	11	12	12	14	13

Table 3b Number of Suicides in England and Wales from 1961–1971. (From Registrar General's Statistical Review of England and Wales, 1971, by courtesy of H.M.S.O.)

Cause of Death		1961	1962	1963	1964	1965	1966	1967	1968	1969	1970	1971
Suicide and self-inflicted injury	M	2980	3215	3261	3130	2899	2783	2708	2695	2523	2271	2263
	F	2151	2299	2378	2363	2192	2145	1961	1889	1803	1669	1682
Poisoning by acid or liquid substance	M	459	618	785	819	792	727	757	776	816	700	750
	F	660	806	1026	1086	1104	1095	1069	1150	1106	1089	1097
Poisoning by gases in domestic use	M	1316	1392	1365	1189	992	930	824	635	476	353	215
	F	1055	1069	998	900	716	663	530	353	314	158	131
Poisoning by other gases	M	93	91	98	107	119	131	127	178	182	153	244
	F	5	5	5	9	9	5	7	29	11	19	23
Hanging, strangulation and suffocation	M	452	460	440	454	390	424	426	460	467	513	467
	F	132	145	106	117	121	122	105	124	130	152	174
Submersion (drowning)	M	227	220	191	181	172	150	149	167	164	170	133
	F	177	172	151	149	147	152	130	130	137	119	129
Cutting and piercing instruments	M	91	67	60	52	58	70	65	95	65	65	74
	F	24	14	16	14	10	17	16	17	20	26	16
Firearms and explosives	M	170	183	149	150	182	168	175	175	144	131	155
	F	11	5	8	6	8	1	13	8	5	12	9
Jumping from high place	M	67	57	49	46	53	57	69	64	85	49	70
	F	33	32	29	46	35	30	36	43	38	45	48
Other and unspecified means	M	105	127	123	122	141	126	115	145	124	138	155
	F	53	50	39	35	42	54	54	35	42	49	55
Late effect of self-inflicted injury	M	—	—	1	—	—	—	1	—	—	—	—
	F	1	1	1	—	—	—	1	—	—	—	—

Table 4a Number of narcotic addicts (including cocaine) coming to the notice of the Home Office between 1935 and 1968.
From Spear, A. B. (1969). *Brit. J. Addict.*, by courtesy of Pergamon Press.

Year	No. of known addicts	Sex M	Sex F	Origin T	Origin N/T	Origin UK	Morphine	Heroin	Cocaine	Pethidine	Methadone	Professional addicts
1935	700 approx.											120 approx.
1936	616	313	300									147
1937	620	300	320									140
1938	519	246	273									143
1939	534	269	265									131
1940	505	251	254									90
1941	503	252	251									91
1942	524	275	249									98
1943	541	280	261									94
1944	559	285	274									93
1945	367†	144	223									80
1946	369	144	225									79
1947	383	164	219									87
1948	395	198	197									119
1949	326	164	162									100
1950	306	158	148									95
1951	301	153	148									77
1952	297	153	144									75
1953	290	149	141									71

Origin: This information was not collected prior to 1958 (except for heroin addicts)

Morphine: Exact numbers not available but the proportion of addicts using morphine has varied from approx. 90% in 1935 to between 60–70% in the years 1950–54

Heroin: Exact numbers not available but the proportion of addicts using heroin has varied from 5% in 1935 to 19% in 1952

Cocaine: Exact numbers not available but less than 10% of the addicts used cocaine

Pethidine: From 1948 to 1954 the proportion of addicts using pethidine varied between 12–19%

Methadone: Exact numbers not available except in 1949 and 1951 when there were 2 and 3 respectively

* Alone, or in combination with other drugs
† Until 1945 the practice had been to include cases for 10 years after the last information (except death)

continued overleaf

Table 4a *continued*

Year	No. of known addicts	Sex		Origin			Drugs used					Professional addicts
		M	F	T	N/T	UK	Morphine	Heroin	Cocaine	Pethidine	Methadone	
1954	317	148	169				179	57				72
1955	335	159	176				176	54	6	64	21	86‡
1956	333	163	170				178	53	6	64	20	99
1957	359	174	185					66	16	92	31	88
1958	442§	197	245	349	68	25	205	62	25	117	47	74
1959	454	196	258	344	98	12	204	68	30	116	60	68
1960	437	195	242	309	122	6	177	94	52	98	68	63
1961	470	223	247	293	159	18	168	132	84	105	59	61
1962	532	262	270	312	212	8	157	175	112	112	54	57
1963	635	339	296	355	270	10	172	237	171	128	59	56
1964	753	409	344	368	372	13	171	342	211	128	62	58
1965	927	558	369	344	580	3	160	521	311	102	72	45
1966	1349	886	463	351	982	16	157	899	441	123	156	54
1967	1729	1262	467	313	1385	31	158	1299	462	112	243	56
1968	2782	2161	621	306	2420	56	198	2240	564	120	486	43

‡Nurses included in 'professional' for first time; hitherto they had been included in 'other'
§From 1958, figures relate only to those persons known to have been taking drugs in the year in question

Table 4b Ages of narcotic addicts known to the Home Office between 1959 and 1968. (From Spear, H. B. (1969). *Brit. J. Addict.*, by courtesy of Pergamon Press).

	1959	1960	1961	1962	1963	1964	1965	1966	1967	1968
Under 20										
(all drugs)	—	1	2	3	17	40	145	329	395	764
(heroin)	—	1	2	3	17	40	134	317	381	729
20–34										
(all drugs)	50	62	94	132	184	257	347	558	906	1530
(heroin)	35	52	87	126	162	219	319	479	827	1390
35–49										
(all drugs)	92	91	95	107	128	138	134	162	142	146
(heroin)	7	14	19	24	38	61	52	83	66	78
50 and over										
(all drugs)	278	267	272	274	298	311	291	286	279	260
(heroin)	26	27	24	22	20	22	16	20	24	20
Age unknown	34	16	7	16	8	7	10	14	7	82

Precise details of age groupings were not included in Annual Reports until 1959

.

Table 5a Total number of notifications received under Dangerous Drugs Act 1968. (From Drugs Branch, Home Office, Romney House, London).

Notifications received	22.2.68– 31.12.68	1.1.69– 31.12.71	1.1.72– 31.12.72	1.1.73– 31.3.73	Gross total
a. First Notifications					
(i) Heroin	2096	1540	557	128	4321
(ii) Methadone	214	740	134	26	1114
(iii) Other Drugs	314	456	118	36	924
(iv) First notification subsequently found not to be addicted	—	560	204	38	802
b. Second and subsequent notifications	1612	4930	1519	381	8442
c. Gross total	4236	8226	2552	609	15603

Table 5b First notifications of heroin addicts, by age and sex. (From Drugs Branch, Home Office, Romney House, London).

Age groups	22.2.68–31.12.68	1.1.69–31.12.71		1.1.72–31.12.72		1.1.73–31.3.73		Gross total
		M	F	M	F	M	F	
Under 20	785	537	104	130	49	31	8	1644
20–34 years	1192	732	135	307	58	71	18	2513
35–49 years	74	23	5	12	1	—	—	115
50 years and over	16	2	—	—	—	—	—	18
Age not known	29	2	—	—	—	—	—	31
Totals	2096	1296	244	449	108	102	26	4321
Previously known	1072	67		—		—		1139
Previously not known	1024	1473		557		128		3182
Totals	2096*	1540		557		128		4321

*Male 1728, Female 368

Table 5c First notifications of methadone addicts, by age and sex. (From Drugs Branch, Home Office, Romney House, London).

Age groups	22.2.68–31.12.68	1.1.69–31.12.71		1.1.72–31.12.72		1.1.73–31.3.73		Gross total
		M	F	M	F	M	F	
Under 20	46	224	46	30	5	10	2	363
20–34 years	115	358	74	73	21	11	2	654
35–49 years	20	9	7	3	—	—	1	40
50 years and over	33	4	2	—	2	—	—	41
Age not known	—	14	2	—	—	—	—	16
Totals	214	609	131	106	28	21	5	1114
Previously known	155	50		—		—		205
Previously not known	59	690		134		26		909
Totals	214	740		134		26		1114

Table 5d First notifications of persons addicted to other dangerous drugs (mainly morphine and pethidine), by age and sex. (From Drugs Branch, Home Office, Romney House, London)

Age groups	22.2.68–31.12.68	1.1.69–31.12.71 M	1.1.69–31.12.71 F	1.1.72–31.12.72 M	1.1.72–31.12.72 F	1.1.73–31.3.73 M	1.1.73–31.3.73 F	Gross total
Under 20	21	115	12	26	3	8	2	187
20–34 years	100	159	24	48	9	16	1	357
35–49 years	39	42	21	15	3	1	—	121
50 years and over	151	35	43	7	7	7	1	251
Age not known	3	3	2	—	—	—	—	8
Totals	314	354	102	96	22	32	4	924
Previously known	218	39		—		—		257
Previously not known	96	417		118		36		667
Totals	314*	456		118		36		924

*Male 189, Female 125

Table 6 Reported experience with drug use for recreational and non-medical purposes by American youth and adults.[1] (Based on Second National Survey (1972) by the American Commission on marihuana and drug abuse.) (By courtesy of *Drugs and Society*)

Drug	Youth (per cent)	Adults (per cent)
Alcoholic beverages[2]	24	53
Tobacco, cigarettes[2]	17	38
Proprietary sedatives, tranquillisers, stimulants[3]	6	7
Ethical sedatives[3]	3	4
Ethical tranquillisers[3]	3	6
Ethical stimulants[3]	4	5
Marijuana	14	16
LSD, other hallucinogens	4·8	4·6
Glue, other inhalants	6·4	2·1
Cocaine	1·5	3·2
Heroin	0·6	1·3

[1]Figures are not additive, so they do not total 100%. Youth includes ages 12–17 (total population 24 905 000). Adults include ages 18 and over (total population 139 774 000)

[2]Within past 7 days

[3]Non-medical use only

Table 7 Psychotropic drug use amongst American students. (From J. Young and J. Brooke Crutchley, by courtesy of *Drugs and Society*).

Year	Author	Population	% Estimate			
			Marijuana	LSD	Amphetamines	Heroin
1965	Harrison	San Francisco State	23	3	—	—
1967	Eels	California Inst. of Technology	20	9	—	—
1967	Devonshire	San Mateo County California Jn College	23	7	—	—
1968	Pearlman	Brooklyn College, New York	27	0	—	1
1969	Blum	5 Californian Colleges	10–23	2–9	11–23	1–2

Harrison, G. (1956). A shocker on use of drugs at SF State. *San Francisco Chronicle*
Eels, K. (1967). *A Survey of Student Practices and Attitudes with respect to Marijuana and LSD* (California Institute of Technology)
Devonshire, C. M. (1967). Associated Press Report
Pearlman, S. (1968). Drug Use and Experience in an Urban College Population. *American Journal of Orthopsychiatry*
Blum, R. (1969). *Students and Drugs*
After J. Young–J. Brooke Crutchley, *Drugs and Society*, Oct. 1972) [13]

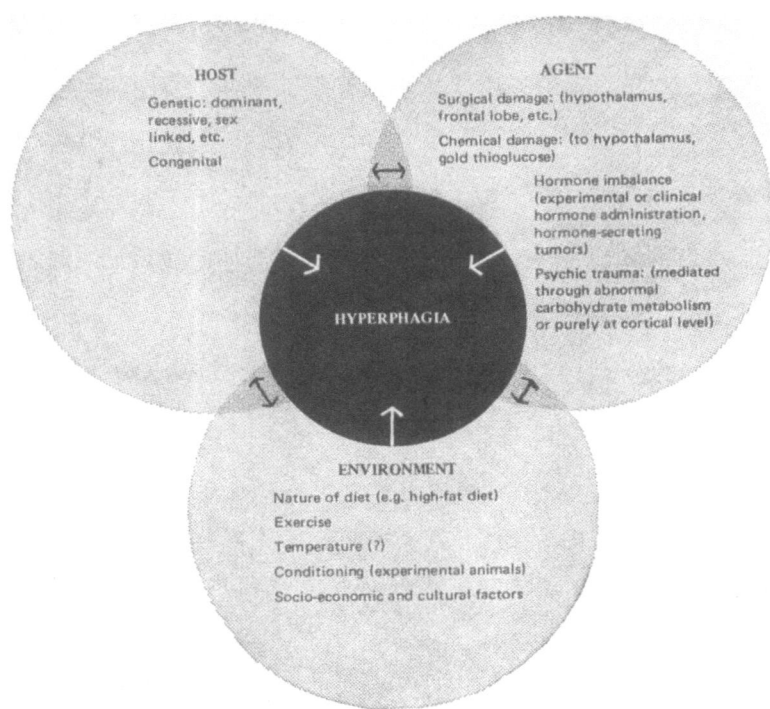

Diagram 1 — A schematic view of constitutional (genetic and congenital), traumatic and environmental factors in the aetiology of obesity.

From Mayer, J. (1959), by courtesy of *Postcard Med.*
Reprinted from *Aspects Of Anxiety*, (1965) (Phildelphia) J. B. Lippincott Company

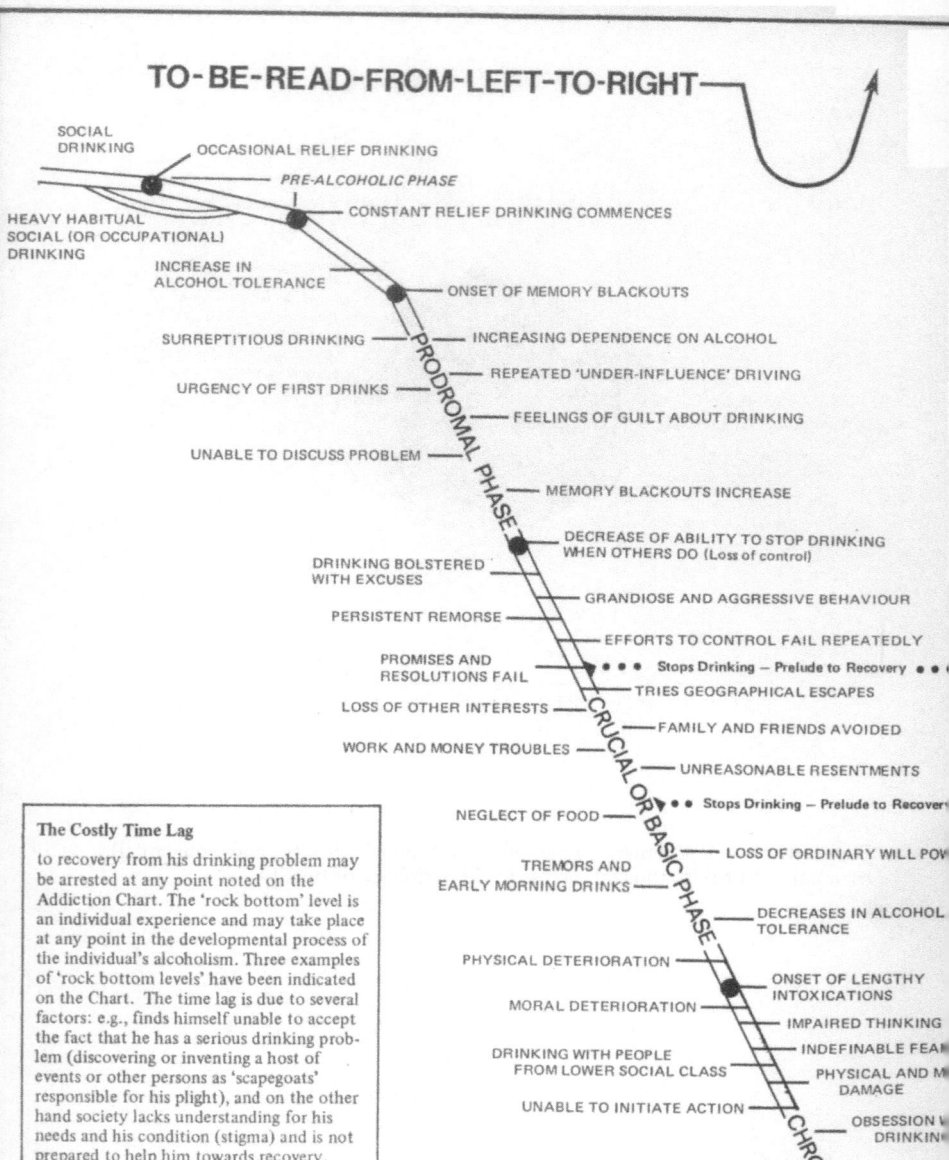

Figure 1.
A TENTATIVE CHART OF ALCOHOL ADDICTION AND RECOVERY

TO-BE-READ-FROM-LEFT-TO-RIGHT

SOCIAL DRINKING

OCCASIONAL RELIEF DRINKING

PRE-ALCOHOLIC PHASE

HEAVY HABITUAL SOCIAL (OR OCCUPATIONAL) DRINKING

CONSTANT RELIEF DRINKING COMMENCES

INCREASE IN ALCOHOL TOLERANCE

ONSET OF MEMORY BLACKOUTS

SURREPTITIOUS DRINKING — INCREASING DEPENDENCE ON ALCOHOL

REPEATED 'UNDER-INFLUENCE' DRIVING

URGENCY OF FIRST DRINKS

FEELINGS OF GUILT ABOUT DRINKING

UNABLE TO DISCUSS PROBLEM

PRODROMAL PHASE

MEMORY BLACKOUTS INCREASE

DECREASE OF ABILITY TO STOP DRINKING WHEN OTHERS DO (Loss of control)

DRINKING BOLSTERED WITH EXCUSES

GRANDIOSE AND AGGRESSIVE BEHAVIOUR

PERSISTENT REMORSE —

EFFORTS TO CONTROL FAIL REPEATEDLY

PROMISES AND RESOLUTIONS FAIL

• • • Stops Drinking – Prelude to Recovery • •

TRIES GEOGRAPHICAL ESCAPES

LOSS OF OTHER INTERESTS —

FAMILY AND FRIENDS AVOIDED

WORK AND MONEY TROUBLES —

UNREASONABLE RESENTMENTS

NEGLECT OF FOOD —

• • Stops Drinking – Prelude to Recover

LOSS OF ORDINARY WILL POW

TREMORS AND EARLY MORNING DRINKS —

DECREASES IN ALCOHOL TOLERANCE

PHYSICAL DETERIORATION —

ONSET OF LENGTHY INTOXICATIONS

MORAL DETERIORATION —

IMPAIRED THINKING

DRINKING WITH PEOPLE FROM LOWER SOCIAL CLASS —

INDEFINABLE FEAR

PHYSICAL AND M DAMAGE

UNABLE TO INITIATE ACTION —

OBSESSION W DRINKIN

CRUCIAL OR BASIC PHASE

VAGUE SPIRITUAL DESIRES —

ALL ALIBI EXHAU

COMPLETE DEFEAT ADMITTED —

• • • De

CHRONIC PHASE

OR. OBSESSIVE DRI

(possibly to point of no reco

The Costly Time Lag

to recovery from his drinking problem may be arrested at any point noted on the Addiction Chart. The 'rock bottom' level is an individual experience and may take place at any point in the developmental process of the individual's alcoholism. Three examples of 'rock bottom levels' have been indicated on the Chart. The time lag is due to several factors: e.g., finds himself unable to accept the fact that he has a serious drinking problem (discovering or inventing a host of events or other persons as 'scapegoats' responsible for his plight), and on the other hand society lacks understanding for his needs and his condition (stigma) and is not prepared to help him towards recovery.

Development period for addiction can be 2 to 25 years. Average 10–15 years

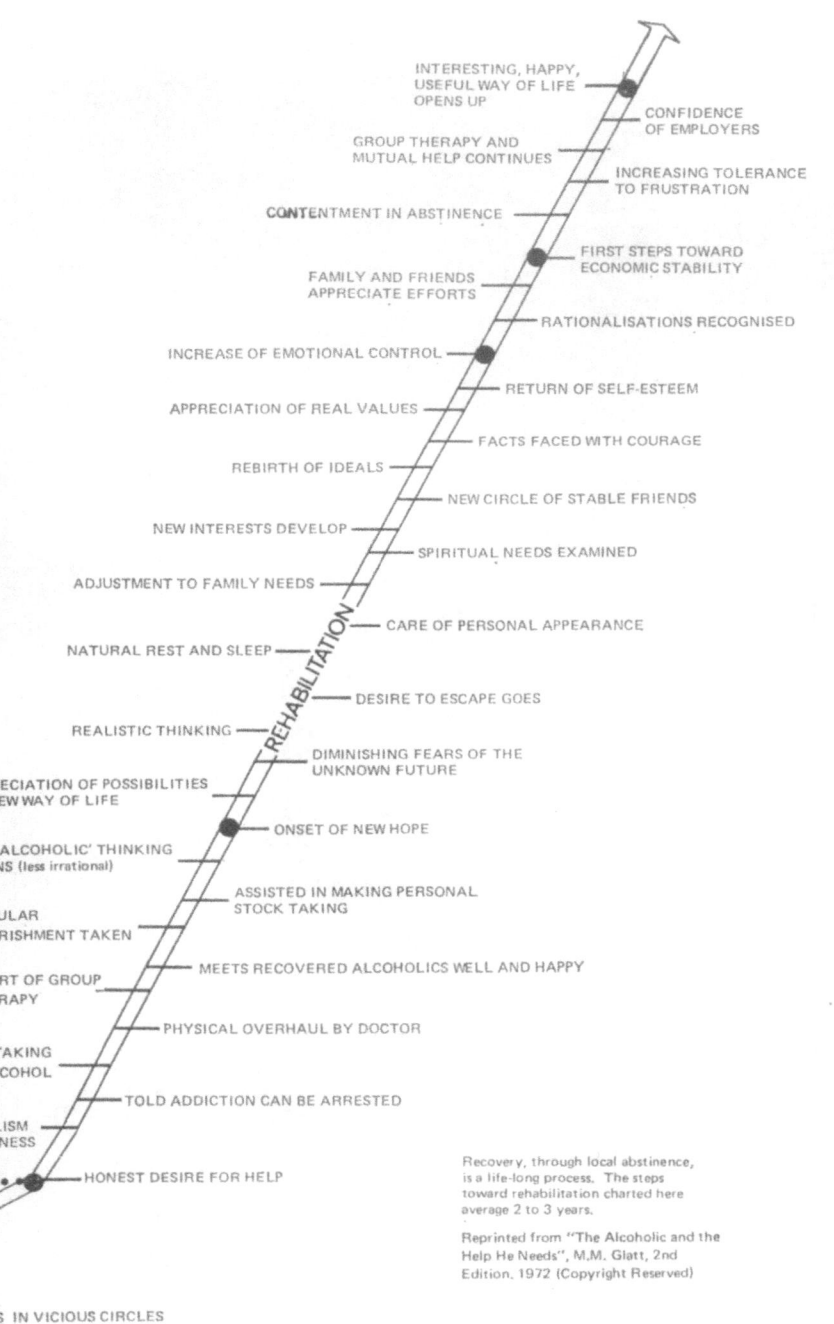

INTERESTING, HAPPY, USEFUL WAY OF LIFE OPENS UP

CONFIDENCE OF EMPLOYERS

GROUP THERAPY AND MUTUAL HELP CONTINUES

INCREASING TOLERANCE TO FRUSTRATION

CONTENTMENT IN ABSTINENCE

FIRST STEPS TOWARD ECONOMIC STABILITY

FAMILY AND FRIENDS APPRECIATE EFFORTS

RATIONALISATIONS RECOGNISED

INCREASE OF EMOTIONAL CONTROL

RETURN OF SELF-ESTEEM

APPRECIATION OF REAL VALUES

FACTS FACED WITH COURAGE

REBIRTH OF IDEALS

NEW CIRCLE OF STABLE FRIENDS

NEW INTERESTS DEVELOP

SPIRITUAL NEEDS EXAMINED

ADJUSTMENT TO FAMILY NEEDS

CARE OF PERSONAL APPEARANCE

NATURAL REST AND SLEEP

REHABILITATION

DESIRE TO ESCAPE GOES

REALISTIC THINKING

DIMINISHING FEARS OF THE UNKNOWN FUTURE

APPRECIATION OF POSSIBILITIES OF NEW WAY OF LIFE

ONSET OF NEW HOPE

'NON-ALCOHOLIC' THINKING BEGINS (less irrational)

ASSISTED IN MAKING PERSONAL STOCK TAKING

REGULAR NOURISHMENT TAKEN

START OF GROUP THERAPY

MEETS RECOVERED ALCOHOLICS WELL AND HAPPY

STOPS TAKING ALCOHOL

PHYSICAL OVERHAUL BY DOCTOR

LEARNS ALCOHOLISM IS AN ILLNESS

TOLD ADDICTION CAN BE ARRESTED

HONEST DESIRE FOR HELP

CONTINUES IN VICIOUS CIRCLES

(possible mental or physical deterioration)

Recovery, through total abstinence, is a life-long process. The steps toward rehabilitation charted here average 2 to 3 years.

Reprinted from "The Alcoholic and the Help He Needs", M.M. Glatt, 2nd Edition, 1972 (Copyright Reserved)

335

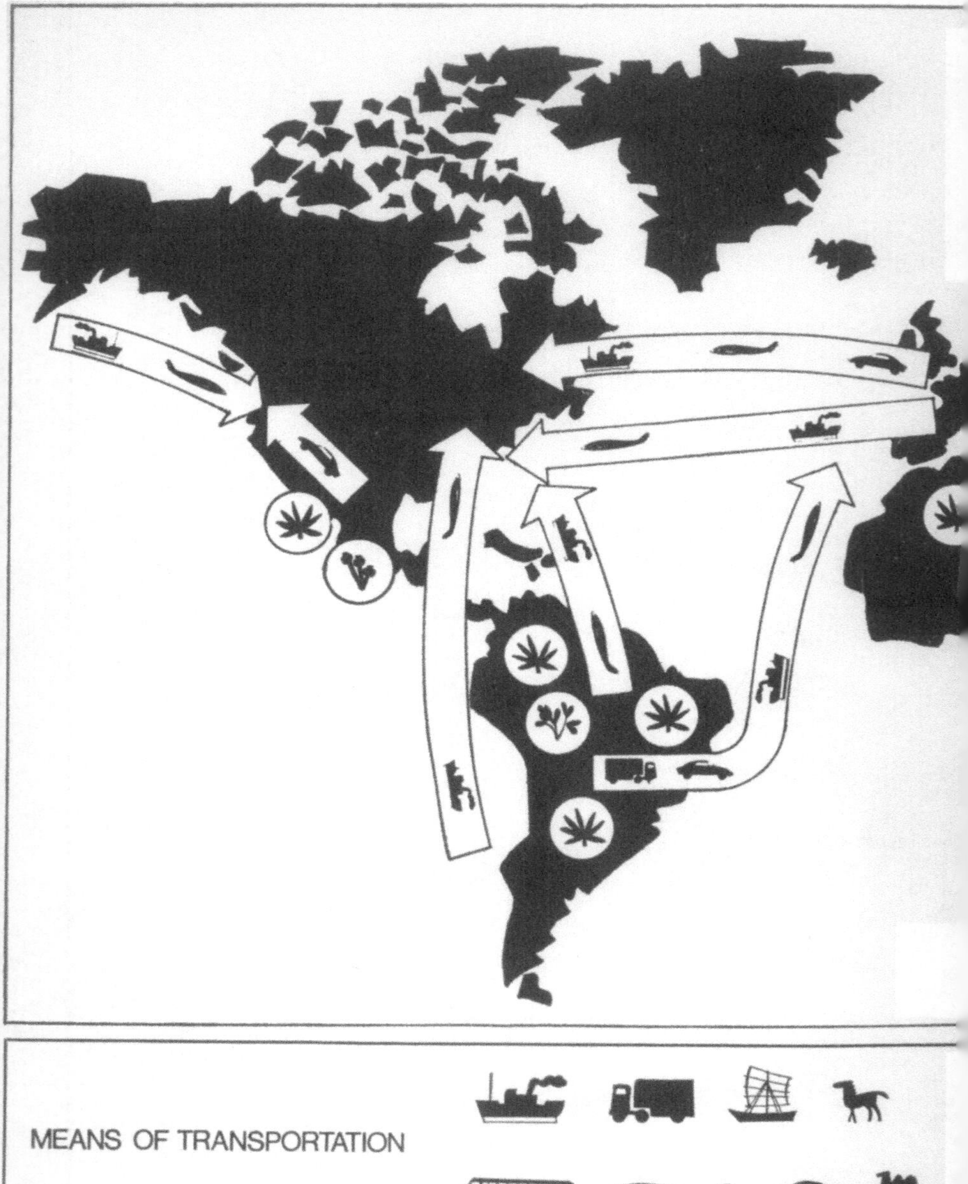

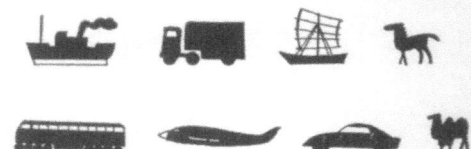

MEANS OF TRANSPORTATION

Adapted from "The Drug Abuse Manual"
published by Smith, Kline and French

**Figure 2 PRINCIPAL TRADE ROUTES
OF ILLICIT DRUGS**

336

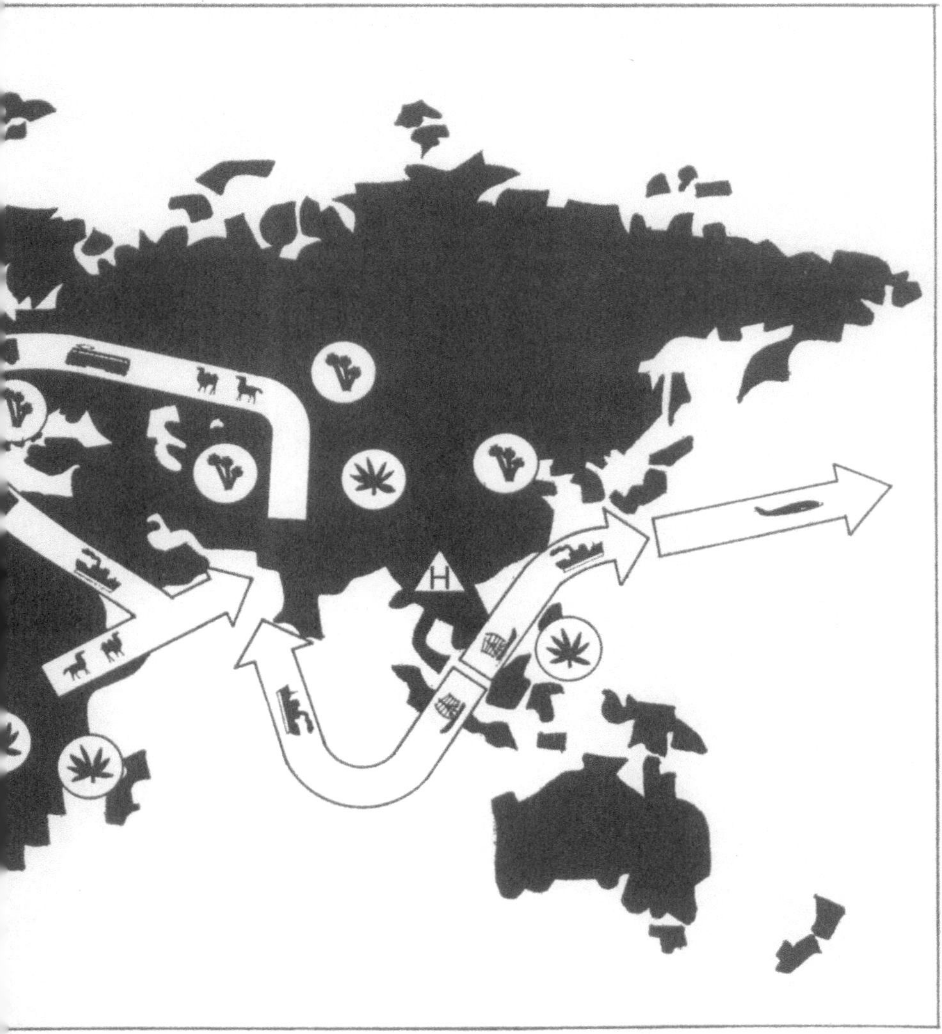

CIT
TIVATION

-called "Chinese heroin" used in
n probably stems mainly from the
n triangle" between Burma, Laos and
nd — and is normally transported from
o Europe via Bangkok and Hong Kong.

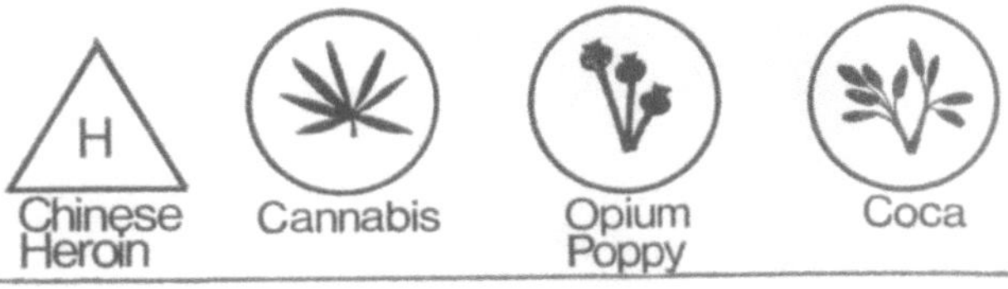

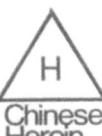

Chinese
Heroin

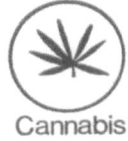

Cannabis

Opium
Poppy

Coca

INDEX

Index